RADIOGRAPHY IN VETERINARY TECHNOLOGY

RADIOGRAPHY IN VETERINARY TECHNOLOGY

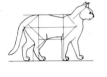

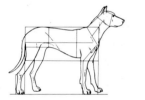

Lisa M. Lavin, C.V.T., A.A.S.
Medical Institute of Minnesota
Bloomington, Minnesota

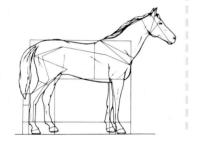

W. B. SAUNDERS COMPANY
A Division of Harcourt Brace & Company
Philadelphia   London   Toronto   Montreal   Sydney   Tokyo

W.B. Saunders Company
A Division of Harcourt Brace & Company

The Curtis Center
Independence Square West
Philadelphia, Pennsylvania 19106

Library of Congress Cataloging-in-Publication Data
Lavin, Lisa M.
    Radiography in veterinary technology / Lisa M. Lavin.
        p.   cm.
    Includes index.
    ISBN 0-7216-6686-8
    1. Veterinary radiography. I. Title.
    [DNLM: 1. Radiography—veterinary. 2. Technology, Radiologic-
-veterinary. SF 757.8 L412r 1994]
SF757.8.L38 1994
636.089′60757—dc20
DNLM/DLC   93-26133

RADIOGRAPHY IN VETERINARY TECHNOLOGY   ISBN 0-7216-6686-8

Printed in the United States of America

Last digit is the print number: 9   8   7   6   5   4   3   2   1

Content reviewed by

Daniel Feeney, D.V.M.

Professor of Radiology
College of Veterinary Medicine
University of Minnesota
St. Paul, Minnesota

With contributions by

Susan L. McClanahan, R.T.(R.)

Radiation Specialist II, X-Ray Unit Leader
Department of Radiation Control Section
State Department of Health
and University of Minnesota Veterinary Hospital
Minneapolis, Minnesota

Quality Assurance/Quality Control

To God Be The Glory . . .

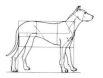

P R E F A C E

A radiograph is an image recorded on a special film consisting of shadows formed by structures and objects in the path of the x-ray beam. A radiograph is in essence a "shadowgraph."

One does not need to be a student of physics to grasp the concepts of radiography. Radiography requires the comprehension of key, integral concepts that form a cerebral foundation. This foundation can then be a building block for further understanding and the subsequent production of high quality radiographs.

Radiography is like no other realm in veterinary technology. Unlike a urinalysis or a blood analysis, the product of radiography can be considered as a piece of art work. Technical staff members can take pride in the results of their efforts.

Much confusion exists about a number of key areas of radiography. These areas include the physics of radiography, patient positioning, and technique evaluation. These areas are presented extensively in this text. To generate better understanding of the material, theoretical concepts are explained in a practical manner. One of the outstanding features of this text is its simplicity, with the intention to minimize confusion concerning the subject of radiography.

This book will act not only as a learning aid, but also as a reference resource. Licensed technicians may find this material to be a bridge between what was learned in school and what is applied in practice.

The primary goal in veterinary radiography is to produce radiographs of diagnostic quality on the first attempt. This goal serves three purposes: (1) to decrease exposure to the patient and veterinary personnel, (2) to decrease the cost to the client, and (3) to produce diagnostic data for rapid interpretation and treatment of the patient. The purpose of this text, therefore, is to provide information on veterinary radiographic technique to achieve this goal.

It is not by trial and error that we achieve quality . . . but a conscious understanding of the variables that transform image into art.

Lisa M. Lavin

A C K N O W L E D G M E N T S

I wish to express my sincere gratitude to the many people who were so generous with their time, patience, and prayer upon the completion of this work.

I am particularly indebted to the administration, faculty, staff, and students of the Medical Institute of Minnesota for technical and moral support. Without them, this text would not be possible. Special thanks to my former student and a talented artist, Barb Fair, who is responsible for the majority of the artwork in this text.

In am thankful for the editorial assistance of Daniel Feeney, professor of radiology, College of Veterinary Medicine, University of Minnesota. Dr. Feeney served not only as an editor, but a mentor as well. Valued assistance was also received from the University of Minnesota department of radiology's faculty and staff.

A large portion of the material in Part II originated in the University of Minnesota Veterinary Teaching Hospital, department of radiology. I am grateful for the 5 years of experience with the staff of this department and for their continued support. Special thanks are extended to Susan L. McClanahan for her contributions and to Michelle Mero for her photographic expertise.

This text would never have been completed if it were not for the steadfast support, encouragement, and guidance of Selma Ozmat of the W.B. Saunders Company.

My deep appreciation is also extended to my family. I am especially grateful to my sister and best friend Sherre — thank you for your loyal friendship, prayer, and unconditional love. Thanks are also extended to Bruce Cunliffe, who served many roles in the completion of this work. Dr. Cunliffe was an outstanding supportive and patient friend.

Although this text is a careful collection of specialized knowledge, the errors are my own and I would appreciate having my attention drawn to them.

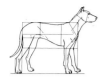

CONTENTS

PART I   RADIOGRAPHIC THEORY AND EQUIPMENT

PART II RADIOGRAPHIC POSITIONING

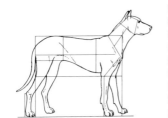

RADIOGRAPHIC THEORY AND EQUIPMENT

X - R A Y
P R O D U C T I O N

OBJECTIVES
Upon completion of this chapter, the reader should be able to:

- Define x-rays
- Define electromagnetic radiation
- List and describe the two characteristics of electromagnetic radiation
- Describe the anatomy of an atom
- State the significance of the wavelength of x-rays
- List the seven physical properties of x-rays
- Describe how x-rays are generated
- Name the man who discovered x-rays

GLOSSARY

ANODE: A positively charged electrode.

ATOM: A basic part of matter made up of a nucleus and a surrounding cloud of electrons.

ATOMIC NUMBER: The number of protons in an atom's nucleus.

CATHODE: A negatively charged electrode.

ELECTROMAGNETIC RADIATION: A method of transporting energy through space, distinguished by wavelength, frequency, and energy.

ELECTROMAGNETIC SPECTRUM: Electromagnetic radiation grouped according to wavelength and frequency.

ELECTRON: A negatively charged particle that travels around the nucleus.

EXCITATION: A process in which an electron is moved to a higher energy level within the atom.

FLUORESCENCE: The ability of a substance to emit visible light.

FREQUENCY: The number of cycles of the wave that pass a stationary point in a second.

GAMMA RAYS: Electromagnetic radiation emitted from the nucleus of radioactive substances.

INFRARED RAYS: Electromagnetic radiation, beyond the red end of the visible spectrum, characterized by long wavelengths.

IONIZATION: A process in which an outer electron is removed from the atom so that the atom is left positively charged.

NEUTRON: A neutral particle located in the nucleus of an atom.

PHOTONS: A bundle of radiant energy (synonymous with **quanta**).

PROTON: A positively charged particle located in the nucleus of an atom.

QUANTA: A bundle of radiant energy (synonymous with **photons**).

RADIANT ENERGY: Energy contained in light rays or any other form of radiation.

RADIOGRAPH: A visible photographic record on film produced by x-rays passing through an object.

SHELL: An electron's orbital path and energy level.

ULTRAVIOLET RAYS: Electromagnetic radiation, beyond the violet end of the visible spectrum, characterized by short wavelengths.

VACUUM: An area from which all air has been removed.

WAVELENGTH: The distance between two consecutive corresponding points on a wave.

X-RAYS: A form of electromagnetic radiation similar to visible light but of shorter wavelength.

X-RAY BEAM: A number of x-rays traveling together through space at a rapid speed.

DEFINITION OF X-RAYS

Knowledge of the nature and behavior of x-rays is the first step in understanding the production of a **radiograph**. The veterinary radiographer does not need to have detailed knowledge of the underlying radiologic physics, but a basic understanding of certain principles is necessary for the production of quality radiographs.

X-rays are defined as a form of electromagnetic radiation similar to visible light but of much shorter wavelength. **Electromagnetic radiation** is a method of transporting energy through space and is distinguished by its wavelength, frequency, and energy. Essentially, there are two characteristics of electromagnetic radiation: particles and waves.

We will first consider the wave. All **radiant energy** travels in a wave form along a straight path and is measured by its wavelength. In a series of waves, the distance between two consecutive corresponding points on a wave is called the **wavelength** (Fig. 1.1). Electromagnetic radiation that has a short wavelength has a high frequency. Electromagnetic radiation that has a long wavelength has a low frequency. **Frequency** is measured by the number of cycles of the wave that pass a stationary point per second (cycles per second).

The higher the frequency, the more penetrating power the energy has through space and matter.

All forms of electromagnetic radiation are grouped according to their wavelength and frequency in what is called the **electromagnetic spectrum**. Examples of electromagnetic radiation are radio waves, television waves, radar, **infrared rays**, the visible spectrum of light, **ultraviolet rays**, x-rays, and **gamma rays** (Fig. 1.2).

Electromagnetic radiation behaves as a particle as well as a wave. **Atoms** consist of small particles called **protons**, **neutrons**, and **electrons**. An atom has a nucleus with a surrounding cloud of electrons (Fig. 1.3). The nucleus of an atom contains protons, which are positively charged, and neutrons, which are neutral. Electrons, which are negatively charged, travel around the nucleus in specific orbits, which are called **shells**.

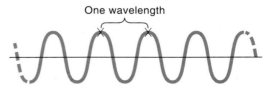

■ **FIG. 1.1** Wavelength motion showing two corresponding points on consecutive waves.

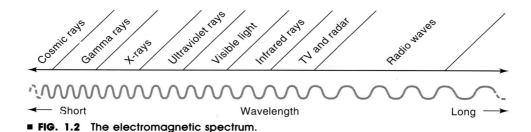

■ FIG. 1.2 The electromagnetic spectrum.

X-rays are produced when charged particles (electrons) are slowed down or stopped by the atoms of a target area. This process occurs inside the x-ray tube to create an **x-ray beam**.

An x-ray beam is composed of bundles of energy that travel in a wave. These bundles of energy or **quanta** are referred to as **photons**. The photons have no mass or electrical charge. Photons consist of pure energy and are transported or "carried" by the wave.

Electromagnetic radiation can carry a wide range of energies. The energy of the radiation is proportional to the wavelength. The shorter the wavelength, the greater the energy. Therefore, in radiography, x-rays, having a shorter wavelength, penetrate farther than rays having longer wavelengths.

PHYSICAL PROPERTIES OF X-RAY ELECTROMAGNETIC RADIATION

The physical properties of x-ray electromagnetic radiation, listed below, have diagnostic, medical, and research application:

1. Wavelength is variable and is related to the energy of the radiation.

2. Travel is in a straight line. Direction can be altered, but the new path is also in a straight line.

3. Because of the extremely short wavelength, x-rays are able to penetrate materials that absorb or reflect visible light. They are gradually absorbed the farther they pass through an object. The amount of absorption depends on the **atomic number** and the physical density of the object and the energy of the x-rays.

4. Certain substances are **fluorescent**; that is, they can emit visible light. Crystalline substances such as calcium tungstate or rare-earth phosphors fluoresce (emit light) within the visible spectrum after absorbing electromagnetic radiation of a shorter wavelength (i.e., x-rays).

5. X-rays produce an invisible image on photographic film that can be made visible by processing the film.

6. X-rays have the ability to excite or ionize the atoms and molecules of the substances, including gases, through which they pass. **Excitation** is a process in which an electron is moved to a higher energy level within the atom. Energy is required to initiate this change. **Ionization** is a process in which an outer electron is completely removed from the atom so that the atom is left positively charged. This process requires more energy than excitation.

7. X-rays can cause biologic changes in living tissue. A biologic change occurs either by direct action of excitation and ionization on important molecules in cells or indirectly as a result of chemical changes occurring near the cells. Affected cells may be damaged or killed.

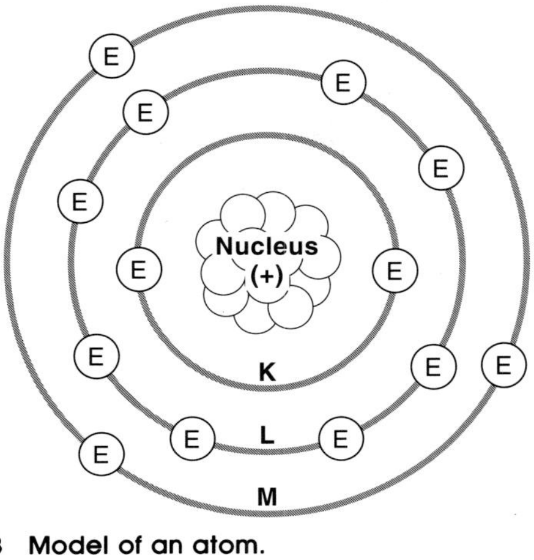

■ FIG. 1.3 Model of an atom.

GENERATION OF X-RAYS

X-rays are generated when fast-moving electrons (small particles bearing a negative charge) collide with any matter. This is best achieved in an x-ray tube. The x-ray tube consists of two electrodes, a **cathode** and an **anode**. Each electrode has an opposite electrical charge. As electrons, having a negative charge at the cathode, are attracted to the positive pole (anode) in the tube, they collide with the positively charged target. This collision results in the production of x-radiation and a great amount of heat. Heat is the result of the interaction of the electrons and the atoms in the target. In fact, in diagnostic x-ray tubes, 99% of the energy from fast-moving electrons is converted into heat and 1% into x-ray energy.

DISCOVERY OF X-RAYS

On November 8, 1895, Wilhelm Conrad Roentgen discovered x-rays, a contribution to science that will remain invaluable.

A professor of physics, Roentgen was the director of the new Physical Institute of the University of Würzburg, Germany. "Gas" tubes were being used at the time to conduct experiments with cathode rays. A **vacuum** was created in the tube by pumping out the air, and a current of electrons was passed through the tube. The tube consisted basically of a cathode (negative electrical charge) and an anode (positive electrical charge). The difference in electrical charge potential between the two electrodes caused the electrons to accelerate toward the tube end, where they interacted with the glass, producing x-rays.

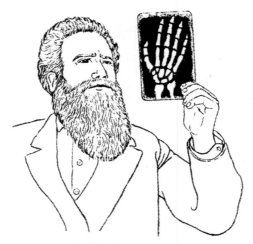

■ FIG. 1.4 Roentgen viewing a radiograph of his wife's hand.

Roentgen then wrapped the glass tube with dark paper, and, during activation, he saw a greenish illumination from a piece of cardboard across the room. The cardboard was painted with a fluorescent material called barium plantinocyanide. This fluorescent material had been used previously to detect cathode rays. Upon this discovery and further investigation, Roentgen presented a written report to the Society of Physics and Medical Sciences at the University of Würzburg on November 28, 1895. With his findings, he also submitted a radiograph of the hand of his wife, which he had produced with his own x-ray tube (Fig. 1.4).

By 1896, thousands of manuscripts and many books on x-rays were published. X-rays were used immediately for medical and surgical diagnosis. And by as early as April 1896, changes in skin color due to exposure to x-rays, similar to a sunburn, were reported. This discovery of skin color changes resulted in the use of x-rays for radiation therapy.

In recognition of Roentgen's discovery, he was awarded the Nobel Prize in 1901. This was the first Nobel Prize awarded in the field of physics.

Interestingly, a professor Goodspeed in Philadelphia had made the discovery of x-rays in 1890 but did not recognize their medical significance.

BIBLIOGRAPHY

Ball JL, Moore AD: *Essential Physics for Radiographers.* Blackwell Scientific, Boston, 1980.

Durez Y, Sieband MP, Jacobsen AF: *Production of X-rays— Applications to Medical Radiography.* University of Wisconsin, Madison, 1978.

Eastman Kodak Company: *Kodak: The Fundamentals of Radiography,* 12th ed. Rochester, NY, 1980.

Johns HE, Cunningham JR: *The Physics of Radiology,* 4th ed. Charles C Thomas, Springfield, IL, 1983.

Sprawls P: *The Physical Principles of Diagnostic Radiology.* University Park Press, Baltimore, MD, 1977.

ANATOMY OF THE X-RAY MACHINE

CHAPTER OUTLINE

- THE X-RAY TUBE
- X-RAY PRODUCTION
- CATHODE
- ANODE

- POSSIBLE AREAS OF TUBE FAILURE
- TECHNICAL COMPONENTS OF THE X-RAY MACHINE

OBJECTIVES

Upon completion of this chapter, the reader should be able to:

- State the purpose of the x-ray tube
- List the five elements necessary for x-ray production
- Describe the anatomy of the x-ray tube
- State the purpose and construction of the cathode
- State the basic construction of the anode
- State the reasons for the use of tungsten, molybdenum, and copper in the construction of the x-ray tube
- List methods of heat dissipation within the x-ray tube housing
- List and describe the two types of anodes
- Define heel effect

- Define and describe the focal spot
- Define the line-focus principle
- List the possible areas of x-ray tube failure
- List the electrical components of an x-ray machine
- State the purpose of the autotransformer, step-up transformer, line-voltage compensator, step-down transformer, and timer switch
- State and define the methods of rectification
- Describe x-ray tube rating and the three-phase generator
- List the components of the x-ray machine and console

GLOSSARY

ACCELERATION: The increase in speed over time.

ACTUAL FOCAL SPOT: The area of the focal spot consisting of a coiled wire that is perpendicular to the surface of the target.

ALLOY: A mixture of metals.

ANODE: A positively charged electrode, which acts as a target for the electrons from the cathode. Electrons interacting with the anode produce heat and x-rays.

ARCING: A phenomenon in which metal deposits on the inner wall of the envelope act as a secondary anode, thereby attracting electrons from the cathode.

AUTOTRANSFORMER: Provides a variable, yet predetermined, voltage to the high-voltage step-up transformer. It acts as the kilovoltage selector.

CATHODE: A negatively charged electrode that provides a source of electrons.

COLLIMATOR: A restricting device used to control the size of the primary x-ray beam.

CONSOLE: The control panel of the x-ray machine.

EFFECTIVE FOCAL SPOT: The area of the focal spot visible through the x-ray tube window and directed toward the x-ray film.

FILAMENT: Part of a low-energy circuit in the cathode that, when heated, releases electrons from their orbits.

FOCAL SPOT: The small area of the target with which electrons collide on the anode.

FOCUSING CUP: A recessed area where the filament lies, directing the electrons toward the anode.

FULL-WAVE RECTIFICATION: Creates a nearly constant electrical potential across the x-ray tube, converting the positive electrical current pulses to 120 times per second compared with the normal 60 times per second.

GLASS ENVELOPE: A glass vacuum tube that contains the anode and cathode of the x-ray tube.

HALF-WAVE RECTIFICATION: A method of converting alternating to direct current in which half of the current is lost.

HEEL EFFECT: A decrease of x-ray intensity on the anode side of the x-ray beam due to the anode target angle.

KILOVOLTAGE: The amount of electrical energy being applied to the anode and cathode to accelerate the electrons from the cathode to the anode (1 kilovolt (kV) = 1000 volts (V)).

KILOVOLTAGE PEAK (KVP): The peak energy of the x-rays, which determines the quality (penetrating power) of the x-ray beam.

LINE-VOLTAGE COMPENSATOR: Adjusts the incoming line voltage to the autotransformer so that the voltage remains constant.

MILLIAMPERAGE (MA): The amount of electrical energy being applied to the filament. Milliamperage describes the number of x-rays produced during the exposure.

MOLYBDENUM: A metal commonly used in focusing cups because of its high melting point and poor conduction of heat.

PENUMBRA: Partial outer shadow of an object being imaged by illumination.

RECTIFICATION: Process of changing alternating current to direct current.

ROTATING ANODE: An anode that turns on an axis to increase x-ray production while dissipating heat.

STATIONARY ANODE: A nonmoving anode, usually found in dental and small portable radiography units.

STEP-DOWN TRANSFORMER: Reduces the x-ray machine input voltage from 110 or 220 V to 10 V to prevent the filament of the cathode from burning out.

STEP-UP TRANSFORMER: Increases the incoming voltage of 110 or 220 V to thousands of volts (i.e., kilovolts).

TARGET: Anode.

TIMER SWITCH: Controls the length of exposure.

TUNGSTEN: A common metal used in the filament of a cathode.

VALVE TUBES: Allow the flow of electrons in one direction only. Commonly called self-rectifiers.

X-RAY TUBE: A mechanism consisting of an anode and a cathode in a vacuum that produces a controlled x-ray beam.

THE X-RAY TUBE

X-rays are generated in an **x-ray tube.** The purpose of the x-ray tube is to produce a controlled x-ray beam. The tube must be responsive to manual control so that both the amount and the penetrating power of the radiation produced are accurately controlled. To better understand the x-ray tube, we need to consider what is necessary for the production of x-rays.

X-ray Production

The following elements are necessary for x-ray production:

1. A source of electrons.
2. A method of accelerating the electrons.
3. An obstacle-free path for the passage of high-speed electrons.
4. A target in which the electrons can interact, releasing energy in the form of x-rays.

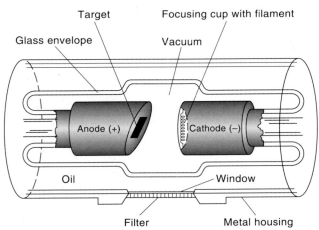

FIG. 2.1 X-ray tube construction.

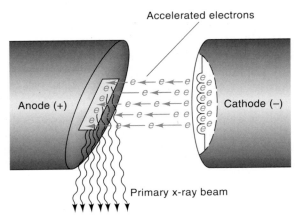

FIG. 2.2 Flow of electrons from the cathode to the anode.

5. An envelope (tube) to provide a vacuum environment, eliminating the air molecule obstacles for the electron stream and preventing rapid oxidation of the elements.

The x-ray tube consists of a **cathode** side (with a negative electrical charge) and an **anode** side (with a positive electrical charge) encased in a **glass envelope**, which is evacuated to form a vacuum (Fig. 2.1).

In the tube, a stream of fast-moving electrons are produced at the cathode and are directed to the anode. As the electrons collide and interact with the atoms of the **target** on the anode, a great amount of energy is produced; 1% of this energy is in the form of roentgen radiation (x-rays), and 99% is released in heat. A thin window area, located on the dependent portion of the tube, acts as a doorway for the exit of the x-rays. The entire tube is encased in a metal housing to prevent the escape of stray radiation and to protect the glass envelope from physical damage.

Cathode

The purpose of the cathode is to provide a source of electrons and to direct these electrons toward the anode (Fig. 2.2). The cathode consists of a coiled wire **filament** that emits electrons when heated. The filament in most x-ray tubes measures approximately 0.2 cm in diameter and 1 cm in length. It is mounted on rigid wires that support it and carry the electrical current used to heat the filament. The filament of the cathode is very similar to the filament of a light bulb (Fig. 2.3A, B). When a filament is heated, electrons are held less tightly by the nucleus of the atoms of the metal. In other words, the electrons become excited. When the energy level exceeds the binding energy, a cloud of electrons is formed and made available to travel to the anode.

The filament is constructed of **tungsten** because of its high melting point (3370°C) and high atomic number. The atomic number is the number of protons in the nucleus of an atom. This number is matched by an equal number of electrons traveling around the nucleus. A high atomic number is proportionate to the potential electron availability. A metal of this type is

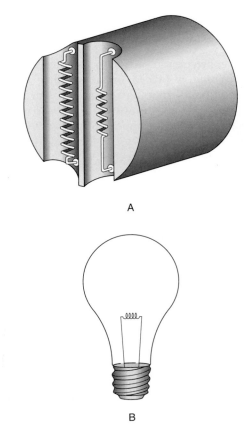

FIG. 2.3 **A,** Cathode filament construction showing a small (fine) and large (coarse) filament within the focusing cup. **B,** Light-bulb containing a filament similar to the filament within the focusing cup of an x-ray tube.

also necessary because of the great amount of heat produced at the filament. Some x-ray tubes, usually those used in small portable and mobile equipment, have a single filament. Most modern tubes have two filaments mounted side by side. One is smaller than the other, each having a different capacity for heat and electron emission.

The filament is located in a concave cup called the **focusing cup**. The focusing cup is made of **molybdenum** because it has a high melting point and is a poor conductor of heat. As a result of the shape and electrical charge of the focusing cup, the electrons are confined and directed toward the anode side of the tube.

The filament is heated by a low-energy circuit. The amount of energy in the circuit is referred to as **milliamperage (mA)**. As the milliamperage is applied and the filament is heated, electrons are released from their atomic orbits. The quantity of electrons produced is dependent on the heat of the filament. Because of its negative electrical charge, the electron cloud is attracted to the anode side of the tube. In order to create an impact great enough to produce x-rays, the electron stream must be accelerated. **Acceleration** of the electrons is controlled by the **kilovoltage** applied between the anode and the cathode. More is said about milliamperage and kilovoltage in Chapter 4.

Anode

The basic construction of the anode consists of a beveled target that is placed on a cylindric base. The target is composed of tungsten, which can withstand and dissipate high temperatures. The base of the target is usually made of copper. Copper acts as a conductor of heat and draws the heat away from the tungsten target. Temperatures in excess of 1000°C occur during x-ray production. If the heat were not removed efficiently, the metal of the target would melt and the tube would be useless. At the energies used in diagnostic radiography, about 99% of the energy released at the impact of the electrons is in the form of heat. Only 1% of the energy is in the form of x-rays.

Other methods of cooling the x-ray tube are used. One such method is surrounding the glass tube with oil within the metal housing. The oil transfers the heat away from the anode. For tubes designed for heavy-duty radiography, the oil in the tube housing is often circulated through a heat exchanger.

In specialized radiography, targets other than of tungsten are used. Molybdenum is an example of such a material, which is used for mammography in a human application of radiography.

Types of Anodes

The construction of the anode varies greatly. This variance is the main factor that differentiates one x-ray tube from another. The difference in anode type is

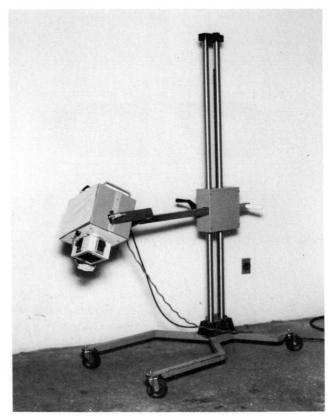

■ **FIG. 2.4** Portable x-ray unit.

associated with the maximum level of heat dissipation possible. The two main types of anodes include the **stationary anode** and the **rotating anode**.

Stationary Anode. Stationary or "fixed" anodes are found in dental and small portable radiography units. These units have a relatively small capacity for x-ray production (Fig. 2.4). As shown in Figure 2.5, the tungsten target area of the stationary anode is embedded on a cylinder of copper, with the face of the target angled down toward the window. The angle may range from 15 to 23 degrees, altering the "focal spot" size. The focal spot is the small area of the target with which the electrons collide. More will be said about the focal spot presently.

The primary limitation of the stationary anode is its inability to withstand large amounts of heat. Repeated bombardment by electrons and subsequent heat production can damage the target. Damage commonly seen from the repeated bombardment of electrons is a pitting of the target surface. Once a target has been damaged in such a way, the x-rays produced from that area will scatter in undesirable directions (Fig. 2.6). Radiographs produced by an x-ray tube that has a pitted target area appear lighter than expected.

With the rapid development of increasingly powerful generators, temperature requirements have far exceeded the capabilities of the stationary anode. This

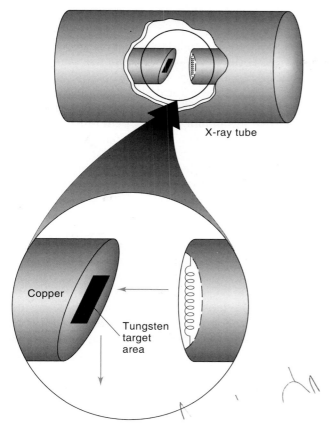

■ **FIG. 2.5** Stationary anode construction.

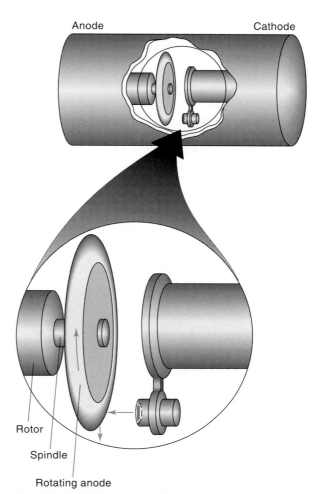

■ **FIG. 2.7** Example of a rotating anode.

limitation provoked a search for a more efficient target area and resulted in the development of the rotating anode.

Rotating Anode. The rotating anode is in the shape of a disk that rotates on an axis through the center of the tube (Fig. 2.7). The disk is approximately 3 inches in diameter and has a beveled edge. It is composed of tungsten or some similar **alloy** that can withstand high temperatures. The spindle on which

the anode is mounted is usually made of molybdenum. Molybdenum dissipates the heat produced at the electron impaction. This heat reduction is necessary to reduce the heat flow to the rotor and bearing mechanism that spins the anode.

The filament is positioned to direct the electron stream at the beveled target area of the rotating disk. The target area in which the x-rays collide remains constant while the anode disk rapidly rotates. The anode rotates approximately 3350 times per minute during the exposure. The rotation continually provides a cooler surface for the electron stream. With the use of a rotating disk, heat is distributed over a larger area, yet still provides a small focal spot.

Spreading the electron stream over a larger area can also be accomplished by decreasing the angle of the target. There is a practical limit to how small the anode angle can be. In a diagnostic x-ray tube, the target is usually angled to about 20 degrees from vertical. A small anode target angle results in an excessive falling off of intensity on the anode side of the x-ray beam. In other words, the x-ray beam will be stronger toward the cathode side than the anode side. This

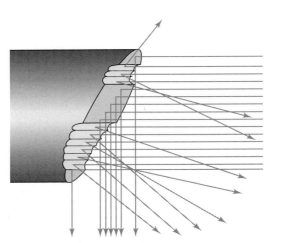

■ **FIG. 2.6** Pitted anode target area showing scatter radiation resulting from the uneven target surface.

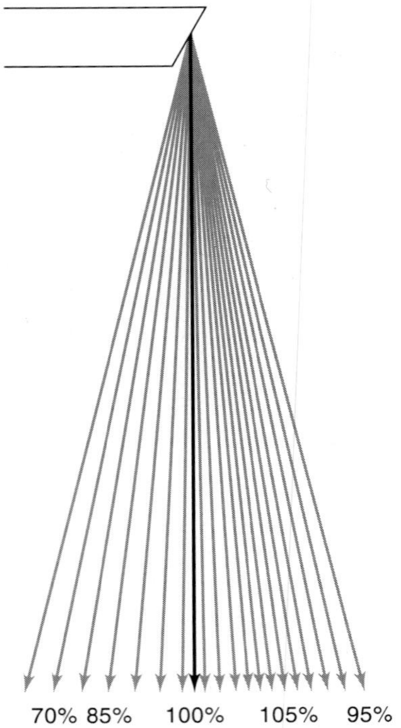

■ FIG. 2.8 Demonstration of the heel effect. The intensity of the primary x-ray beam is not uniform throughout all areas of the beam; the intensity is greater toward the cathode side of the x-ray beam because of the angle of the anode target area.

70% 85%   100%   105%   95%

variation of intensity of the primary x-ray beam is called the **heel effect** (Fig. 2.8). A small anode angle accentuates the heel effect. Decreasing the angle of the target also decreases the field size of the x-ray beam, thereby altering the focal spot.

Focal Spot

The small area of the target with which the electrons collide is called the **focal spot** (Fig. 2.9). The size of

the focal spot has an important effect on the formation of the x-ray image.

X-ray photons collide and leave the entire focal spot area. If the focal spot were the size of a pinpoint, the radiographic image produced would have great image clarity. As the focal spot becomes larger, the "shadow unsharpness" is increased. Any focal spot larger than a pinpoint forms a **penumbra** or halo effect on a radiographic image (Fig. 2.10). Unfortunately, the focal spot size must be larger than a pinpoint in order to withstand the heat generated when the anode is bombarded with electrons. Every focal spot has definite dimensions in most veterinary units, usually covering an area between 1 and 2 mm².

A stationary anode is limited to a larger focal spot to accommodate higher temperatures. The rotating anode has the capacity to have a small focal spot and yet withstand a greater amount of heat.

Effective Focal Spot. If one were to lie on an x-ray table and look into the window of the x-ray tube, the area of the focal spot called the **effective focal spot** would be visible. The **actual focal spot** is the area that is perpendicular to the surface of the target area (Fig. 2.11). The actual focal spot is useless to a radiographer because the effective x-ray beam needs to be directed in a downward angle (toward the x-ray film). However, the actual focal spot size is quite important in determining anode heat capacity.

The actual focal spot does influence the heel effect. As stated previously, the target that has a small angle accentuates the heel effect. More x-rays leave the x-ray tube on the cathode side than the anode side. This will cause a variation in exposure to x-ray film.

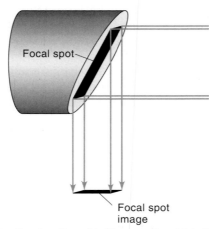

■ FIG. 2.9 The focal spot is the area in which the electrons collide with the target.

Focal spot

Focal spot image

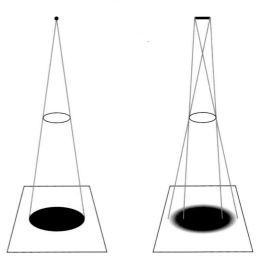

■ FIG. 2.10 Diagram showing the effect of the size of the focal spot on image sharpness—the penumbra effect. A small focal spot produces a sharp image, whereas a larger focal spot causes the penumbra effect, which blurs the projected image.

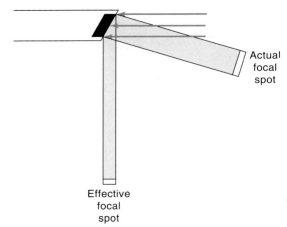

■ **FIG. 2.11** The effective focal spot versus the actual focal spot.

The heel effect can be utilized as an advantage in some circumstances. When radiographing an anatomic area that varies in thickness (e.g., a ventrodorsal abdomen of a dog with a deep thorax), the larger area can be positioned under the cathode side of the tube. The greater intensity toward the cathode side will allow better radiographic exposure of the larger area. The cathode and anode ends of an x-ray tube housing are usually labeled near the area where the main electrical cables are attached.

POSSIBLE AREAS OF TUBE FAILURE

According to current price listings, the x-ray tube can range in cost from $2500 to $30,000. Because of the high replacement cost, the x-ray tube should be cared for properly. The life of a radiographic tube is largely dependent on the manner in which the tube is used. The majority of damaged tubes returned to the manufacturer have been damaged as the result of technical error.

Cathode Failure

The most common cause of x-ray tube failure is filament evaporation. Filament failure can occur in any x-ray tube.

As the tube is fired with normal use, the filament is heated with each exposure. The filament of the cathode is similar to the filament in a light bulb. When a light bulb is "turned on," the filament is heated and emits light. When the filament of the cathode is heated, it emits electrons. With each use, the life of the filament is decreased. The higher the temperature and length of time the filament is heated, the more chance there is for the filament to evaporate. When the filament of the cathode is destroyed, no electron cloud can be produced and, therefore, no flow of electrons is transferred from the cathode to the anode. The film

will remain unexposed and will appear transparent to light after the development procedure.

Current x-ray units have a mechanism that can prolong the life of a tube. This mechanism is known as a "standby current." The standby current preheats the filament to a low temperature when placed in the "on" position. The filament is "on standby" before the exposure is needed. It is not until the pre-exposure button is depressed that the filament is heated to a sufficient temperature to produce an electron cloud.

The pre-exposure switch protects the filament in some respects, but it is important to turn the machine off when not in use. Even the relatively low heat subjected to the filament on standby can be damaging over a long period.

It is also important not to leave the switch in the "ready" position for any extended period. By heating the filament before the exposure for any time longer than necessary, the prolonged high temperature during operation of the filament can promote evaporation as well.

A common problem experienced in practice is depressing the pre-exposure button frequently before actually exposing the film. This problem is the result of not being fully prepared at the time of exposure. It is important to have the proper exposure settings present before final positioning of the animal is done. Animals have the tendency to move out of position at the least opportune time. By presetting the proper technique required for the anatomic area *prior to* the final patient positioning, excess time for animal movement is reduced (Fig. 2.12).

The best practice to lengthen the filament life is to evaluate all aspects of the radiographic procedure before activating the pre-exposure button. Thus, the preheating time or repeated filament preheating is also reduced. By decreasing the amount of time in the pre-exposure phase, the life of an x-ray tube can be increased.

If an x-ray tube has an evaporated filament, it will be apparent not only on the film but also on the machine's control panel. Under normal circumstances, the milliamperage (mA) or milliamperage-seconds (mA-s) meter on the console will move correspondingly to the exposure technique set. In filament failure, no movement of the mA meter needle will be seen.

Anode Bearing Failure

In x-ray tubes that have a rotating anode, the pre-exposure button has two purposes: (1) it heats the filament and (2) it rotates the anode disk at top speed in preparation for the oncoming electrons.

As with other parts of the x-ray tube, bearings in the rotating anode mechanism can be damaged from heat. Unnecessary use of the pre-exposure button can

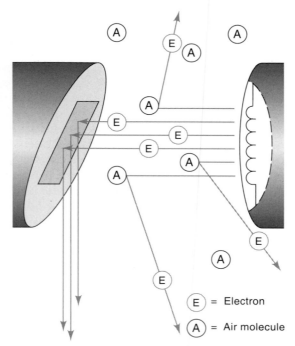

E = Electron

A = Air molecule

■ **FIG. 2.12** Air molecules colliding with the electron stream in a "gassy" x-ray tube.

result in heat accumulation as the anode is spinning. As the heat builds during rotation, the bearings become worn over time and their life is shortened.

Bearing failure can be detected by a change in the noise produced as the anode spins. Usually, the noise increases over time as a result of use and is fostered by thermal overloading of the tube and housing. Eventually, the bearings may decrease anode speed or even stop it. In the case of a slower rotation speed, the anode target will eventually overheat. If the bearings cease to rotate, no noise will be heard when the pre-exposure button is depressed. When the bearings fail, anode target failure is soon to follow.

Anode Target Failure

As stated earlier, the target can be damaged by excessive heat exposure. This can be the result of inadequate heat dissipation or exceeding the melting point during exposure. Damage to the target area is caused by the melting of the surface, resulting in a roughened surface. As electrons hit this rough surface, the intensity of the x-ray beam produced is not uniform in intensity (see Fig. 2.6).

A damaged target can be a major frustration to the radiographer. The x-ray tube remains functional, but the exposures and therefore the film density (blackness) vary among uses. The radiation produced with each exposure is not constant. To prevent damage to the anode, high **kilovoltage peak (kVp)** and low mA-s techniques should be used as often as possible. Exposures made using low mA settings produce fewer

heat units than equivalent exposures made with high mA settings. It is the number of electrons available to the anode impaction that determines the amount of heat produced.

Use of a warm-up procedure is another method to prevent damage to the anode. If heat is introduced to an anode too quickly, the target area will not expand uniformly and may even crack. If warmed gradually, this kind of damage is less likely to occur. Manufacturers specify warm-up procedures in equipment manuals.

Glass Envelope Damage

The glass envelope can become damaged or ineffective in two main ways. The first involves metal deposits that form on the inner lining of the glass, resulting from target overheating. The metal deposits act as a secondary anode and attract the electrons produced at the filament. This phenomenon is called **arcing**. Arcing is often unnoticed until exposure techniques using a higher kVp are used. A tube with such deposits may be effective for quite some time if a lower kVp is used.

The second way a glass envelope can become disabled is by the presence of air within the glass housing. In a "gassy tube," the air molecules interact with the electron stream. This interaction results in a decreased number of x-rays produced at the target area. A gassy tube has little value because of the inability to control the exposure factors necessary for a quality radiograph (Fig. 2.12).

Tube Housing Anomalies

A number of malfunctions can occur in the tube housing, but the problems are rare. Of the various possibilities, two may be of concern in the veterinary practice.

The first possible malfunction involves a shift of the glass envelope within the metal housing. Such a shift may displace the anode target area partially out of alignment with the window, located on the dependent side of the housing. If this were to occur, a portion of the x-ray beam would be absorbed by the metal housing. This would result in a partially exposed radiograph.

The second potential problem is an oil leak out of the metal housing. As stated previously, the oil acts as insulation and assists in heat dissipation. Once the oil is depleted, overheating and eventual destruction of the tube are imminent.

TECHNICAL COMPONENTS OF THE X-RAY MACHINE

Every x-ray apparatus consists of more than the x-ray tube. The x-ray machine comprises many complex mechanisms that allow the radiographer to produce quality radiographs consistently and accurately.

Electrical Components

As described in the beginning of the chapter, the filament in the cathode needs to be heated. Once the filament is heated and an electron cloud is available, there must be a source of power to push the cloud toward the anode target area. These two events not only have to occur, they must be controlled. In order to control the power, time, and amount of release from the x-ray beam, transformers, timers, and generators are necessary.

High-Voltage Circuit

The purpose of the high-voltage circuit is to provide the high electrical potential necessary to transport the electron stream from the cathode to the anode. The high-voltage circuit comprises two transformers: the **autotransformer** and the **step-up transformer**.

The step-up transformer increases the incoming voltage of 110 or 220 V to thousands of volts (kilovoltage). An extremely high potential (kilovoltage peak or kVp) is necessary to transport the electron stream at a fast enough speed to produce x-rays at the anode target impact. The average table-based x-ray machine has a range of 40 to 120 kVp, whereas most portable x-ray machines have a range of 60 to 90 kVp.

In order to control the amount of kVp potential across the x-ray tube, the kVp selection switch on the x-ray machine's control panel is connected to the autotransformer. The autotransformer mechanism is placed between the kVp selector and the high-voltage transformer (Fig. 2.13). The purpose of the autotransformer is to provide a variable yet predetermined voltage to the high-voltage step-up transformer. The high voltage can be preselected at the autotransformer before the exposure is made. Thus, it can be said that the autotransformer is the kVp selector.

Associated with the autotransformer is the **line-voltage compensator**. This mechanism adjusts the incoming line voltage to the autotransformer so that the primary coil voltage remains constant. This compensation is done automatically in newer x-ray units.

Low-Voltage (Filament) Circuit

The purpose of the filament circuit is to provide the electricity (amperage) necessary to heat the filament. Remember that it is the amount of heat at the filament that determines the number of electrons that are available to travel toward the anode. Because the tungsten filament has little resistance to excessive heat, minimal energy is needed to achieve an adequate temperature for electron emission. A simple **step-down transformer** is placed between the cathode filament and the x-ray machine input voltage. The average incoming line voltage to most x-ray machines is 110 or 220 V. This extreme voltage would cause the filament to vaporize instantly. The step-down transformer reduces the voltage of the incoming line to approximately 10 V.

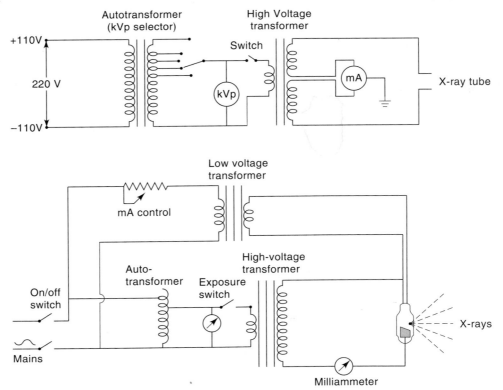

■ **FIG. 2.13** Autotransformer electrical circuit.

The step-down mechanism is connected to the mA control of the x-ray machine's control panel. Control over the amperage in the cathode filament is directly proportional to the number of x-rays produced over a given period.

Timer Switch

A mechanism is needed to control the amount of time during which high voltage is applied across the x-ray tube. By controlling the time of high-voltage transfer, we are thereby controlling the duration of x-ray generation. The device used to control the length of exposure is the **timer switch**.

Exposure time is an important variable in veterinary radiography. Because of the chance of motion due to animal movement, shorter exposure times are necessary. Exposure times of 1/30 of a second (0.3 second) or shorter are needed to decrease the potential for motion on the finished radiograph.

Rectification

When an alternating 60-cycle voltage is applied to the x-ray machine, electrons flow from the cathode to the anode only when the positive deflection of the cycle is applied to the anode. As stated in Chapter 1, all electromagnetic radiation travels in a wave form. During the negative half of every cycle, no electrons are generated within the x-ray tube.

Rectification is the process of changing an alternating current to a direct current. The x-ray tube may perform its own rectification and is known as **half-wave rectification**. As a machine performs its own rectification, one half of the current is lost and there is a marked increase in heat at the anode. If the anode becomes too hot, it is possible that it may form an electron cloud and pass a current from the anode to the cathode. If an electron beam is accelerated toward the filament at the cathode from the anode, severe damage can result. Damage as severe as filament vaporization can occur. Because of this, valve tubes or silicon rectifiers are used to play the role of a rectifier.

Rectifiers allow the flow of electrons in one direction only. The use of **valve tubes** or **self-rectifiers** prolongs the life of the x-ray tube. However, the efficiency of a self-rectified system and that of valve tube or solid-state rectification are not appreciably different.

Half-wave rectification is also possible by placing two rectifiers in a series within the tube. The two sequential rectifiers prevent a reverse flow of the current and subsequent overheating of the cathode. This method has provided some protection of the x-ray tube but has not enabled the use of more of the electrical current (Fig. 2.14A). This type of rectification is employed in most portable and small dental units.

It is possible to convert the alternating current

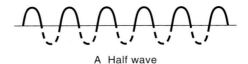
A Half wave

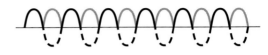
B Full wave

■ **FIG. 2.14** Half-wave rectification (*A*); full-wave rectification (*B*).

into a direct current without losing any amount of electricity. **Full-wave rectification** creates a nearly constant electric potential across the x-ray tube at all times (Fig. 2.14B). By adding four valve tubes or silicon rectifiers to the high-voltage circuit, efficiency of the electrical potential is increased by 100%. The electrical current pulses 120 times per second, as opposed to 60 times per second obtained with half-wave rectification. Full-wave rectification results in twice the x-ray production and gives the advantage of decreased exposure times.

X-ray Tube Rating

X-ray tube rating is based on four factors: (1) focal spot size, (2) target angle, (3) anode speed, and (4) electrical current, single or three-phase operation. The effect of focal spot size, target angle, and anode speed on the x-ray tube efficiency is discussed in previous sections. This section is dedicated to the maximum usage of the electrical supply, which increases the x-ray tube rating.

Each type of x-ray tube has an individual tube rating. X-ray tube ratings dictate the maximum combinations of kVp, mA, and time that can be safely used without overloading the tube. This rating is expressed in kilowatts. Remember that a watt is the unit of electric power, with the kilowatt being a 1000 watts.

Both electrical and thermal limitations exist for a given x-ray tube. To increase the x-ray–producing potential of the x-ray tube, the electrical current potential must be increased. In the United States, commercial electrical power ranges from 115-V to 230-V, 60-cycle alternating current. As discussed in the section on rectification, electrons flow from the cathode to the anode only when the positive deflection of the electrical cycle is applied to the anode. In order to increase the potential power of the electrical supply, a generator is used.

Three-Phase Generator

Most modern table-based x-ray machines have a three-phase generator. Three-phase generators produce an almost constant electrical potential difference between the anode and the cathode. This type of generator produces this almost constant electrical current by superimposing three single-phase currents so that they are 120 degrees out of phase. In other words, each phase is 120 degrees behind the other phase, and there are no deep valleys between the electrical pulses (Fig. 2.15).

The advantages of an x-ray tube with a three-phase generator versus a single-phase generator are:

1. More power is available to the x-ray tube per unit time and therefore allows for shorter exposure.

2. Intensity of the x-radiation generated is considerably higher.

3. Radiation quality is greater because it contains less low-energy x-rays.

4. Tube utilization is more efficient because the target is not subjected to bombardment of low-energy electrons, which create only heat in the anode target area.

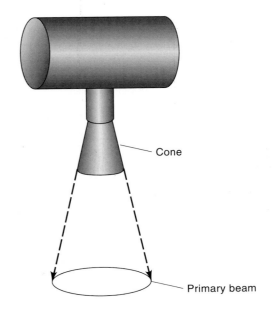

■ **FIG. 2.16** Example of cone collimation.

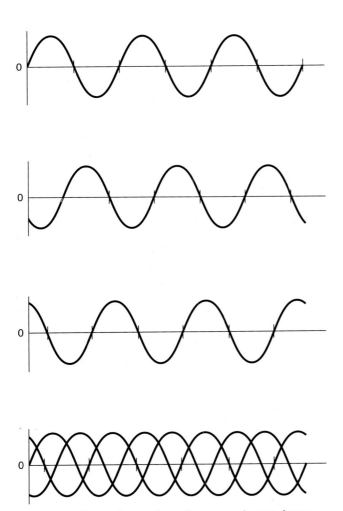

■ **FIG. 2.15** Three-phase alternating current wave forms.

The Collimator

A **collimator** is a restricting device utilized to control the size of the primary x-ray beam. The beam emerges from the x-ray tube in a diverging manner. If uncontrolled, the beam could extend to considerable width. Most x-ray machines incorporate some sort of x-ray beam restriction in order to limit the beam to the essential size. Collimation serves to prevent unnecessary irradiation of the patient or of persons involved in restraining the patient and to reduce scatter radiation as well.

Many of the older or simpler x-ray machines incorporate a lead plate or cone over the aperture of the tube to alter the size of the x-ray beam (Fig. 2.16). Each plate or cone has a different-sized circular hole that alters the size of the window from which the x-rays emerge. Because of the cones, collimation is often described as "coning down."

A more versatile method of collimation is by means of adjustable lead shutters, which are permanently attached to the tube housing, correlating with the tube window. A collimator with lead shutters usually incorporates a light source (Fig. 2.17). The light facilitates visualization of the field size and accurate positioning of the x-ray beam. The collimator light is often difficult to visualize in a brightly lit room and may be most effective in subdued room light.

Knobs located on the collimator allow for adjustment of the field size. It is a good guideline always to use the smallest field size possible for any radiograph. A small field size decreases the amount of scatter radiation.

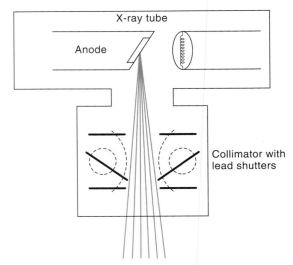

■ **FIG. 2.17** Collimator with lead shutters.

The Tube Stand

The tube stand is the apparatus that supports the x-ray tube during radiographic procedures. The design of the stand varies immensely, differing in forms of suspension. Examples of models range from small table-top stands to larger mobile or overhead ceiling tract stands (Fig. 2.18A, B).

For veterinary purposes, the stand should be durable and sturdy. Some lighter stands that are available are easily moved or damaged by boisterous animals. A shaky stand is a common culprit of motion artifact on a radiograph.

The Control Panel

The control panel or **console** consists of many knobs and switches necessary for the operation of the x-ray machine. It is essential that the radiographer be familiar with all components on the face of the panel and understand that not all control panels are alike (Fig. 2.19). The following is a list of mechanisms found on most x-ray consoles:

1. *On/off switch.* Provides a closure to the electrical circuit to allow the flow of electricity necessary for subsequent exposure.

2. *Voltage compensator.* The voltmeter allows manual adjustment of the transformer to allow for inconsistent electrical output from the main electrical line. The line voltage should be checked whenever the machine is turned on.

3. *Kilovoltage selector.* Most modern x-ray machines are calibrated so that the desired value of kilovoltage can be selected. However, in a number of smaller x-ray units, the kilovoltage control is automatically linked with a certain milliamperage.

4. *Milliamperage selector.* This component lets the radiographer select the desired current to the cathode filament. This method of selection varies among x-ray machines.

5. *Timer.* This mechanism allows the radiographer to preselect the time of each exposure. The timer varies greatly among various models of x-ray

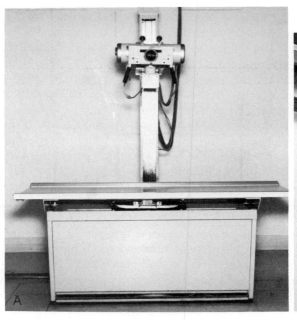
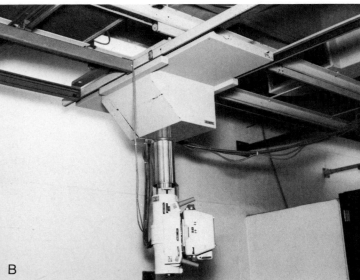

■ **FIG. 2.18** **A,** Example of a fixed tube stand construction. **B,** Example of a ceiling-mounted x-ray unit.

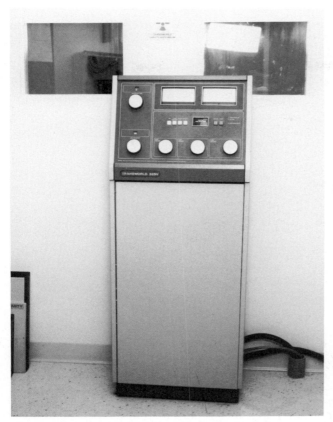

■ **FIG. 2.19** X-ray machine/console anatomy.

6. *Exposure button.* The exposure button is on the face of or attached to the control panel by a length of cable. In either case, the button should be in a position to allow the person making the exposure to be at least 2 m from the tube housing. Many x-ray machines operate on a two-stage button. Two stages are necessary for the cathode filament to be activated and heated to produce the electrons necessary for the exposure. Depression of the first half of the button activates the filament and rotating anode, if present, and, after a few seconds, the button is fully depressed to complete the circuit for exposure.

7. *Warning light.* Most control panels have a light that illuminates when an exposure is made and x-rays are being emitted.

BIBLIOGRAPHY

Ball JL, Moore AD: *Essential Physics for the Radiographer.* Blackwell Scientific, Boston, 1980.

Christensen EE, Curry III ES, Dowdy JE: *An Introduction to the Physics of Diagnostic Radiology,* 2nd ed. Lea & Febiger, Philadelphia, 1978.

Gillette EL, Thrall DE, Lebel JD: *Carlson's Veterinary Radiology,* 3rd ed. Lea & Febiger, Philadelphia, 1977.

Gray JE: *Quality Control in Diagnostic Imaging.* Aspen, Rockville, MD, 1983.

Hendee WR, Chaney EL, Rossi RP: *Radiologic Physics, Equipment and Quality Control.* Year Book Medical, Chicago, 1977.

Kay RS: Modern x-ray tubes. Vet Tech September:575–577, 1992.

Terpogossian MM: *The Physical Aspects of Diagnostic Radiology.* Hoeber Medical Division, Harper & Row, New York, 1967.

Thompson TT: The abuse of radiographic tubes. Radiographics 3:397–399, 1983.

machines. Examples of timers include a clockwork timer, a synchronous timer, and an electronic timer. The advantage of the timer is to have the ability to use a short exposure time with accuracy.

RADIATION
SAFETY

OBJECTIVES

Upon completion of this chapter, the reader should be able to:

- List the tissues most sensitive to radiation-induced damage
- State which personnel are prohibited from radiographic procedures
- State the two types of damage that can occur to tissue from exposure to radiation
- Define maximum permissible dose (MPD) and name the organization that is responsible for setting dose limits
- List and define the units of radiation exposure for absorption
- State the MPD for occupationally exposed personnel

- List and describe the three types of personal exposure dosimeters
- State the three primary methods in which personnel are exposed to radiation during radiography
- List the practical methods that personnel can employ to reduce personal exposure during radiography
- State the proper maintenance protocol for protective apparel
- State the risks and safety measures necessary with use of fluoroscopy

GLOSSARY

DOSIMETER: A device used to measure radiation exposure to personnel.

DOSIMETRY: Various methods used to measure radiation exposure to personnel.

FILM BADGE: A method of dosimetry consisting of a plastic holder with a radiation-sensitive film in a lightproof package.

FLUOROSCOPY: A special radiographic diagnostic method in which a "live view" of the internal anatomy is possible.

GENETIC DAMAGE: Effects of radiation occurring to the genes of reproductive cells.

GRAY (Gy): The unit of absorbed dose imparted by ionizing radiations to matter. One Gray equals 100 rads

HEMOPOIETIC: Anatomic areas where red blood cells are produced.

LEUKOPOIETIC: Anatomic areas where white blood cells are produced.

MAXIMUM PERMISSIBLE DOSE: The maximum dose of radiation a person may receive in a given time period.

POCKET IONIZATION CHAMBER: A method of dosimetry consisting of a charged ion chamber and electrometer, which can be read immediately to determine the amount of exposure.

PRIMARY BEAM: The path that the x-rays follow as they leave the tube.

SECONDARY RADIATION: Commonly called scatter radiation, caused by interaction of the primary beam with objects in its path.

SIEVERT (Sv): The dose of radiation equivalent to the absorbed dose in tissue. One Sievert equals 100 rem.

SOMATIC DAMAGE: Damage to the body induced by radiation that becomes manifest within the lifetime of the recipient.

THERMOLUMINESCENT DOSIMETER (TLD): A method of dosimetry consisting of a chamber containing special compounds that become electrically altered by ionizing radiation.

INTRODUCTION

During every laboratory/diagnostic procedure, safety should be a primary objective. Radiography is no different.

It is a scientific fact that ionizing radiation is a hazard. With the use of diagnostic x-rays in veterinary medicine, the exposure to stray radiation is a common occurrence. However, following proper safety precautions can limit the exposure to radiation.

The veterinarian must establish and maintain a radiation safety program for the protection of the patient, the client, and the technical staff. Safe operating procedures for each facility should include (1) an adequate technique chart or comparable system, (2) positioning aids, (3) protective clothing and other protective barriers, (4) personnel dosimetry devices, (5) emergency procedures for malfunctioning x-ray equipment, and (6) quality control measurements and tests.

All radiographic equipment, including radiation protection devices, must meet state regulation requirements. These regulations can vary within each state. Regulations can usually be obtained from the state Department of Health.

The radiographer should keep one important concept about ionizing radiation in mind:

Radiation should be respected . . . not feared.

HAZARDS OF IONIZING RADIATION

All living cells are susceptible to ionizing radiation damage. Affected cells may be damaged or killed. Cells that are most sensitive to radiation are rapidly dividing cells (e.g., growth cells, gonadal cells, neoplastic cells, and metabolically active cells). Therefore, persons under the age of 18 years and pregnant women should *not* be involved in radiographic procedures. Other tissues that are readily sensitive to radiation include bone, lymphatic, dermis, **leukopoietic** and **hemopoietic** (blood forming), and epithelial tissues.

A vast amount of knowledge has been collected over the years concerning the effects of radiation on the body. Two types of biologic damage can occur from overexposure to radiation: somatic damage and genetic damage.

Somatic damage is a term that describes damage to the body that becomes manifest within the lifetime of the recipient. Radiation can produce immediate changes in the cell, although the damage may not be apparent for some time. Because the body has the ability to repair itself, cell damage may never be appreciated or visible. Damage is more extensive when the body is exposed to a single massive dose of radiation than to smaller, cumulatively equivalent repeated exposures. As mentioned, body cells are not equally sensitive to radiation, and the healing process varies among cell types. Examples of somatic damage include cancer, cataracts, aplastic anemia, and sterility.

Genetic damage from radiation occurs as a result of injury to the genes (DNA) of reproductive cells. Ionizing radiation can damage chromosomal material within any cell. The result of the damage is determined by the cell type (i.e., somatic cell or reproductive cell). Damage to reproductive cells can result in the effect known as gene mutation. Genetic damage is not detectable until future generations are produced. The offspring of irradiated persons may be abnormally formed because of changes in the hereditary material, resulting in the altering of the individual phenotype (physical appearance). The mutation may be lethal or may only be a visible anomaly. The gene mutation may also lay latent or recessive until the second or third generation.

Mortality from radiation is caused by exposure to extremely high levels of radiation. Exposure to a large, single dose of radiation, as from a hydrogen bomb, is necessary to cause rapid death. A single exposure to a dose of 300 rad (radiation absorbed dose; see later) or more has been shown to be lethal to humans. Further information on death due to radiation exposure can be found in a radiobiology textbook. A technologist working in a practical situation, following proper safety protocol, should never receive this level of radiation. Because the body has the ability to repair itself, accumulative smaller doses of radiation are sublethal.

Theoretically, there is no amount of radiation that is nondamaging. Even under the best conditions, some exposure to ionizing radiation will occur. Therefore, it is the responsibility of radiographers to limit the exposure of ionizing radiation to patients, clients, and themselves. The exposure received by any individual should never exceed the maximum permissible dose.

MAXIMUM PERMISSIBLE DOSE

The **maximum permissible dose (MPD)** is of great interest to the radiographer. The MPD is the maximum dose of radiation that a person may receive in a given period. The concept of MPD was introduced to denote an amount of irradiation that does not involve a significantly greater risk to the health of radiation workers so as to influence future generations as well as the individuals occupationally exposed. The MPD helps to determine if procedures and equipment are adequate to provide the degree of protection necessary to stay within the stated limit.

The National Committee on Radiation Protection and Measurements (NCRP) defines the maximum permissible dose (MPD) for occupationally and nonoccu-

pationally exposed persons. The NCRP is a nonprofit organization, chartered by Congress, consisting of scientific committees composed of persons who are considered experts in a particular area.

The NCRP has issued a practical approach to radiation safety in the workplace. The program that has been developed is known as ALARA (as low as reasonably achievable). The process of ensuring that radiation exposures are ALARA may be viewed as an ongoing series of decisions about possible radiation protection actions. A practical approach to the implementation of ALARA in a medical setting must provide a framework for a standard radiation protection program. Thus, certain rules and regulations have been designed to achieve ALARA in the veterinary workplace.

The NCRP and most state health codes permit occupationally exposed persons to restrain and position animal patients manually for radiography when absolutely necessary. However, some state health codes prohibit manual restraint of animals during diagnostic radiography by occupationally exposed personnel. Thus, the animal owner or the staff personnel who are not routinely involved in radiographic procedures have to be used for this purpose.

Another option customary in some states is chemical restraint and positioning devices only (e.g., anesthesia, sandbags, adhesive tape).

Radiation Exposure Units

In order to quantify the amount of radiation received, radiation exposure units are stated in two catagories:

1. **Absorbed dose** is the quantity of energy imparted by ionizing radiations to matter per unit mass of the matter. The unit of absorbed dose is the **gray** (Gy). This replaces the previously used unit which is known as the *rad* (1 Gy = 100 rad).

2. **Dose equivalent** is the quantity obtained by multiplying the absorbed dose in tissue by the quality factor. This equation accounts for the differing biologic effectiveness of equal absorbed doses and other modifying factors. The unit of dose equivalent is the **Sievert** (Sv). The Sievert supersedes the rem, which was previously employed for this purpose (1 Sv = 100 rem).

State and federal restrictions dictate that occupationally exposed individuals over the age of 18 years and wearing monitoring devices can receive up to 0.05 Sv per year from occupational and background exposure.

Any person under the age of 18 is prohibited from the radiographic suite during exposure unless ordered by a medical doctor. Those under the age of 18 are still growing and are more susceptible to radia-

T A B L E   3 . 1

Maximum Permissible Dose (per Calendar Year)

	OCCUPATIONALLY EXPOSED OVER 18 YEARS OF AGE	NON-OCCUPATIONAL, OVER 18 YEARS OF AGE
Whole body	0.05 Sv (5 rem)	0.005 Sv (0.5 rem)
Individual organs and tissues	0.5 Sv (50 rem)	0.05 Sv (5 rem)
Lens of the eye	0.15 Sv (1.5 rem)	0.03 Sv (3 rem)

tion damage. Nonoccupationally exposed persons can receive 10% of this figure (0.005 Sv/year). The MPD for the general public is set at a much lower level because they will not be monitored and they are not trained to recognize and avoid accidental exposure (Table 3.1).

To learn about the specific requirements and regulations on radiation protection in veterinary medicine, booklets can be purchased for a small fee from NCRP.* Suggested readings include NCRP #36, *Radiation Protection in Veterinary Medicine* (also see the Bibliography at end of this chapter).

PATIENT EXPOSURE

The risk of radiation exposure to the patient has been in question by animal owners and veterinary personnel for some time. This chapter is devoted to the discussion of radiation risk to people but is not intended to ignore the risks to animals. Animal patients are just as susceptible to irradiation damage as humans, but, because veterinary personnel are likely to be involved in many more radiographic procedures than one patient, the risk to the animal is, in general, less severe. However, the veterinary radiographer should always be conscious of the radiation risk to the fetus and gonads of breeding animals. Shielding of the gonads of breeding animals is possible and recommended (Fig. 3.1). Unnecessary and excessive radiography should always be avoided to any patient in general.

PERSONNEL MONITORING DEVICES

The actual amount of irradiation received by those engaged in radiography can be monitored (**dosime-**

---

*NCRP Publications, 7910 Woodmont Avenue, Bethesda, MD 20814.

try). Personal exposure monitoring devices (**dosimeters**) should be worn by personnel at all times during radiographic procedures. The monitors are sent regularly to a federally approved laboratory, where they are processed and the dosage received is reported. The exact routine adopted by each practice may vary and depends on the amount and nature of the radio-

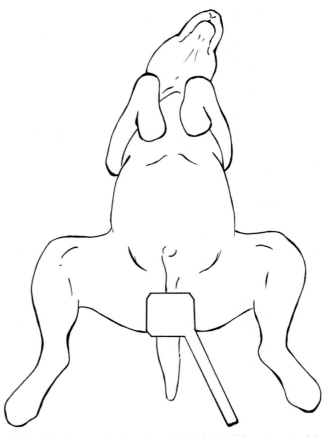

■ **FIG. 3.1** Example of a gonad shield; in this case used to shield the testicles of a male dog.

Various types of radiation monitoring devices are used in veterinary medicine. The **film badge** is the most common type today (Fig. 3.2). A film badge consists of a plastic holder that contains a radiation-sensitive film in a lightproof packaging. The film is sensitive to beta, gamma, and x-radiation of various energies. The films are developed and evaluated by measuring the blackening, due to exposure, on the film. The film badge is worn on the belt, hand, or collar, depending on the anatomic area considered to be most at risk (e.g., gonads, extremities, or thyroid). The same badge is worn for a week, month, or quarter. The length of time depends on the sensitivity of the film and the amount of radiation to which personnel are exposed. Film badges are available in several forms, such as ring badges, wrist badges, and clip-on badges. Film badge dosimetry service can be ordered through several federally approved laboratories (Table 3.2).

Other forms of radiation detectors include the **pocket ionization chamber** and **thermoluminescent dosimeter (TLD)**. The pocket ionization chamber is the same size and shape as a pen and fits conveniently in the pocket of the wearer. It consists of an ion chamber and an electrometer. The chamber is charged before use, and subsequent exposure to radiation discharges the ions. The discharge of the ions is proportional to the amount of radiation received. The exposure can be read immediately from the elec-

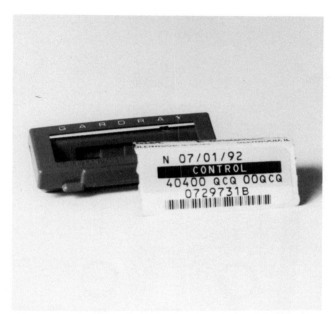

■ **FIG. 3.2** Example of a radiation detection device called a film badge. A film badge consists of a plastic holder containing radiation-sensitive film.

graphic examinations performed. The preferred practice is to wear a dosimeter for a period of 1 month, which is then submitted for evaluation. A replacement dosimeter is issued immediately so that there is no time when the radiographer is not monitored.

T A B L E   3 . 2

Dosimetry Services Meeting National Voluntary Laboratory Accreditation Program (NVLAP) Guidelines*

Radiation Detection Company
162 Wolfe Road
P.O. Box 1414
Sunnyvale, CA 94088
(408) 735-8700

Thermo Analytical, Inc.
TMA/Eberline
5635 Kircher Boulevard NE
P.O. Box 3874
Albuquerque, NM 87109-3874
(505) 345-9931

R.S. Landaurer Jr. & Company
Glenwood Science Park
2 Science Road
Glenwood, IL 60425
(800) 323-8830

Siemens Gammasonics, Inc.
2501 Barrington Road
Hoffman Estates, IL 60195
(800) 666-4552

Teledyne Isotopes
50 Van Buren Avenue
Westwood, NJ 07675
(201) 664-7070

ICN Dosimetry Service
Div. of ICN Biomedicals, Inc.
330 Hyland Avenue
ICN Plaza
Costa Mesa, CA 92626
(714) 545-0100

United States Testing Company
2800 George Washington Way
Richland, WA 99352
(509) 946-8738

*List does not include all organizations that have dosimetry service.

trometer, providing an instant determination of the amount of radiation received. The use of this device in medical diagnostic situations is not recommended.

TLDs contain special compounds (e.g., lithium fluoride and calcium fluoride) that are electrically altered by ionizing radiation. The compounds are available in fine crystals, which are placed in small containers (badges) and worn by personnel. After a period of time, the badge is returned to the dosimetry service for heat processing. When the crystal compounds are heated, they emit light directly proportional to the amount of radiation they have absorbed before heating. TLD dosimetry is considered superior because the measurements can be collected over a long period and can be stored for years without losing information. TLDs can also be reused.

Most dosimetry services supply both film and TLD badges. Currently, film badges cost approximately 25% less than TLD badges.

PRACTICAL APPLICATION OF RADIATION SAFETY

Personnel exposure is a result of (1) exposure to the primary beam, (2) exposure from secondary (scatter) radiation caused by interaction of the primary beam with objects in its path, and (3) exposure from "leakage" radiation from the x-ray tube housing.

Exposure to the **primary beam** is usually the result of technical error. At no time should personnel have any part of their own body in the primary beam, even with proper shielding such as lead aprons and gloves. It is the responsibility of each individual in the radiography suite, at the time of exposure, to ensure his or her own radiation protection.

Beam-limiting devices, such as a collimator, help reduce scatter radiation exposure to the patient and to those assisting with the radiographic procedure.

Radiation exposure due to leakage from the x-ray tube housing is another possibility for radiography personnel. Current regulations for the manufacturing of x-ray tubes require sufficient shielding to minimize exposure to personnel and patients. Normally, a recently manufactured tube head can be considered safe. Unfortunately, many veterinary clinics in the United States still use extremely old x-ray units that have minimal shielding in the tube housing. Such x-ray tubes require additional shielding to decrease the amount of exposure leakage. If the machine is of an older vintage, or if there is a question of radiation leakage, the x-ray tube should be checked by the state Department of Health.

All states have one safety code in common. Each state requires that a minimum of 2.5 mm aluminum filtration of the primary beam be utilized in any diag-

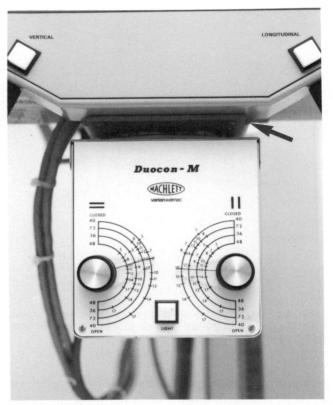

■ **FIG. 3.3** An aluminum filter (*arrow*) is placed between the x-ray tube and the collimator to absorb "soft" x-rays.

nostic x-ray machine that has the capacity of over 70 kilovoltage (kVp). The filter is located between the window of the x-ray tube and the collimator (Fig. 3.3). This filtration essentially eliminates the less penetrating or "soft" x-rays. The soft x-rays, when not filtered, add to the skin exposure of the patient and assisting personnel. Without added filters, the total skin radiation dose of both the patient and the personnel would be increased approximately four times.

Radiation exposure due to **secondary radiation** or **scatter radiation** is produced when the primary beam interacts with objects in its path. Scatter can be produced within the patient, tabletop, floor, or any other object in the path of the primary beam (Fig. 3.4). The amount and direction of scatter depend on the intensity of the beam, the composition of the structure being radiographed, the kVp level, and the thickness of the patient.

Scatter is produced in all directions and travels in straight lines. A large portion of scatter travels in an upward path toward the torso and head of the restrainer. Personnel involved in the radiographic procedure should have as much distance as possible between them and the primary beam at all times. Looking away from the primary beam during exposure will minimize radiation to the lenses of the eye. At no time should personnel lean over or sit on the x-ray

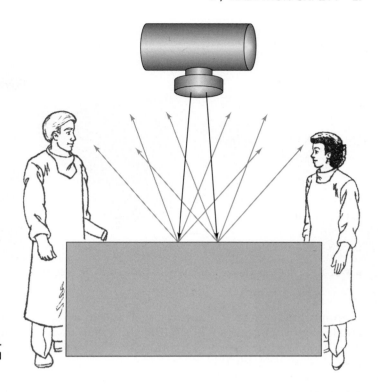

■ **FIG. 3.4** Example of scatter radiation due to the interaction of the primary x-ray beam with the tabletop and patient.

table (Fig. 3.5). Provided that the recommended precautions are observed, most animals can be radiographed without anyone's receiving a significant amount of radiation.

Chemical restraint of the animal should be considered whenever possible to minimize exposure to employees in the workplace. (Note: Some states forbid

humans from restraining animals in veterinary radiography.) Ideally, the animal should be sedated and positioned with supporting devices (Fig. 3.6A,B). The operator is then shielded by the wall of the control booth or behind a leaded screen during exposure.

If chemical restraint is not possible, certain safety measures must be observed. All personnel should wear

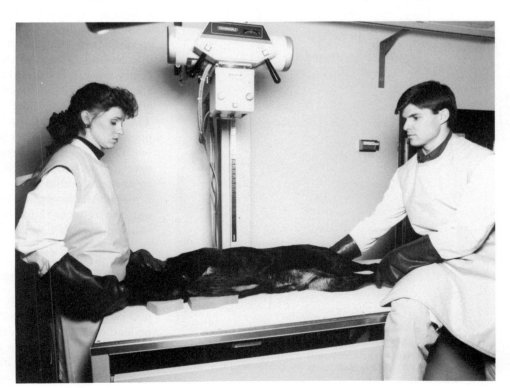

■ **FIG. 3.5** Incorrect posture for manual restraint. At no time should a restrainer sit on the x-ray table during exposure.

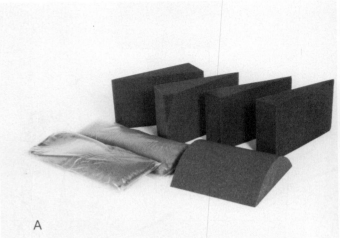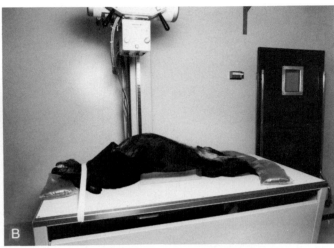

■ **FIG. 3.6 A,** Examples of various positioning aids. **B,** A sedated patient held in place with the assistance of positioning aids.

the appropriate protective apparel, such as lead aprons and lead gloves having a 0.5 mm lead equivalent thickness. Mobile lead screens with a lead glass window or leaded plastic shields that hang from the ceiling are also available. The lead glass window or lead plastic shield permits observation of the patient, yet provides adequate protection from exposure. Lead walls are useful but are an expensive method of protection (Fig. 3.7).

When restraining an animal on the x-ray table, personnel should stand in an upright position at the end of the table. In this way, the distance between the source of scatter radiation and the restrainer is increased (Fig. 3.8A,B). The restrainer should never be exposed to the primary beam of radiation, even if shielded (Fig. 3.9). The lead apparel will usually reduce the dose of scatter radiation significantly; however, only a fraction of the higher energy of the primary beam will be absorbed.

A common artifact seen on veterinary radiographs is the appearance of fingers or entire hands holding an animal in position (Fig. 3.10). This artifact is considered "illegal" and should be avoided.

No individuals, other than the operator and necessary restrainers, should be present when exposures are being made. If restraint by humans is used, it is good practice to rotate personnel that are required. This practice decreases the possibility of one or two persons exceeding their MPD.

One of the best ways to minimize radiation exposure in the workplace is to avoid the occurrence of retakes. It should be the radiographer's goal to achieve a quality radiograph on the first attempt. This not only reduces radiation exposure to the patient and restrainers, it is cost-effective and saves time.

Maintenance of Protective Apparel

Proper care of protective apparel is essential to continued radiation safety. Lead aprons and gloves are made of lead-impregnated rubber and other materials that have an equivalent range of thickness from 0.25 to 1.0 mm lead. Regulations in veterinary radiography require 0.5 mm of lead equivalent in the aprons and

■ **FIG. 3.7** A portable lead wall with a leaded glass window. The lead wall is designed to allow the radiographer to remain in the x-ray room during exposure by protecting him or her from radiation exposure.

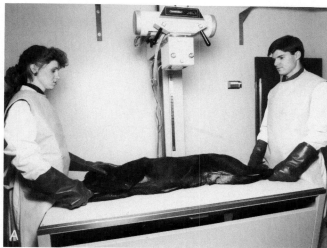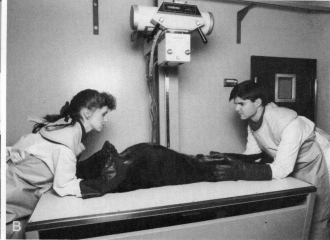

■ **FIG. 3.8 A,** Appropriate posture for manual restraint during exposure. **B,** *Improper* posture for manual restraint during exposure.

gloves because the restrainer is often very close to the primary beam.

The shielding material is constructed to allow agility to the wearer. Therefore, cracks can result from improper handling and storage. Aprons should be hung vertically over a round surface (not less than 3 cm in diameter) or laid flat when not in use. Gloves should be placed on vertical holders that allow air to circulate throughout the inside (Fig. 3.11A,B,C). Another method that will allow air circulation is to place metal soup cans, with both ends cut out, in the gloves. With the cans in place, the gloves can be laid horizontally on a flat surface. This circulation of air is necessary to eliminate the moisture that can accumulate in the gloves.

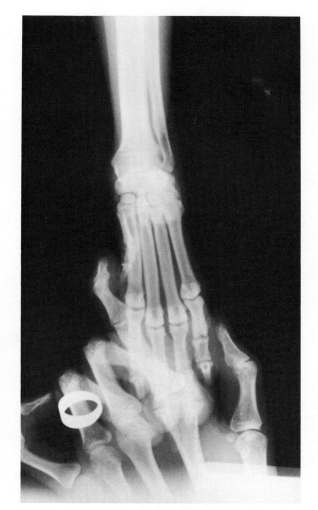

■ **FIG. 3.10** Radiograph of a forelimb of a canine patient with a human hand holding the limb. This type of restraint should be considered forbidden; human anatomy should never be viewed on a veterinary radiograph.

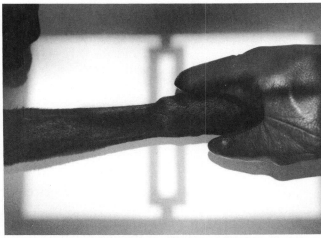

■ **FIG. 3.9** A poor radiation safety practice. Hands should never be positioned within the field of the primary x-ray beam, even with lead gloves on.

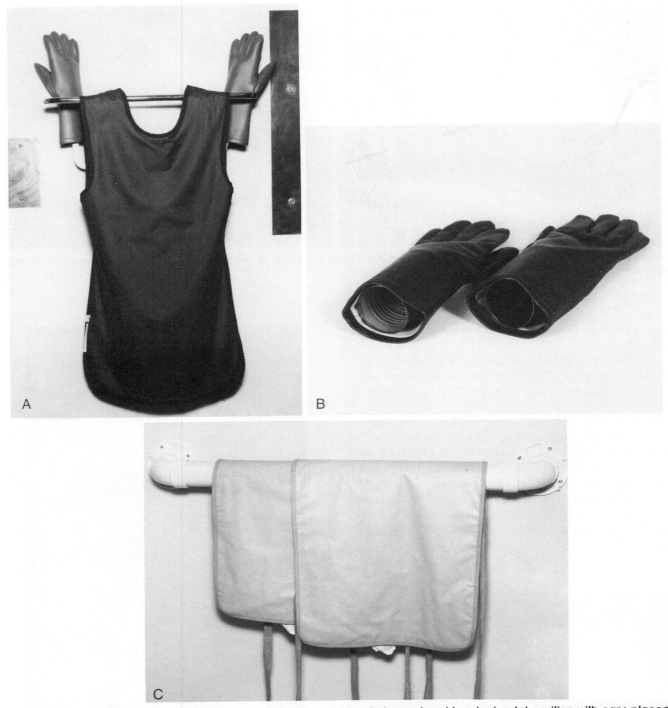

■ **FIG. 3.11** **A,** Vertical storage of lead aprons and gloves. **B,** Lead gloves stored in a horizontal position with cans placed inside to allow air circulation. **C,** Lead aprons draped over a "homemade" hanger. The hanger consists of a cylindric tube that is 4 inches or greater in diameter.

Lead aprons and gloves should be inspected periodically for damage. Every time the apparel is worn, a visual inspection should be made. Obvious tears, cracks, or signs of deterioration should be investigated further. The aprons and gloves should be manually checked on a quarterly basis. A manual inspection includes feeling the internal and external surfaces for defects or irregularities. The most conclusive inspection method is taking a radiograph (or a fluoroscopic study, if available) of all protective apparel. If any cracks are present in the lead lining, it will be apparent on a radiograph. After processing, the film should

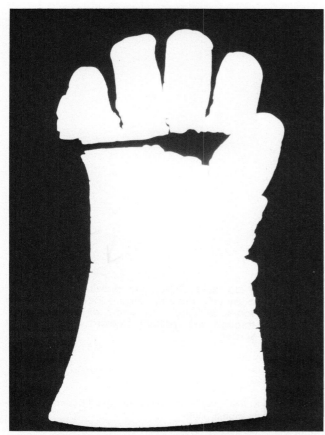

■ **FIG. 3.12** Radiograph of a lead glove showing a crack in the lead lining.

- Always wear protective apparel designed to absorb secondary radiation effectively (0.5 mm lead thickness).
- Ensure maximum life of protective apparel with proper use and care.
- Never permit any part of the body to be within the primary beam *whether shielded or not.*
- Use collimation whenever possible to decrease field size and scatter radiation.
- Use a 2.5-mm aluminum filter to remove soft x-rays from the primary beam.
- Do not direct the x-ray beam directly at any personnel or an adjacent occupied room.
- Never hand-hold the x-ray tube.
- Wear film or TLD badges near the collar, outside of the lead apron, to monitor radiation exposure.
- Plan the radiographic procedure carefully to avoid unnecessary retakes.
- Maintain darkroom chemicals in good operating condition.
- Have the x-ray machine calibrated annually by a qualified service representative.
- Keep an exposure log that identifies the patient, the type of study performed, and the exposure values.
- Adhere to the radiation safety codes for your state.
- Remember that patience is an important virtue.

Additional Radiation Safety Rules for Fluoroscopy

Fluoroscopy is employed for special radiographic diagnostic studies when a "live view" of the internal anatomy is necessary. The primary x-ray beam of the fluoroscope is directed through the animal onto a view screen (Fig. 3.13). A primary use of fluoroscopy is for evaluation of the alimentary function. This is observed by the passage of barium sulfate (a radiopaque contrast medium) through the stomach and intestines. Because sedation or general anesthesia affects normal bowel activity, manual restraint is usually necessary.

During fluoroscopy, a continuous stream of x-rays is emitted while the machine is activated. Because of the high levels of radiation and the need for manual restraint, special safety rules must be followed:

- Never use fluoroscopy in the place of radiography.
- Always use protective aprons, gloves, and shields.
- Keep the collimator beam as small as possible.
- Never palpate the anatomic area that is being viewed while the machine is activated.
- Follow all rules that apply to the use of a regular x-ray machine.

remain relatively clear. If there are any breaks in the lead of the apron or glove, an increase in density (blackness) will appear on the film surface (Fig. 3.12).

If the apron is defective within the main body area, it should be discarded. If the defect is located near the hem or shoulder area, it can be marked with a permanent marker and checked more frequently. A person wearing a defective lead apron or glove is potentially being exposed to radiation at the area of the defect. To prevent unnecessary exposure, this safety test should be performed at least annually.

RADIATION SAFETY RULES — A CHECKLIST
- Remove all unnecessary personnel from the radiographic suite during exposure.
- Never permit persons under the age of 18 or pregnant women in the radiographic suite while in use.
- Rotate personnel who assist in radiographic procedures to minimize exposure.
- Use mechanical restraints whenever possible (e.g., sandbags).
- Use chemical restraint whenever possible (anesthetize or tranquilize).

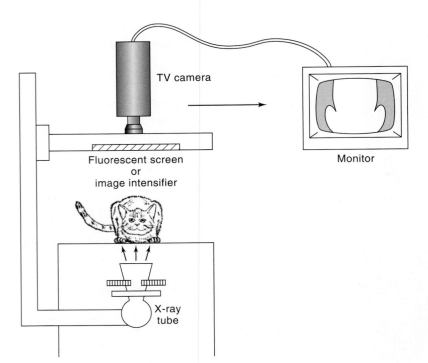

TV camera

Fluorescent screen
or
image intensifier

X-ray
tube

Monitor

■ **FIG. 3.13** Schematic drawing of a fluoroscopy unit. The x-ray tube is located under the table, with the x-ray beam directed upward, through the patient, toward a fluorescent screen.

BIBLIOGRAPHY

Burkhart RL: *A Basic Quality Assurance Program for Diagnostic Radiology Facilities.* HEW Publication (FDA) 83-8218, Rockville, Md, 1983.

Burkhart RL: *Patient Radiation Exposure in Diagnostic Radiology Examinations: An Overview.* HHS Publication (FDA) 83-8217, Rockville, Md, 1983.

Gray JE, Winkler NT, Stears J, Frank ED: *Quality Control in Diagnostic Imaging.* Aspen, Rockville, Md, 1983.

McKinney WE: *Radiographic Processing and Quality Control.* JB Lippincott, Philadelphia, 1988.

Minnesota Department of Health Advisory Work Group: *Rules Governing Sources of Ionizing Radiation.* Mayo Clinic, Rochester, Minn.

NCRP: *Radiation Protection in Veterinary Medicine (#36).* Bethesda, Md, 1970.

NCRP: *Structural Shielding Design and Evaluation or Medical Use of X-rays and Gamma Rays of Energies up to 10 MeV (#49).* Bethesda, Md, 1970.

EXPOSURE FACTORS

OBJECTIVES

Upon completion of this chapter, the reader should be able to:

- State the variable that controls the quality of an x-ray beam
- State the variable that controls the quantity of an x-ray beam
- Define the role of milliamperage in the production of x-rays
- Define the role of time in the production of x-rays
- List the advantages of the use of high milliamperage settings
- State the equation used to determine mA-s

- Define the role of kilovoltage in the production of x-rays
- List the effects of increased kilovoltage on the x-ray beam
- Define Santes' rule, and use the equation given a measurement in centimeters
- State the effect of distance on the intensity of an x-ray beam
- Define the inverse square law
- Describe how radiography works

GLOSSARY

CALIPER: A device used to measure the thickness of anatomic parts.

CONTRAST: The measurable difference between two adjacent densities.

DENSITY: The degree of blackness on a radiograph.

EXPOSURE TIME: The period of time during which x-rays are permitted to leave the x-ray tube.

INVERSE SQUARE LAW: The intensity of the radiation varies inversely as the square of the distance from the source.

KILOVOLTAGE: Related to thousands of volts. Describes the electrical potential (difference) between the cathode and the anode; is responsible for accelerating the electrons from the cathode to the anode; and relates to the penetrating power of the x-rays.

KINETIC ENERGY: The energy related to motion.

MILLIAMPERAGE-SECONDS (mA-s): The number of x-rays produced over a given period. Calculated by multiplying the milliamperage by the time.

MILLIAMPERE: One thousandth of an ampere. A measure of electron current to the filament, which has a direct relationship to the number of x-rays produced.

SANTES' RULE: A method of estimating kilovoltage in relation to area thickness: (2 × thickness in cm) + 40 = kilovoltage.

SOURCE-IMAGE DISTANCE (SID): Formerly called **focal-film distance (FFD)**, the distance between the source of x-rays and the image receptor or film.

THERMIONIC EMISSION: The process of releasing electrons from their atomic orbits by heat.

A REVIEW

In order for an x-ray tube to produce x-rays, suitable electrical currents must be supplied to both the cathode filament and the field between the cathode and the anode.

The *quality* of an x-ray beam is determined by its penetrating power. Radiation of shorter wavelength has increased penetrating power and is said to have increased penetrating ability.

The *quantity* or intensity of the x-ray beam is defined as the amount of energy flowing per second through a unit area perpendicular to the direction of the beam. Simply stated, it is the number of x-rays traveling from the x-ray tube toward the image receptor in a period of time.

The quantity and quality of the x-ray beam are affected by various factors.

Milliamperage and Time

Electrons are produced by heating the cathode filament. By passing a calibrated electrical current through the low-tension circuit of the x-ray machine, the metal of the filament is heated and electrons are released. The process of "boiling off" the electrons from their atomic orbits is known as **thermionic emission**. The "free" electrons form a cloud around the filament. The number of electrons in the electron cloud is directly proportional to the temperature of the filament (Fig. 4.1).

The electrical current that heats the filament is measured in **milliamperes** (one thousandth of an am-

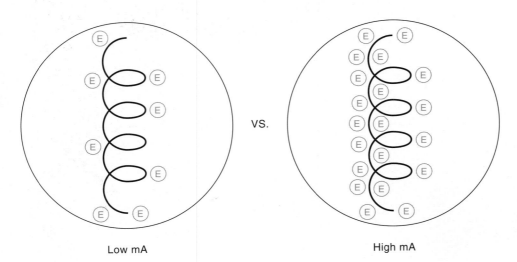

VS.

Low mA   High mA

■ **FIG. 4.1** Drawing showing the effect of mA placed on the filament; the mA setting is proportionate to the number of electrons produced.

pere). As the milliamperage (mA) is increased, the number of electrons available is increased. The number of x-rays produced at the anode impaction is dependent on the size of the electron cloud. The mA, therefore, affects the intensity of the x-ray beam and is the measure of quantity of x-radiation produced.

The total quantity of x-rays produced during a given exposure is also dependent on the length of exposure. That is, there is a direct relationship between mA and the length of exposure (time). The period during which the x-rays are permitted to leave the x-ray tube is termed the **exposure time** and is measured in fractions of seconds. The number of electrons and the period of time set for their release determine how many x-rays are available. Therefore, the quantity of x-rays required for a given exposure is best expressed as the product of the mA and the time in **milliamperage-seconds (mA-s)**.

Milliamperage-seconds can be calculated using the following equation:

$$ma \times time \ (in \ seconds[s]) = mA\text{-}s$$

EXAMPLES:

20 mA × ½ (s) = 10 mA-s
100 mA × ¹⁄₁₀ (s) = 10 mA-s
200 mA × ¹⁄₂₀ (s) = 10 mA-s
300 mA × ¹⁄₃₀ (s) = 10 mA-s

There are advantages to the use of high mA settings. As seen in the examples a higher mA setting allows for a shorter time setting with the same number of x-rays produced. By using a shorter time setting, the possibility of motion occurring on a radiograph is decreased. Motion is considered the most common artifact in veterinary radiography ("Murphy's law" of veterinary radiography states that an animal will move at the moment the exposure is made). A shorter exposure time also decreases the exposure to restraining personnel. It is therefore advantageous to use the highest mA setting possible.

Another advantage of a higher mA setting is the greater amount of x-rays produced. A suitable mA-s setting is dependent on the thickness and type of tissue being radiographed. A machine with high mA capability allows examination of thicker anatomic areas of the patient.

X-ray machines vary according to their mA potential. Machines that have a higher mA capacity are more powerful and have increased diversity of use in practice. There are smaller x-ray machines, however, that have a constant mA capability with no provision for alteration. Other small units have variable settings in the range of 10 to 30 mA. Larger, more expensive equipment may have a maximum mA value as high as 1600 (Figs. 4.2 and 4.3; see Fig. 2.4).

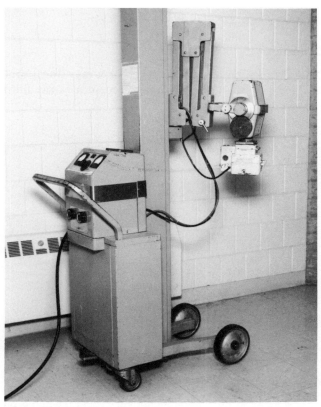

■ **FIG. 4.2** Mobile x-ray unit.

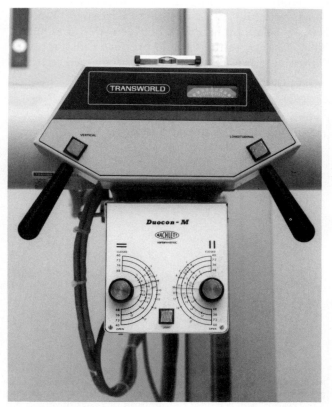

■ **FIG. 4.3** Fixed x-ray unit.

Kilovoltage

During an exposure, the anode is maintained at a high positive electrical potential relative to the cathode. Because of this difference in electrical charge, the electron cloud at the filament is formed into a narrow beam and accelerates toward the anode at a very high speed. The **kinetic energy** of the electrons when they reach the target is proportional to the potential difference placed between the anode and the cathode. The potential difference between the anode and the cathode, or the **kilovoltage**, is measured in kilovolts (thousands of volts, or kV).

Another term commonly used for the kilovoltage is kilovoltage peak (kVp). The word "peak" indicates the maximum energy available at that kilovoltage setting. The higher the kilovoltage, the faster the electrons are accelerated. This acceleration increases the energy of the x-rays produced at the electron collision with the anode target.

A change in kilovoltage has a number of effects. First, it results in a change in penetrating power of the x-ray beam. When the kVp is raised, new, shorter wavelength x-rays are produced.

The kVp determines the quality of the x-ray beam and, thus, its ability to penetrate tissue. Higher kVp settings produce more penetrating beams, with a higher percentage of radiation reaching the film (Fig. 4.4).

Higher kVp settings allow for lower mA-s settings, which generally call for shorter exposure time. An inverse relationship exists between kVp and mA-s. The following settings would produce radiographs of comparable density if other factors remained constant:

60 kVp and 4.0 mA-s (10 mA × 0.4 s)
70 kVp and 2.0 mA-s (10 mA × 0.2 s)
80 kVp and 1.0 mA-s (10 mA × 0.1 s)
90 kVp and 0.5 mA-s (5 mA × 0.1 s)

(Note: Although the techniques provide a comparable density, the radiographic contrast is affected, which will alter the appearance of an image. **Contrast** and **density** are discussed in Chapter 5.)

The kVp can be estimated utilizing an equation known as **Santes' rule**. Santes' rule uses the thickness of the area of interest to be radiographed to calculate the kVp needed. Santes' rule states:

$$(2 \times cm \ [\text{measurement thickness}]) + 40 = kVp$$

Measurement of an anatomic area is taken with a **caliper** and is measured in centimeters (Fig. 4.5). The number 40 represents the distance from the x-ray tube's focal spot (source of x-rays) to the image receptor (x-ray film) in inches and is referred to as the **focal-film distance (FFD)** or **source-image distance (SID)**. The SID will be discussed presently.

The sum of Santes' rule is the kVp necessary for an exposure with the film on the tabletop, without the use of a grid or film Bucky tray system. Santes' rule supplies the radiographer with a starting point that can be modified for the grid, cassette tray, or other variable.

EXAMPLE:

Dr. Smith has requested an abdominal radiograph on a Labrador retriever. The measurement of the lateral view was 16 cm.

$$(2 \times 16) + 40 = 72 \ kVp$$

Distance

The distance between the source of x-rays (focal spot of the x-ray tube) and the image receptor (x-ray film)

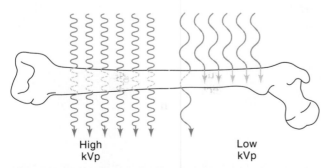

■ **FIG. 4.4** Drawing showing the effect of the kVp level on penetration. High kVp settings produce a more penetrating x-ray beam, with a higher percentage of x-rays reaching the film.

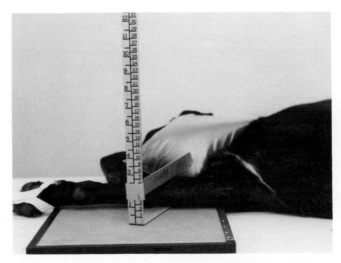

■ **FIG. 4.5** Example of a caliper, the instrument used to measure the thickness of an anatomic area. The measurement is taken in centimeter increments, using the scale on the left side of the caliper. This patient measures 14 cm.

also affects the intensity of the image produced. As the SID is decreased, the intensity of the x-rays is increased.

To demonstrate this phenomenon, take a flashlight into a room with little or no light. Stand approximately 3 m away from a wall, and shine the light at the wall. Keeping the light aimed at the same point, walk toward the wall. Notice how the light intensity increases as the distance between the light and the wall decreases. Exactly the same thing happens with x-rays.

In the same respect, as the SID is increased, the intensity of the x-radiation is decreased. Increasing the distance from the radiation source reduces the intensity of the beam according to the **inverse square law**.

X-rays obey the laws of light in that they diverge from the point source. The intensity of the beam varies inversely according to the square of the distance (Fig. 4.6). A change in distance is similar to a change in mA in its effect on the overall intensity of the beam. In other words, radiographic density is affected by a change in distance.

When the SID is changed, the total amount of x-rays must be increased or decreased in order to make a comparable exposure employing the new distance. This can be done by changing the mA-s, which governs the rate in which the x-ray tube produces x-radiation. When a different distance is used, the adjustment of the mA-s can be calculated as follows:

$$\text{old mA-s} \times \frac{(\text{new SID})^2}{(\text{old SID})^2} = \text{new mA-s}$$

$$10 \text{ mA-s} \times \frac{(150 \text{ cm})^2}{(75 \text{ cm})^2} = \frac{40}{1} = 40 \text{ mA-s}$$

When the SID is changed, image detail is changed. As any SID is decreased, image sharpness is decreased. This topic is discussed later.

The SID is an important exposure factor. Whenever possible, the SID should be kept constant. The most common SID in veterinary practice ranges from 36 to 40 inches (90 to 100 cm). The distance is usually noted on the x-ray tube stand or is measured with the tape mounted on the side of the tube housing. It is important to verify the correct SID before every radiograph because of the effect of the SID on radiographic film density.

HOW RADIOGRAPHY WORKS: A REVIEW

X-rays are generated in an x-ray tube. The tube consists of a cathode side (with a negative electrical charge) and an anode side (with a positive charge). In the tube, a stream of fast-moving electrons is attracted and directed from the cathode to the anode. As the electrons collide and interact with the atoms on the anode target, a great amount of energy is produced; 1% of this energy is in the form of x-radiation.

The cathode consists of a wire filament that emits electrons when heated. The temperature of the filament is controlled by the milliamperage (mA) setting on the console of the machine. As the mA is increased, the temperature of the filament is increased and the filament produces more electrons. The period of time during which the electrons (x-rays) are permitted to leave the x-ray tube is measured in fractions of seconds (s). The number of electrons available and the time period set for their release determine how many x-rays are available. The milliamperage-seconds (mA-s) thus controls the total number of x-rays produced.

The anode, which attracts negatively charged electrons, is constructed at an angle so that the x-rays produced are directed downward (toward the film) through a window in the metal housing of the x-ray tube.

The electron speed necessary to create a high-energy impact is achieved by applying thousands of volts (kVp) across the anode and cathode field. High voltage produces x-rays with greater penetrating power and intensity. The kVp thus controls the penetrating power of the x-rays.

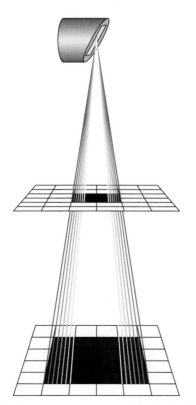

■ **FIG. 4.6** The inverse square law: The intensity of the primary x-ray beam is inversely proportionate to the source-image distance. The intensity of the primary beam projected on a given perpendicular plane is reduced to one quarter by doubling the distance from the point source.

This version of how radiography works is abridged, and some confusion may remain. The following section is intended to demonstrate a simplified version of how the variables work together to form a radiograph of good quality.

HOW RADIOGRAPHY WORKS: A DIFFERENT LOOK

Imagine yourself in a grocery store, with a grocery cart and ready to go. Your purpose, however, is not to shop for the week's food but to knock down a large pile of tomato juice cans stacked in a pyramid. The pyramid is located in the center of the store and stands 10-feet tall. To accomplish your goal, you have only the cart and all the muscle you can muster.

With a running start, you head for the pyramid. Despite your running speed and strength, you are unable to knock down all of the cans of tomato juice—only a few are displaced. The grocery cart is stopped in its tracks, and you are thrown into the produce aisle. Among the canned goods, you decide to put something inside the cart to increase its weight. Perhaps the momentum of a heavy cart pushed with great force will knock down the pyramid. You fill the cart with cans of beans (Fig. 4.7). Straining with effort, you slowly push the cart toward the stack of juice cans. Because of the extreme weight in the cart, your strength is insufficient to break through the pyramid.

Feeling a bit dismayed, you sit once again. But with sudden inspiration, you remove half of the beans from the cart and again race toward the stack of juice cans. The sufficient weight and your adequate strength enable you to topple the entire pyramid.

In order to apply this parable, it is necessary to examine the facts. To topple the pyramid, you needed a certain number of cans of beans in the cart and sufficient strength to push the cart through. The beans represent the amount of electrons (number of x-rays) or mA-s, the muscle power pushing the cart represents the kVp, and the pyramid represents the

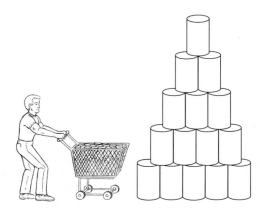

■ **FIG. 4.7** Bean scenario illustrated (see text).

patient. If there is insufficient weight in the cart (milliamperage-seconds), it is impossible to knock down all of the cans of juice (the tissue of the patient) regardless of the amount of pushing power (kilovoltage).

Similarly, regardless of the amount of weight in the cart, it is impossible to penetrate the pyramid if there is inadequate strength. The necessary amount of muscle and beans always depends on the size of the pyramid. The amount of milliamperage-seconds and kilovoltage required for a given patient depends on the density of the anatomic part being radiographed.

BIBLIOGRAPHY

Ball JL, Moore AD: *Essential Physics for Radiographers.* Blackwell Scientific, Boston, 1980.

Cunliffe-Lavin LM: Radiographic technique: A ray of hope. Vet Tech J 12:444, 1991.

Curry TS, Dowdy JE, Murry RC: *Christensen's Physics of Diagnostic Radiology,* 4th ed. Lea & Febiger, Philadelphia, 1990.

Douglas SW, Herrtage ME, Williamson HD: *Principles of Veterinary Radiography,* 4th ed. Bailliere Tindall, Philadelphia, 1987.

Eastman Kodak Company: *Kodak: The Fundamentals of Radiography,* 12th ed. Rochester, NY, 1980.

Morgan JP, Silverman S: *Techniques of Veterinary Radiography,* 4th ed. Iowa State University Press, Ames, 1987.

RADIOGRAPHIC QUALITY

5

OBJECTIVES

Upon completion of this chapter, the reader should be able to:

- Define radiographic density
- List the factors that affect radiographic density
- Define contrast, radiographic contrast, and subject contrast
- List and describe the exposure factors that affect contrast and density
- Define scatter radiation and its effect on the radiographic image
- Describe a grid and its purpose in radiography
- Define grid focus and its significance

- Describe grid cutoff, its radiographic appearance, and the various ways it is produced
- List the variables that contribute to grid efficiency
- List and describe the various grid types and their advantages and disadvantages
- Describe the correct care of a grid
- Define radiographic detail
- List and describe the factors that affect radiographic detail

G L O S S A R Y

BACKSCATTER: Process of scattering or reflecting radiation in the opposite direction intended. Radiation that is reflected from behind the image plane back to the image.

CONTRAST: The measurable difference between two adjacent densities.

CROSSED GRID: Two parallel or two focused grids that are set at right angles to each other. Also called **crisscross grid**.

ELONGATION: Distortion of anatomic structures when the image appears longer than actual size owing to the x-ray beam not being directed perpendicular to the film surface.

FOCUSED GRID: A grid with a parallel center lead strip with strips on either side radiating out progressively inclined at greater angles.

FORESHORTENING: Distortion of anatomic structures when the image appears shorter than actual size due to the plane of interest not being parallel to the film surface.

GEOMETRIC DISTORTION: Variation in normal size and shape of anatomic structures due to their position related to the x-ray source and film.

GEOMETRIC UNSHARPNESS: Loss of detail due to geometric distortion

GRID: A device made of lead strips imbedded in a spacing material, placed between the patient and the film, designed to absorb non–image-forming radiation.

GRID CUTOFF: A progressive decrease in transmitted x-ray intensity caused by the grid lines absorbing primary x-rays.

GRID EFFICIENCY: The ability of a grid to absorb non–image-forming radiation in the production of a quality radiograph.

GRID FACTOR: The amount the exposure needs to be increased to compensate for the grid's absorption of a portion of the primary beam.

GRID FOCUS: The distance from the source of x-rays and the grid in which the grid is effective without grid cutoff.

GRID RATIO: The relation of the height of the lead strips to the distance between them.

LINEAR GRID: Grid in which the lead strips are parallel to each other.

LINES PER CENTIMETER: The number of lead strips per centimeter area.

MAGNIFICATION: Distortion of anatomic structures when the image appears larger than actual size.

POTTER-BUCKY DIAPHRAGM: A mechanical device that consists of a focused grid within a diaphragm, which moves the grid across the x-ray beam during the exposure.

PSEUDOFOCUSED GRID: A grid with parallel lead strips that are progressively reduced in height toward the edges of the grid.

RADIOGRAPHIC CONTRAST: The density difference between two adjacent areas on a radiograph.

RADIOGRAPHIC DENSITY: The degree of blackness or "darkness" on a radiograph.

RADIOGRAPHIC DETAIL: The definition of the edge of an anatomic structure on a radiograph.

RADIOGRAPHIC QUALITY: The ease with which details can be perceived on a radiograph.

SCATTER RADIATION: Non–image-forming radiation that is scattered in all directions owing to objects in the path of the x-ray beam.

SUBJECT CONTRAST: The difference in density and mass of two adjacent anatomic structures.

UNFOCUSED GRID: A grid with lead strips that are parallel to one another and at right angles to the film. Also called parallel grid.

I N T R O D U C T I O N

A radiograph without quality is similar to a story without meaning. To produce a quality radiograph, predetermined aspects of quality must be understood by the radiographer. Comprehension of the aspects of quality is essential to a complete understanding of how radiography works.

Radiographic quality refers to the ease with which details can be perceived on a radiograph. We must obtain as much diagnostic information as possible about the internal structures of the patient. Radiographic quality is dependent on radiographic density, contrast, and geometric factors that affect detail. The intention of this chapter is to define diagnostic image characteristics and how to obtain them (Fig. 5.1).

RADIOGRAPHIC DENSITY

Radiographic density is defined as the degree of blackness or "darkness" on a radiograph. Black areas on a developed radiograph are produced by deposits of metallic silver in the film emulsion resulting from exposure to x-rays and subsequent processing. A radiograph that consists of many black areas and is very dark when viewed has high density.

An important concept to remember is that *x-rays make radiographic film black*. The degree of blackness on a radiograph is dependent on the amount of x-rays reaching the film. Density is influenced by the quantity and quality of the x-ray beam as well as the type and thickness of the tissue under examination.

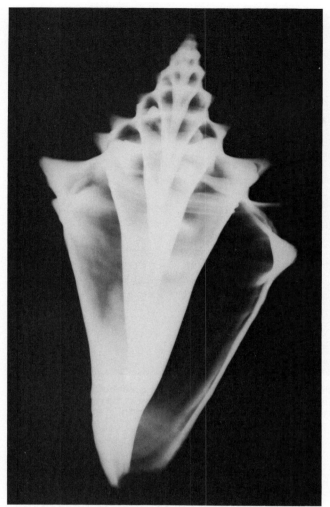

■ **FIG. 5.1** Radiograph of a seashell showing contrast, density, and detail characteristics.

Factors Affecting Radiographic Density

Greater radiographic density may be produced by increasing the (a) total number of x-rays that reach the film, (b) penetrating power of the x-rays, (c) developing time, or (d) temperature of the developer. (Film development is discussed in Chapter 7.)

As discussed in Chapter 3, the number of x-rays leaving the x-ray tube is determined by the milliamperage-seconds (mA-s). As the mA-s is increased, more x-rays reach the patient and film, and radiographic density is increased. In the same respect, raising the kilovoltage (or kVp) of the x-ray beam increases radiographic density as well. As the kVp is increased, the penetrating power of the x-rays is increased, resulting in more x-rays reaching the film. The radiograph becomes darker as more x-rays reach the film.

Radiographic density is also influenced by the thickness and type of tissue being radiographed. Body parts that have greater thickness absorb more x-rays,

resulting in a lighter image on the radiograph. Radiographic density is inversely proportional to tissue density. In other words, if the density or thickness of tissue doubles, the number of x-rays reaching the film is approximately halved. For example, the body of a 150-pound Saint Bernard will absorb many more x-rays than the body of a 75-pound Labrador retriever. Assuming that the same amount of x-rays were used for the Saint Bernard as required for the Labrador, the radiograph of the Saint Bernard would lack adequate radiographic density. The area of the film where the body of the Saint Bernard was located would be too white and would lack sufficient radiographic density to be diagnostic. In comparison, the radiograph of the Labrador would have adequate density because the correct exposure levels were selected for its body thickness (Fig. 5.2A, B).

The body of an animal has many different types of tissues as well. Compare an animal's bone to its surrounding muscle. We can conclude that the bone has higher tissue density compared with that of the muscle. Because of the tissue density difference, more x-rays will be absorbed by the bone. The area of film under an anatomic area with high tissue density will be lighter (less radiographic density). In other words, the area of the film where the bone was located will remain relatively white compared with the muscle tissue surrounding it. Because x-rays have varied penetrability, the total number of x-rays reaching the film is partially dependent on the tissue density. Simply stated, the higher the tissue density, the lower the radiographic density (Fig. 5.3).

CONTRAST

Contrast is defined as the visible difference between two adjacent radiographic densities. Contrast is divided into two separate categories: radiographic contrast and subject contrast. To avoid confusion, we will define each contrast-associated term and how both influence the outcome of a radiograph.

Radiographic Contrast

Radiographic contrast is the density difference between two adjacent areas on a radiograph. When the density difference is great, the radiograph is said to have high contrast or a short scale of contrast. That is, a radiograph with high contrast exhibits many black-and-white tones. For example, a radiograph with white bone and a black background has high contrast (Fig. 5.4A).

A radiograph that exhibits many grays and a small density difference between two adjacent areas has low contrast or a long scale of contrast. An increased number of gray tones between the white and black tones on

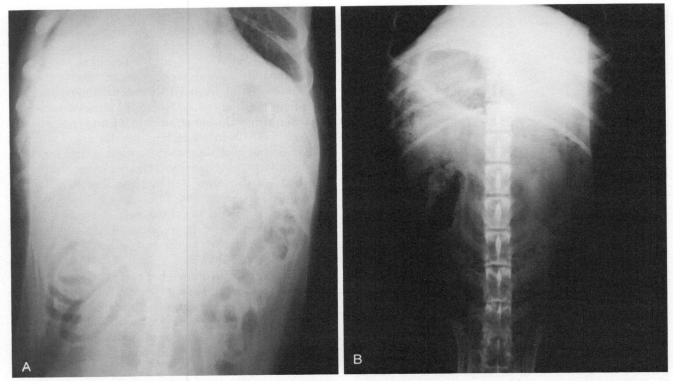

■ **FIG. 5.2 A, B** These two radiographs have been exposed with the same exposure factors. *A* is a ventrodorsal view of the abdomen of a Saint Bernard. *B* is a ventrodorsal view of the abdomen of a Labrador retriever. Because of the great difference in size of the Saint Bernard and the Labrador retriever, there is a marked difference in radiographic density. *A* exhibits much less radiographic density than *B*.

a radiograph constitutes a long scale of contrast. In other words, it takes a *long* time to get from black to white on the radiograph. The type of contrast desired for each radiograph is dependent on the anatomic area (Fig. 5.4B). General guidelines for desired contrast are listed in Table 5.1.

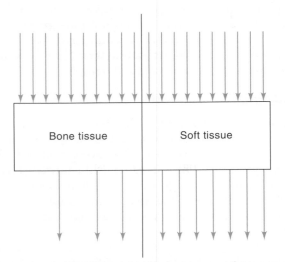

■ **FIG. 5.3** Drawing illustrating the influence of tissue density on radiographic density. Bone tissue is almost twice as dense as soft tissue.

Of course there are extremes in contrast. It is not desirable to have a radiograph with too high or too low contrast (Fig. 5.5). A good radiograph should have a suitable range of differentiated radiographic densities (blacks, whites, and grays) so that the eye can easily see the detail.

Radiographic contrast is influenced by (1) subject contrast, (2) kVp level, (3) scatter radiation, (4) film type, and (5) film fog.

Subject Contrast

Subject contrast is defined as the difference in density and mass between two adjacent anatomic structures. Subject contrast is dependent on the thickness and density of the anatomic part.

As discussed earlier, the body has various tissue densities. Because x-rays cannot penetrate bone tissue as easily as soft tissue, less x-rays will reach the film where the bone is located. Bone will absorb many more x-rays than muscle or fat, assuming both have equal thickness. With appropriate exposure factors, anatomy that has high tissue density can increase the amount of whites and blacks on the radiograph; therefore, high subject contrast increases radiographic contrast (Table 5.2).

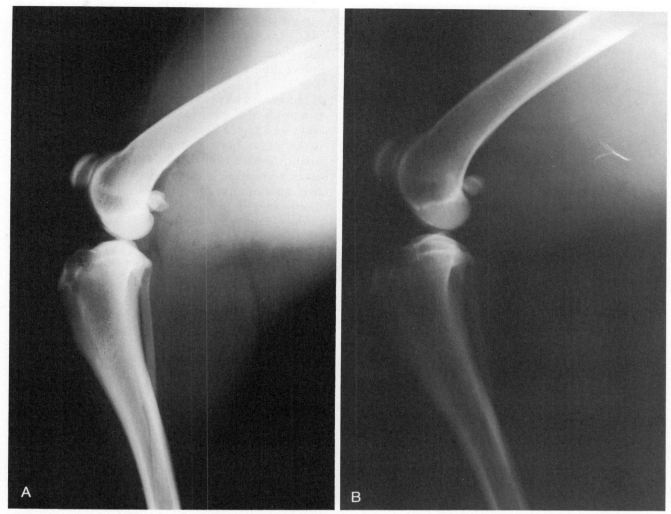

■ **FIG. 5.4** **A,** Radiograph of a lateral view of a canine stifle joint showing a short scale of contrast. The bone tissue of the leg is relatively white compared with the surrounding tissue. **B,** Radiograph of a lateral view of a canine stifle joint showing a long scale of contrast. The entire radiograph—bone and soft tissue—has an overall gray appearance.

EXPOSURE FACTORS

The most common cause of poor contrast on a radiograph is inappropriate exposure factors.

Milliamperage-Seconds

The mA-s may affect contrast only when insufficient or excessive mA-s is used. Remember, the mA-s is the quantity of the x-rays and is the primary factor that affects density. When a correct mA-s setting is utilized,

contrast is primarily dependent on the kVp setting. However, when the mA-s factor is insufficient, the contrast is reduced because the overall density of the radiograph is reduced. If the quantity of x-rays reaching the film is too low, the film will be pale. Close inspection will reveal that dense structures have been penetrated and that the anatomic silhouettes are visible but that the images lack density (Fig. 5.6). Overexposure, due to too much mA-s, will result in increased overall density (overall black appearance) but will have less effect on radiographic contrast (Fig. 5.7).

Kilovoltage

Both contrast and density are affected by kVp. The correct amount of kVp will produce differential x-ray absorption of soft and dense anatomic structures. A change in kVp has a number of effects. An increase in kVp results in an increase in penetrating power of the x-ray beam. When the kVp is raised, shorter-wave-

TABLE 5.1

General Guidelines for Desired Contrast

TISSUE	CONTRAST	EXPOSURE FACTOR (kVp)
Bone	High	Low
Soft tissue	Low	High

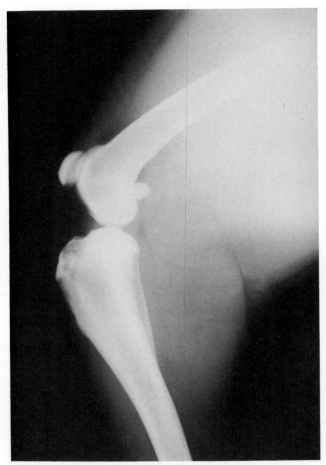

■ **FIG. 5.5** Radiograph of a lateral view of a canine stifle joint showing extremely high contrast.

length x-rays are produced, which raises penetration power. As the penetration is increased, radiographic contrast is altered as a result of scatter radiation. More will be said about scatter radiation presently.

If the kVp is too low, the resulting radiograph will have a "soot and whitewash" (gray and white) appearance and the anatomic image will be imperceptible. The image will lack adequate density because the x-rays were unable to penetrate the patient. Therefore, the area on the radiograph where the patient was posi-

tioned will remain white because insufficient x-rays reached the film. This will result in a white image against a black background. The contrast within the radiographic image will lack contrast; there will be no distinct difference between the anatomic organs (Fig. 5.8).

Increased kVp causes excessive scatter radiation. As a result of the increased penetrating power of the x-rays with high kVp, more x-rays will reach the film. As the x-rays, having a high kVp, travel through the patient, fewer x-rays are absorbed or scattered and a higher percentage of them reach the film. If the x-rays have sufficient penetrating power, the radiographic cassette and its components do not stop them and scatter radiation results (Fig. 5.9).

SCATTER RADIATION

Non–image-forming radiation that is scattered in all directions resulting from objects in the path of the beam is called **scatter radiation.** Scatter radiation is undesirable for a number of reasons. Because inappropriate areas of the film are being exposed, contrast is decreased.

Scatter radiation primarily originates from the patient, but there are other sources as well. Materials such as the table and film tray also act as sources of scatter. Radiation arising from such sources behind the image plane may be scattered back to the image. This phenomenon is referred to as **backscatter.** Limiting the size of the x-ray beam so that the field does not exceed the image receptor is the most effective way of reducing backscatter. In addition, many cassettes contain lead-foil backing to prevent backscatter from reaching the film.

Because kVp controls penetration and, to a degree, the amount of scatter radiation, it is the primary exposure factor that controls contrast. Radiographic examinations rely on correct kVp levels to produce desired contrast. How then is it possible to radiograph thick body parts without excessive scatter radiation? A mechanism known as a grid is necessary to reduce the scatter radiation with the use of high kVp needed for thick body parts.

GRID

A **grid** is a device placed between the patient and the radiographic film that is designed to absorb non–image-forming x-rays (scatter radiation). A grid is composed of alternating strips of lead and spacer material. The lead strips are approximately 0.5 mm in thickness and number between 500 and 1500 on edge. The spacer material usually consists of fiber, aluminum, or plastic because these materials have low x-ray absorption ability. The strips are encased in a protec-

T A B L E 5 . 2
Subject Contrast

	Least Dense	High Penetration	Appears Black
1. Gas			
2. Fat			
3. Water			
4. Bone			
5. Metal			
	Most Dense	Low Penetration	Appears White

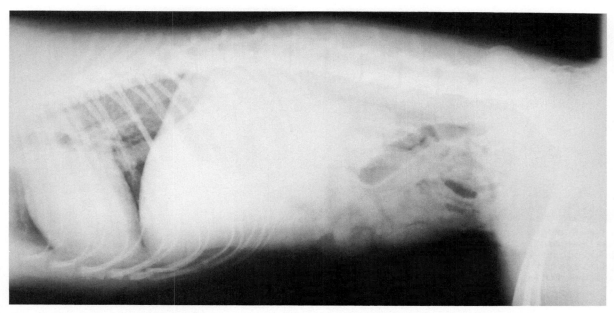

■ **FIG. 5.6** Radiograph of a lateral view of the abdomen that was exposed with an insufficient amount of mA-s.

tive cover (usually aluminum) to provide strength and durability (Fig. 5.10). The lead strips are aligned with the primary x-ray beam in a manner that allows the desirable x-rays to reach the film. The lead absorbs a considerable amount of the x-rays not traveling in the direction of the primary beam. The spacer material permits most of the primary x-rays (desirable x-rays) to pass through to the film (Fig. 5.11).

A grid may be (a) placed directly on top of a cassette, (b) built into a cassette, or (c) placed directly under the x-ray table between the patient and the cassette. Some grids are designed to be placed under-

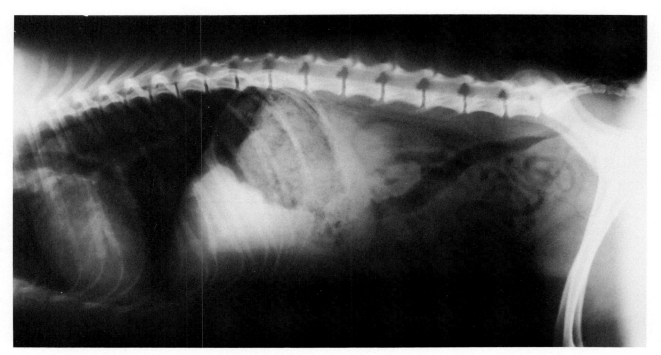

■ **FIG. 5.7** Radiograph of a lateral view of the abdomen that was exposed with too much mA-s. Note that the radiograph is too dark, yet the contrast is not altered drastically.

FIG. 5.8 Radiograph of a lateral view of the abdomen that has been exposed with an insufficient amount of kVp. The radiograph has very little contrast within the abdominal cavity because of the lack of penetration of the x-rays. The lack of penetration resulted in a lack of radiographic density.

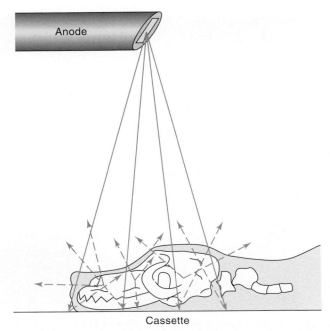

FIG. 5.9 Drawing of a canine skull being exposed with too much kVp. As a result of the excessive kVp, a large amount of scatter radiation is produced.

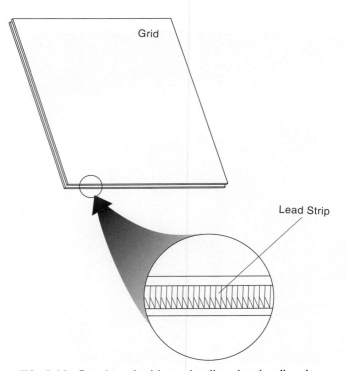

FIG. 5.10 Drawing of grid construction showing the structure of the lead strips and radiolucent interspacers.

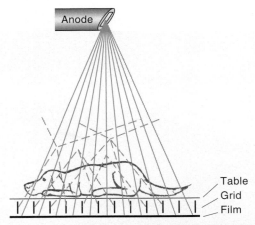

FIG. 5.11 Drawing showing grid device being used to absorb the scatter radiation caused by an interaction of the x-ray beam with an object in its path. Notice that the lead strips are placed parallel to the primary x-ray beam to allow the desirable x-rays to reach the film.

neath the x-ray tabletop, above the cassette tray, so that the lead strips run parallel to the length of the table. The cassette tray is discussed further.

Grid Focus

The lead strips of the grid may vary in size and angle, but each grid has a center point where the central x-ray must be centered. This central point is called the focal point (or focal line in linear grids). Ideally, the focal spot of the x-ray tube should coincide with the focal point (or focal line) of the grid, and the central ray of the x-ray beam should intersect with the center of the grid perpendicularly.

The distance from the source of x-rays (x-ray tube) and the grid is called the **grid focus** and is usually specified by the manufacturer. If the grid is used outside this specified range, **grid cutoff** may occur. Cutoff is a progressive decrease in transmitted x-ray intensity near the edge of the grid caused by the grid lines absorbing primary x-rays. Radiographically, the image appears lighter with distinct white lines over the underexposed areas of the film (Fig. 5.12). Cutoff is caused by the malalignment of the grid lines and the x-ray beam. This cutoff can occur for many reasons, ranging from improper centering of the x-ray tube over the grid, to tilting the tube laterally or tilting the grid itself, to having a focused grid upside-down.

Grid Efficiency

The purpose of a grid is to reduce the amount of scatter radiation and increase the quality of the radio-graphic image. It is important that the lead lines be barely detectable on the finished radiograph, but this may not always be possible. Thick lead strips break up a radiographic image more readily than do thin lead strips. The thicker the lead strips, the more radiation that is absorbed before reaching the film. As the lead strips become thinner and closer together within a grid, they are less perceptible on a radiographic image. However, less radiation is absorbed because of the decreased lead content per lead strip.

Grids vary in size and efficiency. The dimensions of a grid are usually 2 cm larger than the radiographic film sizes. The height, thickness, and number of lead strips determine the **grid efficiency**. The relation of the height of the lead strips to the distance between them is the **grid ratio**. For example, if the height of the lead strip is six times the width of the interspace, the grid ratio is 6:1. As the grid ratio increases, the efficiency of the grid increases. A 12:1 grid can absorb more scatter radiation than a 6:1 grid because of the greater size of the lead strips (Fig. 5.13).

Grids are also produced with a varying number of lead strips per centimeter. A grid is not only identified by its ratio but by its **lines per centimeter**. More lines per centimeter means that the lines are more narrow. This is an important consideration for several reasons. If a grid is used in a stationary manner, narrow grid lines would be less objectionable as they appear on a radiograph. As the lead lines decrease in width, however, the grid is less efficient in the absorption of higher-energy scatter radiation. Very fine grids are made with 40 lines per centimeter. (Note: 40 lines per cm = 60 − 100 lines to the inch.)

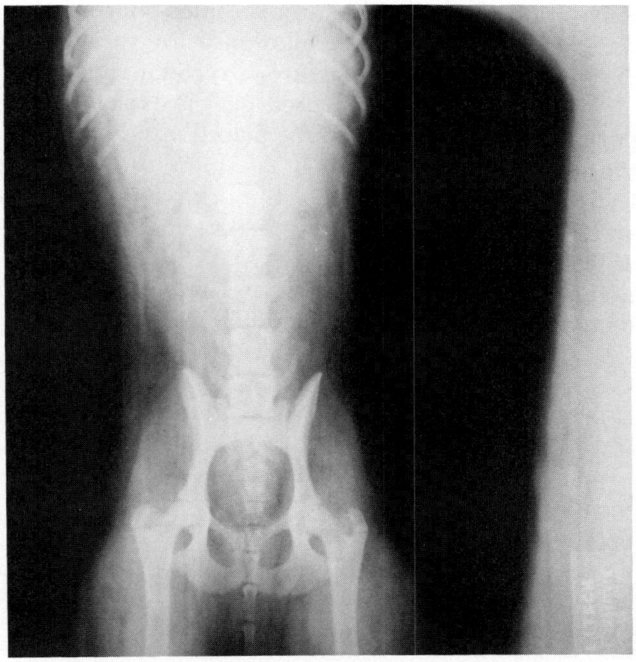

■ **FIG. 5.12** Example of a radiograph with grid cutoff. Note the prominent horizontal lines and overall lack of radiographic density.

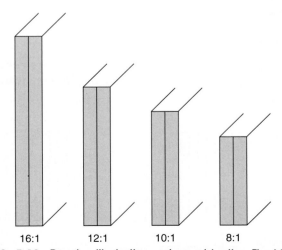

16:1   12:1   10:1   8:1

■ **FIG. 5.13** Drawing illustrating various grid ratios. The high-ratio grids absorb more scatter radiation as a result of the smaller angle allowed for the x-rays to pass toward the film.

Grid Factor

It is inevitable that the lead strips of the grid will absorb a portion of the primary x-ray beam. In order to compensate, the exposure must be increased with the use of a **grid factor**. See Chapter 9 for the radiographic techniques used to compensate for the variable grids.

Grid Pattern

Grid pattern refers to the orientation of the lead strips in their longitudinal axis. It is the pattern of the grid that we see from the top view. The two basic patterns are linear and crossed (Fig. 5.14A, D).

Linear Grid

The **linear grid** is patterned with the lead strips parallel to each other in their longitudinal axis. The parallel grid lines allow primary x-rays through to the film but absorb x-rays not traveling in a perpendicular path to the film. Most table-type x-ray units are equipped with linear grids. The advantage of a linear grid is that it allows the radiographer to angle the x-ray tube along the length of the grid without loss of primary radiation from grid cutoff.

Crossed Grid

A **crossed** (or **crisscross**) **grid** consists of two superimposed linear grids. The grid ratio of crossed grids is equal to the sum of the ratios of the two linear grids. For example, a crossed grid made up of two 5:1 linear grids has a ratio of 10:1. The advantage of this grid is that the maximum amount of scatter radiation is absorbed. The grid absorbs scatter traveling not only "east and west" but "north and south" as well. The biggest disadvantage of a crossed grid is that it cannot be used with oblique techniques requiring angulation of the x-ray tube.

Focused Versus Unfocused Grids

Both linear and crossed grid patterns are designed to be focused or unfocused. A **focused grid** is made up of

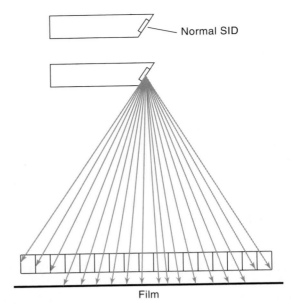

■ **FIG. 5.15** Grid cutoff due to a decreased distance between the anode and the grid (source-image distance (SID)). A portion of the primary x-ray beam toward the edges of the film is being "cut off" or absorbed by the grid.

lead strips that are angled slightly so that they focus at the central point of the grid (Fig. 5.14B). The lead strips of a focused grid radiate from the center strip, which is parallel to the central x-ray. In other words, beginning from the center lead strip, the slats on either side are progressively inclined at a greater angle. This angling of the grid lines allows for the diverging peripheral x-rays to pass through the grid (Fig. 5.15). Such grids are to be used at a specified source-image distance (SID), with some allowance for variation in distance from the manufacturer's recommendations.

Positioning of the focused grid is extremely important. The grid must not be placed upside-down. If the grid is displaced in such a fashion, the radiating lead slats will absorb most of the primary x-ray beam and will result in an underexposed radiograph. This is an example of grid cutoff (Fig. 5.16). The construction of a focused grid must be precise, and it tends to be more expensive than a parallel grid.

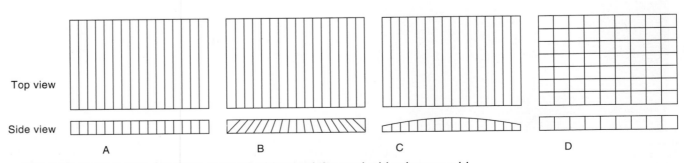

■ **FIG. 5.14** **A, B, C, D** Parallel grid, focused grid, pseudofocused grid, crisscross grid.

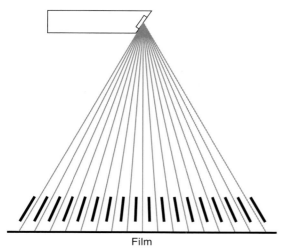

■ **FIG. 5.16** The diverging lead strips of a focused grid allow the diverging x-ray beam to pass through to the x-ray film.

An **unfocused** or **parallel grid** is one in which the lead strips are parallel when viewed from a cross section. Because they are focused at infinity, they do not have a convergent line. These grids can be used effectively only with very small x-ray fields or with long focal-grid distances (focal spot to grid distance).

When a parallel grid is utilized with a short focal-grid distance, the outer diverging portion of the primary beam tends to hit the lead slats. The x-rays hitting the lead slats are absorbed rather than passing between them. This is likely to result in an underexposure of the edge of the radiograph. This is the result of grid cutoff (Fig. 5.17). Grid cutoff will occur to a certain extent with a parallel grid at any focal-grid distance. But this artifact can be minimized by utilizing the grid according to the manufacturer's recom-

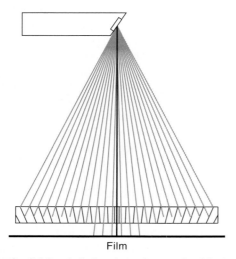

■ **FIG. 5.17** Grid cutoff due to a focused grid placed upside-down between the source of x-rays and the film.

mended focal-grid distance. Because the parallel grid does not have as intricate a construction as other types of grids, the cost is slightly less.

Pseudofocused Grid

The **pseudofocused grid** is a combination of the parallel and focused grids. It was produced to obtain a perfectly uniform parallel grid, yet alleviate the absorption of the primary radiation at the edge of the x-ray beam. This was achieved by a progressive reduction in the height of the lead strips toward the edge of the grid (Fig. 5.14C).

Potter-Bucky Diaphragm

The previous discussion of grids is limited to stationary grids that are permanently fixed under the x-ray table or mounted to a cassette. There is a mechanism, however, that can mechanically move the grid across the x-ray beam at a uniform speed. The device consists of a focused grid within a diaphragm that travels back and forth during exposure. The value of a moving grid lies in filtering scatter radiation while eliminating the grid lines from the finished radiograph.

The **Potter-Bucky diaphragm** ("Bucky") is normally placed directly under the x-ray table or in a vertical wall-mounted unit (Fig. 5.18). As stated, the grid is positioned so that the lead strips run parallel to the length of the table or wall unit. This device is used extensively in human radiography, and its use is recommended in specialized large animal facilities that are equipped to radiograph a horse or cow.

A Bucky system is not recommended for portable x-ray equipment. Suitable connections and power are lacking in a portable unit. Because the Bucky apparatus is mechanical, it can break down. Judgment is required to determine the need for a Bucky system in a new veterinary installation for small animal use.

Care of Grids

Grids are delicate and very expensive. If a grid is dropped on edge, it can be damaged permanently. Once the lead strips become bent or warped, a permanent artifact will be present on all radiographs taken with that grid. Grids that are attached to cassettes are more prone to this type of injury. Grids that are installed in a Potter-Bucky diaphragm system are well protected under the tabletop and generally need little care.

RADIOGRAPHIC DETAIL AND DEFINITION

Radiographic detail and definition are terms used to describe image sharpness, clarity, distinctness, and

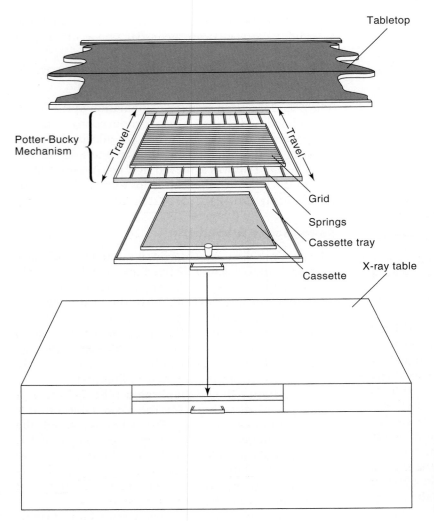

Tabletop

Potter-Bucky Mechanism

Travel

Travel

Grid

Springs

Cassette tray

Cassette

X-ray table

■ **FIG. 5.18** Diagram of the x-ray table, grid, Potter-Bucky diaphragm, and cassette tray with cassette. Note that the direction of the grid lines run with the length of the table and that the travel of the grid is in a transverse direction during exposure.

perceptibility. Detail is the feature of the radiograph that describes the definition of the edge of an anatomic structure. It is the goal of the radiographer to obtain as much diagnostic information as possible about the internal structures of the patient. In order to achieve this goal, image clarity is essential. Lack of detail can be a result of several different factors.

Geometric Unsharpness

Geometric unsharpness can be attributed to many factors. To prevent confusion, each is discussed individually.

Loss of detail due to some geometric distortion can be the result of a large focal spot size or a decreased source-image distance (SID), as discussed in Chapter 3. As the focal spot size increases, the "shadow sharpness" decreases. In the same respect, as the SID increases, the image sharpness increases.

Motion can be another cause of geometric unsharpness. When an animal, x-ray tube, or x-ray film moves during exposure, blurring of the image results (Fig. 5.19). Patient motion is the most common artifact in veterinary radiography (remember another "Murphy's Law" of veterinary radiography: the animal will move at the least opportune time). Sedation is sometimes helpful to decrease the chance of motion on a radiograph.

Geometric unsharpness due to the screens and film is another possibility. The screens are located inside the cassette to transform x-rays into light. Certain screen/film combinations are designed to produce radiographs with high detail and some with low detail. Screens and film are discussed in Chapter 6.

Geometric Distortion and Magnification

X-rays, like visible light, travel in straight lines that diverge from a central projection. All geometric anomalies that occur with visible light also occur with x-rays and can be explained using visible light as an analogy.

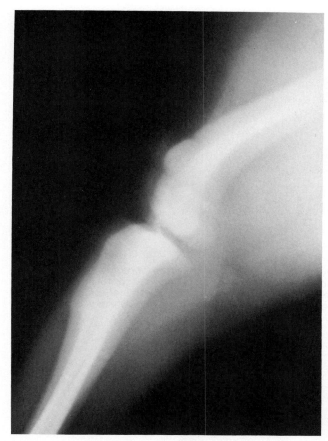

■ **FIG. 5.19** Radiograph illustrating patient motion.

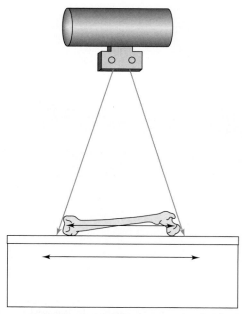

■ **FIG. 5.20** Drawing of correct geometric projection position: the subject should remain parallel to the image receptor (film).

The best way to describe **geometric distortion** is to take the example of your shadow on a sunny day. At 12 o'clock noon, when the sun is directly overhead, your shadow will be directly underneath your body. As time passes and the sun begins to set, the shadow projected by your body will be elongated and distorted. The phenomenon is called geometric distortion.

Geometric distortion of a radiographic image may result in difficulty during interpretation. To alleviate the possibility of any geometric distortion on a radiograph, a basic understanding of the geometric projection of a subject onto the image receptor is necessary.

To maintain an accurate geometric projection, the subject under examination must be parallel to the image receptor (Fig. 5.20). If the anatomic part under examination is not parallel to the image receptor, geometric distortion results. The simplest way to demonstrate this phenomenon is with a flashlight and a subject (an object) in order to project an image on a wall. With the flashlight approximately 1 m from the wall, interpose an object in the path of the light. The shadow of the subject will appear on the wall. When the object is close to the wall, the projected shadow will appear approximately the same size as the subject

and the edges of the image will be distinct. As the subject is moved away from the wall, closer to the flashlight, the image will become progressively magnified and diffuse. The edges of the magnified image become blurred, and the subject becomes almost unrecognizable. Now move one side of the object farther from the wall. Note that the edge farthest from the wall is distorted and magnified. When the subject is not parallel to the wall, the entire image is distorted (Fig. 5.21A, B). This experiment proves two points. When the subject of interest is not close and parallel to the image receptor, the image is distorted and lacks detail.

In the same respect, the focal spot of the x-ray beam must be directly above the object and centered on the point of interest or geometric distortion will result. To illustrate this point, another experiment can be performed with a flashlight and an object projected in its path. This time, instead of moving the subject toward the light source, follow the parallel plane of the wall and move the subject to the left or right. Notice that the shadow image, when not directly under the source of light, becomes elongated and diffuse on one edge of the projected image (Fig. 5.22). This is called **elongation** distortion.

With the same object and light source, perform one more experiment. This time, assume the correct position in the path of the light source with the subject directly centered in the beam of light and the subject positioned parallel and relatively close to the wall. In this experiment, move only one side of the subject away from the wall, keeping the other side stationary.

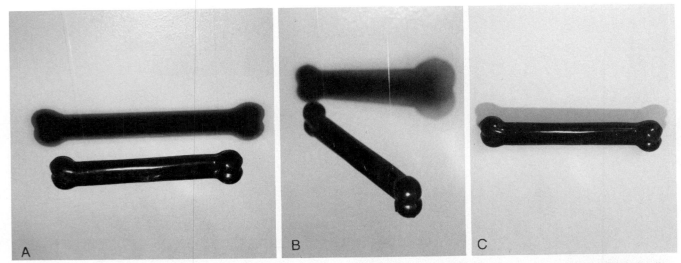

■ **FIG. 5.21** With use of a small light source held perpendicular to a wall and a bone, these photographs illustrate the importance of keeping the subject under radiographic investigation close and parallel to the image receptor. In *A*, the bone is close and parallel to the wall. Note that the image projected on the wall is distorted. In *B*, the bone is farther away from the wall and the image projected on the wall is magnified. *C* exhibits the distortion known as foreshortening, which is a result of the object not being positioned parallel to the wall.

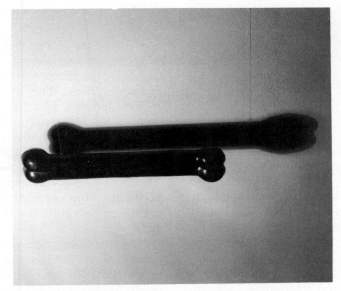

■ **FIG. 5.22** With use of a small light source and a bone, this photograph illustrates the distortion known as elongation. The light source should remain perpendicular to the wall in order to achieve accurate image projection. In this case, the light source was not directly above the bone and the image of the bone was elongated.

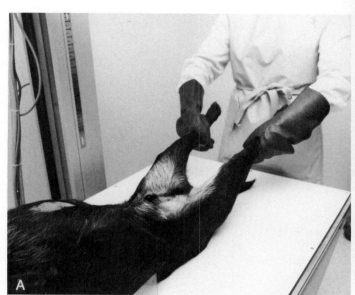
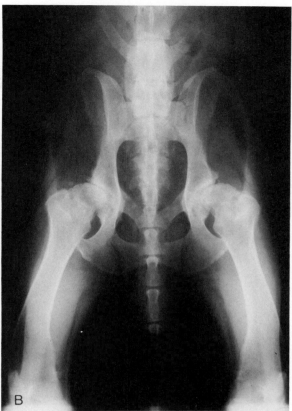

■ **FIG. 5.23** **A,** Dogs with severe hip dysplasia may be difficult to position correctly. The most common problem is the inability to extend the rear limbs properly for the radiograph, which can result in distortion of the image (shown in Fig. 5.23B). **B,** Radiograph showing the distortion known as foreshortening. Note that the femurs appear shorter and that the distal femurs are enlarged.

Notice that the image projected on the wall appears shorter than the actual size of the object. This type of geometric distortion is called **foreshortening** (Fig. 5.21C). This proves the importance of the subject remaining parallel to the plane of the image receptor.

Foreshortening distortion is a common occurrence when radiographing a dog with severe hip dysplasia. The hips of a dog with severe dysplasia are difficult to position because of the bone changes that have occurred within the hip joints. The femurs need to be parallel to the cassette. In a dog with hip dysplasia, it can be difficult, if not impossible, to maneuver the femurs into this position (Fig. 5.23A, B).

BIBLIOGRAPHY

Curry TS, Dowdy JE, Murry RC: *Christensen's Physics of Diagnostic Radiology,* 4th ed. Lea & Febiger, Philadelphia, 1990.

Douglas SW, Herrtage ME, Williamson HD: *Principles of Veterinary Radiography,* 4th ed. Bailliere Tindall, Philadelphia, 1987.

Eastman Kodak Company: *Kodak: The Fundamentals of Radiography,* 12th ed. Rochester, NY, 1980.

Gray JE, et al: *Quality Control in Diagnostic Imaging.* Aspen, Rockville, Md, 1983.

Morgan JP, Silverman S: *Techniques in Veterinary Radiography,* 4th ed. Iowa State University Press, Ames, 1987.

Radiographic Artifacts: Their Cause and Control. JB Lippincott, New York, 1983.

Ticer JW: *Radiographic Techniques in Small Animal Practice,* 2nd ed. WB Saunders, Philadelphia, 1984.

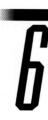

IMAGE RECEPTORS

OBJECTIVES
Upon completion of this chapter, the reader should be able to:

- Describe a cassette
- State the proper care of a cassette
- List the three properties that determine efficiency of a screen
- Describe intensifying screen construction
- List the common phosphor types used in diagnostic intensifying screens
- List and describe the factors that govern screen speed
- Explain how screen speeds are rated
- Define quantum mottle
- Describe the correct method of mounting a screen inside the cassette

- Define and describe fluoroscopy
- Describe proper screen care
- State the purpose of x-ray film
- Describe the composition of x-ray film
- Define a latent image
- List the two general categories (types) of x-ray film
- Describe how film speed is determined
- Define film latitude
- Describe proper film care
- State the significance of film-screen system comprehension

GLOSSARY

AFTERGLOW: The tendency of a luminescent compound to continue to give off light after x-radiation has stopped.

BASE: A transparent flexible polyester support layer of radiographic film.

CASSETTE: A lightproof encasement designed to hold x-ray film and intensifying screens in close contact.

EMULSION: A layer of radiographic film that is made of gelatin containing suspended silver halide crystals.

FILM LATITUDE: The exposure range of a film that will produce acceptable densities.

FLUOROSCOPY: A special radiographic diagnostic method by which a "live view" of the internal anatomy is possible.

INTENSIFYING SCREENS: Sheets of luminescent phosphor crystals bound together and mounted on a cardboard or plastic base.

LATENT IMAGE: An invisible image on the x-ray film after it is exposed to ionizing radiation or light before processing.

NONSCREEN FILM: Film that is more sensitive to ionizing radiation than to fluorescent light.

QUANTUM MOTTLE: An artifact of faster screens resulting in density variation due to random spatial distribution of the phosphor crystals within the screen.

REFLECTIVE LAYER: A layer of an intensifying screen that reflects the light from the phosphor layer toward the film.

SCREEN FILM: Film with silver crystals that are more sensitive to fluorescent light emitted from intensifying screens than to ionizing radiation.

SILVER HALIDE: A compound of silver and bromine, chlorine, or iodine, all of which are in the halogen group of elements.

SUPERCOAT: A clear protective layer on radiographic film.

INTRODUCTION

In the previous chapters, the discussions are limited to the production and action of x-rays. To further understand radiography, we need to discuss how a permanent record is produced using x-rays.

Essentially, a radiograph is formed with light-sensitive film contained in a lightproof encasement. In radiography, the lightproof encasement used most often is called a **cassette** (Fig. 6.1). The general-use cassette is designed to hold a piece of double-emulsion x-ray film sandwiched between two fluorescent sheets of plastic called **intensifying screens**. The intensifying screens are responsible for converting the x-ray radiation into visible light, which creates a **latent image** on the x-ray film. The film is then processed to convert the latent image into a visible image. Remarkably, over 95% of the exposure recorded on the film is due to the light emitted from the intensifying screens. Only 5% of the exposure of the film is due to the ionization of x-rays.

Many different types of image receptors and detectors convert invisible ionizing radiation into a visible image. These detectors and receptors can take many forms and, in turn, facilitate a number of diagnostic procedures that use radiant energy. These procedures include:

1. The exposure of fluorescent materials that convert x-ray radiation into visible light, which can be utilized to expose special film containing silver halide/ bromide crystals (radiography).

2. The interaction of x-rays with charged selenium plates. When exposed, the distribution of the electrical charge is altered, producing a negative image on the plate (xeroradiography).

3. The absorption of x-rays by ionizing chambers to produce voltage pulses, which can be displayed on cathode ray tubes (computed tomography).

4. The injection of a radiopharmaceutical followed by imaging distribution of the radioactivity with a sodium iodide crystal gamma camera (nuclear scintigraphy).

This list is only a sampling of the imaging techniques that utilize radiant energy. We will restrict our attention to fluorescent intensifying screens and silver halide films as image receptors.

THE CASSETTE

In radiography, the cassette is a rigid film holder designed to hold the x-ray film and intensifying screens in close contact. The cassette must be constructed with materials that are light-tight to prevent any unwanted exposure to the film, yet allow penetration of the x-rays.

The first cassettes were constructed with cardboard. This material could not be reused and thus did not pass the test of time. Over the years, cassettes made of aluminum became standard. Aluminum cassettes are still common today; however, improvements have been made to cassette fronts. As mentioned, the front of the cassette must be strong and opaque to light, yet remain radiolucent to x-rays. Examples of available cassette fronts are those made of (1) polycarbonate (Bakelite), (2) aluminum, (3) magnesium, and (4) carbon fiber.

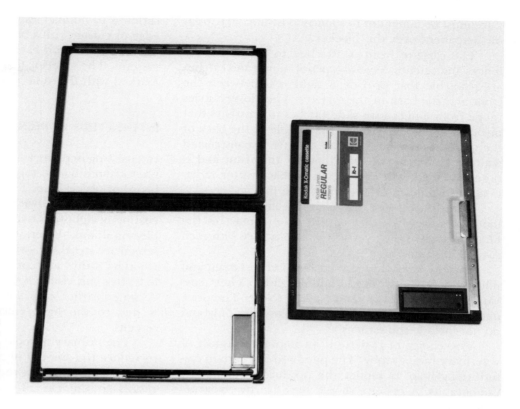

■ **FIG. 6.1** A cassette; one open and one closed. Inside the cassette are two fluorescent screens that sandwich the radiographic film. When closed, the cassette provides a lightproof environment for the film.

Some cassette fronts are color-coded or have a colored dot on the edge to indicate the screen type inside. Color coding allows easy identification when choosing a cassette for each clinical situation. The front may also be marked into four quadrants to facilitate more than one exposure per film. Taking a number of exposures on one film is accomplished by exposing one quadrant while shielding the others with lead rubber strips (Fig. 6.2). An area approximately 3 × 7 cm may also be marked in the corner of the cassette front to indicate the presence of a lead blocker (Fig. 6.3). This lead blocker is present to prevent irradiation of that part of the film needed for identification. (Film identification is discussed in Chapter 7.)

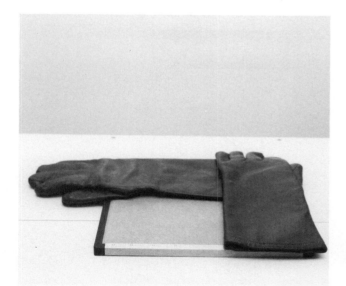

■ **FIG. 6.2** The cassette has been divided into four quadrants so that a number of views can be exposed. Three of the sections are being shielded with lead to prevent exposure until desired. In this case, the quadrants are being shielded with lead gloves. Commercially available lead sheets can be purchased for this purpose as well.

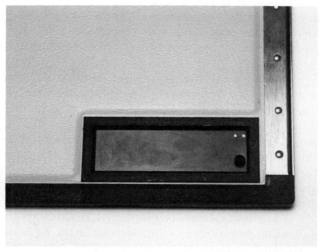

■ **FIG. 6.3** A 3 × 7 cm lead blocker for photographic identification. The blocker prevents exposure to x-rays to this area so that information can be exposed on the film in the darkroom with the use of a photoimprinter.

Care must be taken not to superimpose any vital areas of the patient over this blocker.

The cassette front is attached to the back with hinges and catches. Several types of hinges and catches are available that provide a tight seal between the front and the back of the cassette. The closure styles range from hinges with slide catches to crossbars that pivot on a shoulder rivet in the middle of the back of the cassette. The back of the cassette is constructed with heavier material than that for the front and is normally lined with lead to absorb backscatter radiation that would cause fogging of the film.

Inside the cassette, both sides are lined with felt or foam pressure pads that ensure close contact of the film and screens. Felt versus foam pads vary with each cassette manufacturer.

Cassette sizes vary and correspond to screen and film sizes (in both metric and English). Their cost varies according to size and quality. (Note: The price quotes in most catalogs are for the cassettes only and do not include the screens.)

The choice of cassette is an important aspect of veterinary radiography. The purchase of a certain cassette may help or hinder the production of quality radiographs. A cassette should have sturdy construction, maintain screen-film contact, and be user-friendly in the darkroom.

Cassette Care

As with any expensive piece of equipment, the cassette should be handled with care. In veterinary medicine, cassettes tend to be exposed to some physical abuse. This is especially true in a large animal practice. The most common causes of physical damage are (1) by dropping the cassette on a hard surface and (2) leaking of fluid such as blood or urine into the cassette.

Dropping a cassette on a hard surface can result in a loss of contact between the screens and film. This loss of contact results in a blurred radiographic image. (See Chapter 10 for how to test for screen-film contact.)

Keeping a cassette clean when working with animals is always a challenge. Taking precautions such as placing the cassette in a plastic bag when a "messy" situation is expected will prevent damage to the cassette's exterior and interior. A cassette should be cleaned on a regular basis with mild soap and water. Cleaning the exterior of the cassette when the screens are cleaned (monthly) is usually adequate unless circumstances necessitate a more frequent schedule.

All cassettes should be numbered. In this way, any noticeable defects on a radiograph can be traced to the "problem" cassette. Most intensifying screens, within the cassette, have a serial number imprinted on the screen edge. These numbers are small, however, and difficult to read. The best method of cassette identification is to number each intensifying screen near the edge or corner with a black felt-tip marker. This number will appear on each radiograph taken with that cassette. The exterior (back of the cassette) should be marked with the same number.

INTENSIFYING SCREENS

Intensifying screens are sheets of luminescent phosphor crystals bound together and mounted on a cardboard or plastic base. Two screens are normally inside the cassette to sandwich the x-ray film, which has a coating of light-sensitive emulsion on both sides (double emulsion). When the phosphor crystals in the screen are struck by x-radiation, the crystals fluoresce, whereby x-rays are converted into visible light (Fig. 6.4). It is this visible light that exposes the x-ray film. As stated earlier, over 95% of the exposure to the film is due to the light emitted from the intensifying screens.

The primary purpose of the intensifying screen is to reduce the amount of radiation exposure required to produce a diagnostic radiograph. The use of screens results in the use of lower milliamperage-seconds (mA-s), thus decreasing the dose of radiation to the patient and the chance of motion on the radiograph.

Three properties determine the efficiency of the screen materials:

1. They must have a high level of x-ray absorption.

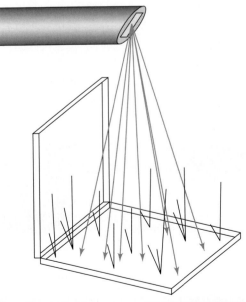

■ **FIG. 6.4** Fluorescent screens emit light when x-rays strike them. This drawing illustrates how the screens "glow" during exposure.

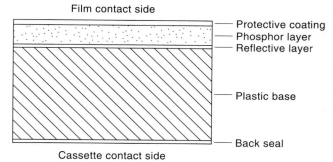

Film contact side

— Protective coating
— Phosphor layer
— Reflective layer

— Plastic base

— Back seal

Cassette contact side

■ **FIG. 6.5** Cross section of an intensifying screen.

2. They must have high x-ray-to-light conversion with suitable energy and color.

3. There must be little or no "afterglow" once radiation has ceased.

Screen Construction

An intensifying screen has four integral layers: (1) a base or support, (2) a reflective layer, (3) a phosphor crystal layer, and (4) a protective coat (Fig. 6.5).

The base serves as a flexible support to attach the phosphor layer to the cassette. The base must have a tough, moisture-resistant surface and not become brittle with extended use.

The reflective layer, which is attached to the base, is made of a white substance such as titanium dioxide. The purpose of the reflective layer is to reflect the light emitted by the phosphor layer back toward the x-ray film. The reflective layer increases the efficiency of the screen so that none of the light photons are lost through the base layer.

The phosphor crystal layer consists of uniformly distributed phosphor crystals held in place with a binder material. It is extremely important that this layer not change in thickness, crack, or discolor with age. Any variance in screen uniformity would alter the amount of light produced when irradiated and would alter the uniform exposure of the film (Fig. 6.6).

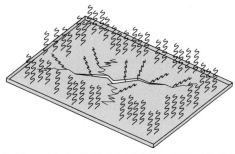

■ **FIG. 6.6** A crack in an intensifying screen. During exposure to x-rays, an irregular light emission results in the area of the screen damage.

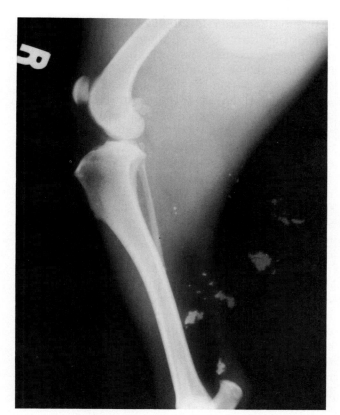

■ **FIG. 6.7** Radiographic artifact that is the result of having dirt within the cassette.

The protective coat is a clear coating placed on the outer surface of the screen and provides the needed protection of the phosphor layer. This layer must be strong enough to resist marks and abrasions and must be easy to clean. Veterinary radiography has many pitfalls, one of which is animal hair. Any foreign material caught in the cassette between the intensifying screen and the film will alter the exposure to the film. The debris on the screen will result in radiographic artifacts (Fig. 6.7). Because of the likelihood of artifacts and the need for subsequent cleaning of screens, the protective surface must be durable and resistant to deterioration.

Phosphor Types

As discussed previously, x-rays have the ability to cause phosphors to emit light. The phosphor chosen for an intensifying screen must absorb x-rays efficiently, have a minimum afterglow, and emit sufficient light of the desired color.

Afterglow is the tendency of a phosphor to continue to give off light after the x-radiation has stopped. This continued phosphorescence can interfere with rapid-succession serial film changers. A serial film changer is employed when a number of films are needed per second. For example, a rapid serial film changer is necessary for angiography to view the action of the heart. With a radiopaque liquid contrast medium injected intravenously, the movement of the fluid through the chambers of the heart can be recorded. A serial film changer has the ability to expose many films per second. If there is any afterglow from the intensifying screen present, it would interfere with the exposure of each successive film.

The absorption rate of the phosphor refers to the extraction of x-ray photons from the beam. The absorption of one x-ray quantum (unit of radiant energy) results in the emission of hundreds of light quanta from the screen. These light photons are more readily absorbed by the x-ray film than are x-ray photons. The more x-ray quanta absorbed, the greater the amount of light produced.

The first phosphor intensifying screen, introduced in 1896 by Thomas Edison, was made of calcium tungstate. Calcium tungstate was chosen because its emission of light is in the blue regions of the ultraviolet spectrum. This was important because of the high sensitivity of silver halide to this spectrum of light. Calcium tungstate has a relatively high x-ray absorption ability and is physically strong, but it is lacking in light conversion efficiency. Despite this one weakness, calcium tungstate screens are still widely utilized today.

New phosphor technology has led to the introduction of phosphors having greater speed. In 1972, a class of phosphors known as the rare-earth elements was developed. The term "rare earth" is used because these elements are difficult and expensive to separate from the earth and from each other, not because they are scarce. The rare-earth group is also known as the lanthanide series because it consists of elements having atomic numbers 57 (lanthanum) through 71 (lutetium).

The x-ray-to-light conversion efficiency of rare-earth phosphors is significantly greater than that of calcium tungstate. The light conversion of a rare-earth screen is four times as great as that of a calcium tungstate screen. The spectral emission of rare-earth phosphors is in the green light part of the spectrum. Because standard x-ray silver halide film will not absorb (i.e., is not sensitive to) light in the green area, a special film that is sensitive to the green spectrum of light must be employed with this type of screen.

Screen Speed

Factors other than phosphor type affect the speed and efficiency of a screen. Many types of screens are available today, all of which are graded by their speed and efficiency. The speed of a screen is governed by crystal size, phosphor layer thickness, reflective layer efficiency, and dyes in the phosphor layer.

Crystal Size

Within certain limits, the larger the crystal, the greater its light emission. An x-ray striking any part of a phosphor crystal causes the entire crystal to fluoresce. Because of the larger flashes of light with larger crystals, less x-radiation is needed to expose the x-ray film (Fig. 6.8). Another way to consider this concept is illustrated in the following scenario.

Imagine that you are standing 10 feet away from a wall that has two mirrors hanging on it. One mirror is 2 inches in diameter and the other is much larger, having a 10-inch diameter. Facing the wall, you shine a flashlight beam at the mirrors. As you examine the light being reflected back at you, you notice that the amount of light from each mirror is not equal. The amount of light reflected from the smaller mirror is significantly less than that from the larger mirror.

The same principle applies to phosphor crystal size. Unfortunately, as the crystal size is increased, the detail of the image is decreased. The result of increasing the speed of the screen by increasing the crystal size is a grainy image. Within certain limits, an increase in crystal size is acceptable and will not compromise radiographic detail excessively. In comparison, smaller crystals produce a film with increased detail but larger amounts of radiation are required.

GENERAL RULES
Large crystals: Faster screens ▪ Less detail ▪ High grain
Small crystals: Slower screens ▪ More detail ▪ Low grain

Phosphor Layer Thickness

The thickness of the phosphor layer is another factor that influences both screen speed and image detail. When the phosphor layer thickness is increased, the x-ray absorption and light emission are increased. There are limits to screen thickness, however. An increase in the thickness of the phosphor layer will result in a decrease in image detail. The image will be blurred as a result of the diffusion or "spreading out" of the light as it travels through the screen from the phosphor crystal where the light originated. Recall that light leaves a central point and diverges outward. Lateral spreading of light is a result of this light divergence (Fig. 6.9).

Reflective Layer Efficiency

As mentioned, the **reflective layer** is positioned between the base and the phosphor layer. The purpose of the reflective layer is to reflect all light emission from the phosphor layer toward the x-ray film. If the reflective layer contains a light-absorbing material, however, a portion of the light produced by the phosphors will be lost. More x-radiation is needed to produce an adequate exposure on the x-ray film. There-

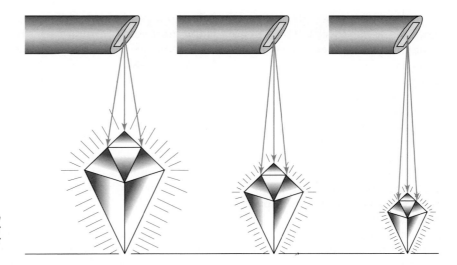

■ **FIG. 6.8** One factor that influences the speed of screens is the size of the phosphor crystals. A large crystal emits a larger amount of light than a smaller crystal.

fore, it is important that the reflective layer material have a high reflective capability and a low absorption capacity.

Dyes in the Phosphor Layer

A light-absorbing dye (pigment) may be incorporated into the binder material of the phosphor layer of some screens. The primary purpose of the dye is to decrease lateral spreading of the light emitting from the phosphor crystals. When the lateral spread of light is reduced, blurring of the radiographic image is decreased. Unfortunately, the light intensity emitted by the screen is also reduced and the speed of the screen is decreased. Common pigments used are yellow, gray, or pink.

Screen Speed Ratings

Because many factors affect screen speed, it is natural to assume that there are many screens to choose from. It might also be assumed that screen speeds can be accurately measured and that screen speed categories are clearly defined. Unfortunately, this is not the case. Screen speed categories are broad and general. Most manufacturers divide screen speeds into three basic categories relative to the screen's light output:

1. *Slow* (also referred to as high definition, ultra-detail, or fine grain). This group of screens is specifically designed for radiographic examinations that require optimal detail and in which exposure time is not critical.

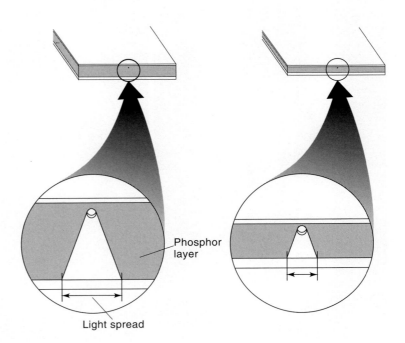

■ **FIG. 6.9** A cross section of two screens; one screen is much thicker than the other. As a result of the difference in thickness, the light spread is much greater with the thicker screen.

Phosphor layer

Light spread

2. *Medium* (also referred to as regular, midspeed, normal, or par speed). This category is the most common in private veterinary practice. Medium-speed screens provide good resolution with relatively low exposures.

3. *Fast* (also referred to as high speed). High-speed screens reduce exposure time or patient exposure or penetrate extremely thick tissue areas where more exposure is needed.

Each manufacturer's screen speed categories do not correlate precisely with one another. For example, manufacturer A may produce a par speed screen that is 10% faster than the par speed screen produced by manufacturer B.

Increased screen speed has led to a radiographic artifact known as **quantum mottle**. This artifact gives a radiograph a spotty or mottled appearance. Quantum mottle occurs because the new, faster screens are so sensitive that only a few x-ray quanta are necessary to produce the desired density on the x-ray film. As the small number of quanta strike the intensifying screen,

not all of the phosphor crystals are struck, thus not all fluoresce. Inconsistent fluorescence from the phosphors results in a density variation (mottling) on a uniformly exposed radiograph. Quantum mottle is a disadvantage of rare-earth screens for brief exposures, but its effects are greatly reduced with correct film-screen combinations.

Screen Speed Summary

In radiography, screen speed is inversely proportional to the exposure required to produce a given effect. That is, a fast screen requires a small exposure, and a slow screen requires a larger exposure. A fast screen has the physical capability to emit more light when struck by x-radiation than does a slow screen given the same exposure (Fig. 6.10A, B).

In the same respect, radiographic detail is inversely proportional to the speed of the screen. A screen that is manufactured to be fast will inherently produce a radiograph with less detail. The cost of fast screens is increased graininess. Although slow screens

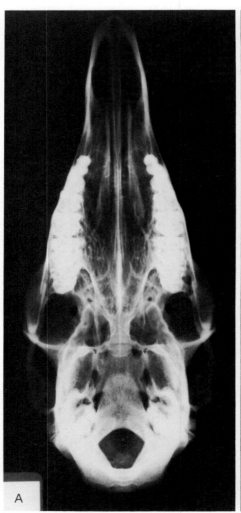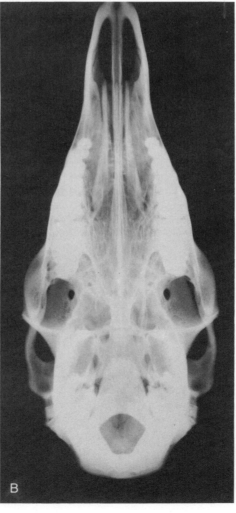

■ **FIG. 6.10** These two radiographs were exposed with identical exposure factors with the use of two different screen types. *A* was exposed with fast screens, and *B* was exposed with slow screens. Note that *A* is properly exposed, whereas *B* is too light. Slow screens need a greater amount of exposure compared with fast screens.

require more x-radiation, the detail is greatly increased (Fig. 6.11A, B).

Mounting Screens in the Cassette

Intensifying screens are usually mounted in pairs in the cassette. Most screens are labeled FRONT and BACK and should be placed in the cassette appropriately. The screen on the front side is slightly thinner than the screen on the back so that the front does not absorb an excessive amount of the x-ray beam and the exposure of light to both sides of the film is even.

Securing the screens in the cassette is vital. Screens should never be loose inside the cassette. Double-sided tape, provided by the manufacturer, should be applied to secure the screens in place. Commercial liquid adhesives should be avoided because certain chemicals can interact with the screens.

Some screens are used singly in a cassette. The utilization of only one screen increases the image resolution but tends to be slower and to need more exposure to achieve a desired product. Single-screen cassettes are employed primarily for extremity radiography in which image detail is critical and must be paired with single-emulsion film.

Specialized Screens: Fluoroscopy

Fluoroscopy is essentially the visualization of a "live" or "real-time" radiographic image. Fluoroscopy is used for a number of purposes:

1. To evaluate the esophagus and upper and lower gastrointestinal tract configuration and function.
2. To assist in surgical procedures (e.g., foreign body removal, cardiac catheterization).
3. To evaluate ventilation mechanics (e.g., trachea, lungs, diaphragm).
4. To evaluate cardiac function.

The main feature of a fluoroscopy unit is its screen. Special crystals such as cadmium sulfide or caesium iodide are in the screen because they emit green light, to which the human eye is most sensitive. The screen is substituted for conventional x-ray film and is placed in the path of the x-ray beam after it has

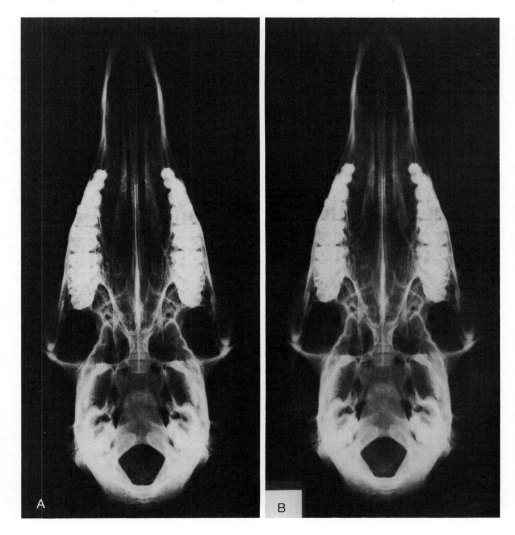

■ **FIG. 6.11** These two radiographs are of the same object but exposed with two different screens. *A* was exposed with the use of ultradetail screens, and *B* was exposed with rare-earth screens. Note the difference in detail of the two radiographs. *A* has a much clearer image than *B*.

passed through the patient. The fluoroscopic screen enables the radiographer to visualize the fluorescent image created by the interaction of x-rays and phosphor crystals as it occurs.

The image viewed is the opposite of an x-ray seen on a view box. The image produced is a "positive" image. The black-and-white areas on the screen are reversed compared with a normal radiograph. The intensity of the light emitted by each part of the screen is proportional to the intensity of the x-rays striking that part of the screen. The visible light pattern corresponds precisely with the x-ray pattern.

Fluoroscopy equipment is installed in a manner opposite that of conventional x-ray equipment. The fluoroscopic screen is suspended above the x-ray table, and the x-ray tube, coupled to the screen, is under the table directed toward the screen (Fig. 6.12). Leaded glass is positioned over the screen so that the image can be viewed without exposing the operator's eyes to radiation.

Today, technology has replaced this type of fluoroscopy unit with an image-intensifying unit. An image intensifier essentially converts and transfers the image on the intensifying screen to a photoelectric surface. Image-intensified fluoroscopy can be observed through an optical lens and mirrors (mirror optics system) or on a television monitor.

At no time should fluoroscopy replace radiography. Not only is there more risk of radiation exposure, but the image created by the fluoroscope has far less resolution. In the past, some veterinary practices employed hand-held fluoroscopy units exclusively in order to save the time and expense of exposing and developing x-ray film. This practice is deemed "illegal" in most states in the United States.

Screen Care

Because of the cost of screens and their sensitivity to damage, the importance of screen care cannot be minimized. Screens should be inspected and cleaned on a regular basis to keep them free of dirt and foreign material. Dust and animal hair are common artifacts in veterinary radiography (Fig. 6.13). Any abrasion, chemical spill, or artifact will be noticeable on all films taken in conjunction with that screen. Incorrect diagnoses have occurred as a result of unsuspected screen artifacts.

Screens should be cleaned in accordance with the manufacturer's instructions to avoid damage to the screen surfaces. For example, a soft brush or pressurized air can remove loose foreign material. The protective coat can be cleaned by careful swabbing of the surface with dampened gauze pads and cleaning solution. Commercial screen cleaning solutions, mild soap and water, or dilute ethyl alcohol is recommended. Commercial solutions have the advantage of possessing antistatic properties.

After being cleaned the cassette should be left open and propped in a vertical position to allow the screens to dry completely before reloading. The vertical position prevents any dust or foreign material from settling inside the cassette. At all other times, the cassette should be kept closed to prevent accidental damage and artifacts. Care should also be taken when loading and unloading film from the cassette to avoid "digs" and scratches on the screen surface. Touching the screens and writing on film that is still in the cassette should also be avoided Damage to the screen surface is permanent and cannot be repaired.

X-RAY FILM

The purpose of x-ray film is to provide a permanent record containing essential diagnostic information. X-ray film provides information not only for present use but for later evaluation as well.

X-ray film consists of a polyester base coated on both sides with a light-sensitive emulsion containing

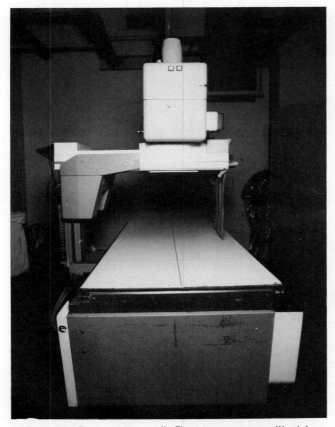

■ FIG. 6.12 Fluoroscopy unit. The x-rays are emitted from under the table and projected on a fluorescent screen above the table. The image is then transferred to a TV monitor.

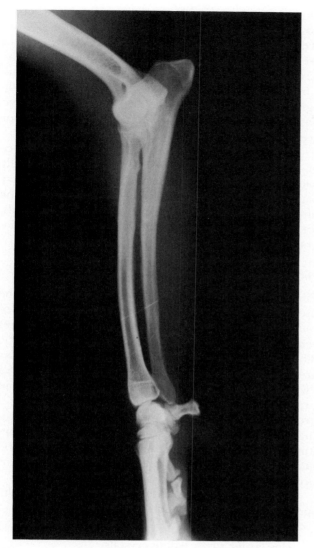

■ FIG. 6.13 Radiograph showing a hair artifact. The hair was trapped inside the cassette during exposure.

silver halide crystals. When visible light or ionizing radiation (x-rays) interacts with the silver halide crystals, an invisible (latent) image is formed. Through processing, this invisible image is converted into a visible image. The final product is a radiograph.

Film Composition

X-ray film has a number of layers, each having individual characteristics and purposes (Fig. 6.14). The transparent polyester **base** provides a flexible support with a thin adhesive subcoating on each side. The adhesive serves to bind the next layer, the emulsion, to the base. **Emulsion** consists of gelatin that contains silver halide microcrystals suspended and dispersed evenly throughout the layer. Gelatin provides reasonable permanence and permits rapid processing because it is easily penetrated by developing solutions.

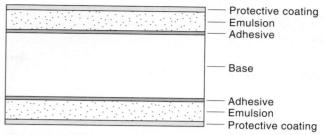

■ FIG. 6.14 Cross section of x-ray film.

Silver halide is a compound of silver and bromine, chlorine, or iodine, which are members of the halogen family of elements. (Silver bromide crystals are common in diagnostic x-ray film.) Viewed through a microscope, the emulsion appears to be filled with tiny grains of sand. These tiny grains are the silver microcrystals suspended in the gelatin — there are billions of crystals per cubic centimeter of emulsion. Over the emulsion is a clear **supercoat** of protective material to decrease the possibility of damage to the fragile emulsion.

Latent Image

As the silver halide crystals absorb energy from visible light or x-rays, a physical change takes place and a latent image is formed. By definition, a latent image is an invisible image on the x-ray film after it is exposed to ionizing radiation or visible light before processing. After processing with a special chemical developer solution, the latent image is converted into a visible image.

The latent image is formed on a screen-type film by the absorption of a light photon by a grain of silver halide. When exposed, the silver halide is converted to metallic silver. The greater the number of silver halide crystals that are converted to metallic silver, the blacker the film will be once developed. The unexposed silver halide crystals are cleared off the film during the fixing portion of the processing procedure. A film that has not been exposed to any ionizing radiation or visible light will be clear after processing because none of the silver halide crystals were converted to metallic silver (Fig. 6.15).

Film Types

The two general categories of film used in diagnostic radiography are screen and nonscreen.

Screen Film

Screen film is manufactured with silver crystals that are sensitive to fluorescent light emitted from intensifying screens and less sensitive to ionizing radiation. This type of film requires less exposure of x-rays to

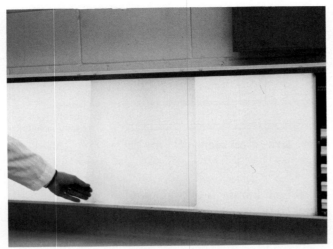

■ FIG. 6.15 Photograph showing a sheet of x-ray film that was unexposed and processed. Because the silver crystals in the film emulsion were never exposed to light or x-rays, all of the unexposed silver crystals were cleared off of the film during the processing procedure.

produce a quality image because of its high sensitivity to fluorescent light.

For many years, screen film has primarily been "blue-sensitive," that is, highly responsive to the ultraviolet, violet, and blue spectrum of light. Today, newer films have been developed that are sensitive to green light as well as to blue. The importance of this is linked to the new generation of intensifying screens known as rare-earth screens. Some rare-earth screens emit primarily a green spectrum of light, whereas calcium tungstate uses phosphors that convert the energy of x-rays into blue light. Because of this variation, it is important to match a suitable film to an appropriate screen.

Nonscreen Film

Nonscreen film is exposed by the direct action of x-radiation. This type of film is manufactured to be more sensitive to ionizing radiation. Because there is no intensification of the x-ray beam, greater exposures are required. However, because intensifying screens are not utilized, there is no loss of detail due to the screens. Resulting radiographs have greater detail. This film is of particular value in bone or dental radiography. But, because of the necessity for greater exposure of nonscreen film, it should be utilized only for areas where tissue thickness is minimal.

One problem with nonscreen film is the absence of a strong protective cover. The film is normally packaged in a light-tight envelope made of heavy paper. Because this paper offers little protection, the film is highly sensitive to pressure from a dog's nails, for example, when extremities are being radiographed.

Film Speed

Film is manufactured with various speeds through the use of different-sized silver halide crystals. Speeds of radiographic films are determined from the exposures required to produce an image with adequate density. The exposure range over which acceptable densities are produced is known as **film latitude.** Film that has a "wide" latitude will accept a significant variation in exposure factors or processing without exhibiting a great change in density. On the one hand, wide-latitude film is considered a "forgiving" film. Narrow-latitude or high-contrast film, on the other hand, requires considerably less change in exposure factors or processing to alter the radiographic density.

To maintain simplicity, we will examine film speed in three basic groups:

FAST FILM (ULTRASPEED):
Has larger silver halide crystals
Requires less exposure by x-rays or fluorescent light from intensifying screens
Produces a grainier image that lacks definition
Has less latitude in exposure factors and processing

TABLE 6.1

Kodak Film Screen Speed Systems: Green Emitting

FILM TYPE	Lanex Fine	SCREEN Lanex Medium	Lanex Regular	Lanex Fast
TML	100	300	400	600
PDG	100	300	400	600
TMG	100	300	400	600
OL	100	250	400	600
OG	100	250	400	600
TMH	—	600	800	1200
PDH	—	600	800	1200

TABLE 6.2

Du Pont Film Screen Speed Systems: Blue Emitting

			SCREEN		
FILM TYPE	Par	High Plus	Quanta Detail	Quanta Fast Detail	Quanta III
Cronex 4	100	200	100	400	800
Cronex 4L	100	200	100	400	800
Cronex 7	—	—	80	250	400
Cronex 7L	—	—	80	250	400
Cronex 10	—	—	80	250	400
Cronex 10L	—	—	80	250	400
Cronex 10T	—	—	80	250	400
Cronex WDR	—	—	—	200	400

MEDIUM FILM (STANDARD OR PAR SPEED):

Is most widely used in veterinary radiography

Represents a compromise between fine grain and speed

Has a medium latitude in exposure factors

SLOW FILM (HIGH DETAIL):

Has smaller silver halide crystals

Requires greater exposure by x-rays or fluorescent light from intensifying screens

Produces an image that is less grainy and has greater definition

Has greater latitude in exposure factors

In veterinary radiography, the most common film is medium speed, also known as standard or par speed. This category represents a compromise between fine detail and speed. Medium-speed film is suitable for a wide range of examinations and acts as a standard by which manufacturers rate other films. Medium-speed film is often the only type of film stocked in a veterinary practice.

Film Care

Because of the delicate nature of x-ray film, specifically in terms of the emulsion layer, film handling and storage are of great importance.

Film boxes should be stored on end so that the film is in a vertical position. If the film is stored in a horizontal position for an extended period or if any pressure is placed on the film, the emulsion on each sheet may blend together. The result may be a "block" of x-ray film that is useless. The temperature of storage is also important. The storage area should be cool (10 to 15°C) and have a low relative humidity (40 to 60%). Excessive heat and humidity can cause the film emulsion to soften, causing the film to stick together and in effect decreasing its shelf life.

Film should not be stored near any source of ionizing radiation or where vapors from formalin, hydrogen peroxide, or ammonia can reach it. These substances can cause fogging.

Close observation of the film expiration date is important. The expiration date is marked on the end of each box. If a number of boxes are stored, the film should be used in sequence to avoid expired film.

FILM-SCREEN SYSTEMS

It is not enough for the technologist to know the speed of the film and screen alone. Knowledge of the film-screen "combination" is vital. The combined speed or "system speed" is what determines the exposure requirements for any given clinical situation. A wide assortment of film-screen combinations is available. The choice of a system depends on the desired image detail and necessary speed requirements. In some instances, the fastest system possible must be employed because of the anticipated studies or because of the relatively low-powered equipment.

A numeric value is assigned to each film and screen type. Unfortunately, each film manufacturer has its own manner of speed evaluation, and these may not correlate. In veterinary practice, a medium-speed system (300 to 400) is the most common because of its versatility. See Tables 6.1 to 6.3 for lists of common film-screen system speeds. To acquire specific information concerning the system speed in a given practice, the film manufacturer should be consulted. In

TABLE 6.3

3M Film Screen Speed Systems: Green Emitting

	SCREEN
FILM TYPE	Trimax 12
Ultradetail	400
Wide latitude	600

general, the numeric value for film-screen combinations ranges from about 25 to 1200. Although these numbers resemble those of the ASA (ISO) system for photographic film, the standards are not as rigid.

BIBLIOGRAPHY

Eastman Kodak Company: *Kodak: The Fundamentals of Radiography,* 12th ed. Rochester, NY, 1980.

Koblik P, Hornof JW, O'Brien TR: Rare earth intensification screen for veterinary radiography: An evaluation of two systems. Vet Radiol 21:224–232, 1980.

Morgan, JP, Silverman, S: *Techniques in Veterinary Radiography,* 4th ed. Iowa State University Press, Ames, 1987.

Radiologic Science for Technologists, 3rd ed. CV Mosby, St. Louis, 1984.

Schmidt RA, Chan HP, Kodera Y, Doi K, Chen CT: Evaluation of cassette performance: Physical factors affecting patient exposure and contrast. Radiology 146:801–806, 1983.

FILM
PROCESSING

OBJECTIVES

Upon completion of this chapter, the reader should be able to:

- List and describe the three qualities of a good darkroom
- Describe an organized darkroom
- State the various methods of darkroom lightproofing
- State the correct safelight to be used with blue-light– and green-light–sensitive film
- List the five basic steps of film processing
- State the primary function of the developer
- List and describe the six developer components
- State the function of the rinse bath
- State the two basic purposes of the fix bath
- List and describe the six components that make up the fix solution
- Describe the methods of recognizing exhausted chemicals

- Explain how biologic growth can be minimized in processing tanks
- List and describe the nine steps in manual processing
- State the two primary advantages of automatic processing
- Describe how an automatic processor works
- List the basic maintenance procedures recommended for an automatic processor
- List the three methods and reasons for silver recovery
- State the importance of film identification, and list the several methods of film identification available
- State the recommended criteria for filing a radiograph

GLOSSARY

ACCELERATORS: Chemicals that increase the pH of the developer and subsequently increase the rate of developing.

ACIDIFIERS: Compounds that accelerate the fixing process and neutralize the alkaline developer.

BUFFERS: Compounds in the fixer that maintain proper pH of the solution.

CLEARING AGENTS: Also called **fixing agents**; a portion of the fixer that dissolves and removes the unexposed silver halide crystals from the film emulsion.

DEVELOPER: A chemical solution that converts the latent image on a film to a visible image by converting the exposed silver halide crystals to black metallic silver.

DEVELOPING AGENTS: Chemical solutions used to convert a latent image on x-ray film to a visible image.

FIXATION: The process by which the unexposed silver halide crystals are removed from the film and the gelatin is hardened.

FIXER: The chemical solution used during fixation.

HARDENERS: Added to the fixing solution or to developers in automatic processors to prevent excessive swelling of the emulsion.

LATENT IMAGE: An invisible image on unprocessed x-ray film after it has been exposed to ionizing radiation or light.

PRESERVATIVES: Prevent rapid decomposition of the developer or fixer.

RESTRAINERS: Often potassium bromide and potassium iodide are used as restrainers or antifoggants. Restrainers limit the action of the developing agent to the exposed silver bromide crystals in the film.

RETICULATION: A darkroom artifact due to variable chemical temperatures that cause irregular expansion and contraction of the film eulusion resulting in a mottled density appearance.

RINSE BATH: A solution (usually water) used to remove excess developer solution prior to the placement of the film in the fix tank.

SOLVENT: Water; dissolves the ingredients of the developer and fixer and diffuses the chemical into the emulsion of the film.

STOP BATH: A solution of acetic acid and water used to "stop" the development of the x-ray film by rapidly neutralizing the alkaline developer solution.

INTRODUCTION

Proper film processing is vital to the production of a quality radiograph. Many believe that the use of appropriate exposure factors is the only component necessary to produce a "good" film. This belief is far from the truth. The production of a good quality radiograph depends on many factors, one of which is film processing. When manual processing was the norm in human hospitals, it was said that 90% of all poor quality radiographs were the result of poor processing. This is still relevant in veterinary radiography. One goal of the radiographer is to eliminate all possible pitfalls that may inhibit quality. A common area for pitfalls is the darkroom. Although quality does not begin in the darkroom, it could very possibly end there.

The basic principles of radiographic processing have remained the same over the years, but technology has made remarkable advances toward automation. However, although an increasing number of veterinary practices use automatic film processing, the majority still process radiographs by hand with tanks to hold the processing chemicals. Both methods of processing are discussed in detail in this chapter.

THE DARKROOM

Three qualities constitute a good darkroom. A darkroom must be (1) clean, (2) organized, and (3) lightproof. Although each individual darkroom may vary in design, all should possess the same qualities. The darkroom should be separate from the radiographic suite and be used for only one purpose: processing exposed radiographs. Ideally, the room dimensions should be no less than 6 × 8 feet (2.6 × 2 m), and the layout should reduce the possibility of film damage. Most of the work performed in the darkroom is performed with minimal illumination. Therefore, it is important that the darkroom be organized so that all of the equipment can be located quickly and easily. And, of course, cleanliness is crucial. This is the only room where both the intensifying screens and the x-ray film are exposed to the air. If the countertops are dirty and soiled with chemicals, it is easy for both to be sucked into the cassette as it is opened and possibly damage the intensifying screens.

Another factor that is often overlooked in the darkroom is climate control. Because the film emulsion is extremely sensitive to heat and humidity, good ventilation and temperature control are mandatory. A

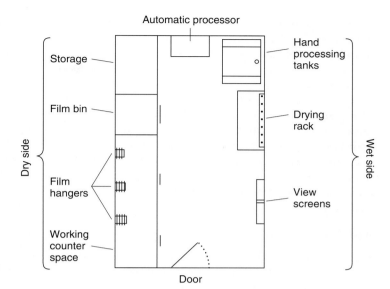

■ FIG. 7.1 A bird's-eye view of a wet side and a dry side of a darkroom.

darkroom should be relatively cool and have low humidity. For specific temperatures and humidity for proper film care, see Chapter 6.

Organization

There should be essentially two sides to the darkroom: a dry side and a wet side (Fig. 7.1).

Dry Side

The dry side of the darkroom is where the cassettes are unloaded and reloaded. A countertop or tabletop should be available to provide a suitable working area large enough to accommodate the largest cassette in an open position. The tabletop should be constructed of a material that allows frequent cleaning, which is necessary to reduce the source of darkroom artifacts

that can potentially get on the film. It must be impossible for chemicals to splash into the dry side. At no time should anything "wet" be brought to the dry side. It is customary to store film under the dry table, either in a cupboard or in a film bin, to allow easy access for reloading cassettes (Fig. 7.2). Film hangers for each size of film should be hung above the table on the dry side on an appropriate bracket. Brackets can be purchased commercially or be constructed inexpensively using large hooks found at any hardware store.

Film hangers are available in two designs: channel hangers and clip hangers (Fig. 7.3). Channel hangers tend to retain water and chemicals and need special cleaning and drying to prevent contamination of the

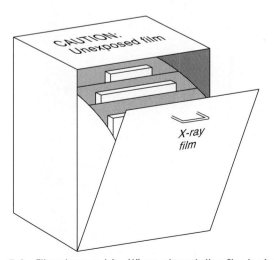

■ FIG. 7.2 Film storage bin. When closed, the film is stored light-tight in a vertical position.

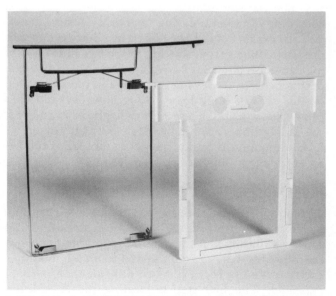

■ FIG. 7.3 A clip film hanger versus a channel film hanger.

dry side. Films must also be removed from the channel hangers to be dried. However, clip hangers are more fragile than the channel type. When the clips are used frequently over a period of time, they become weak and lose the ability to "stretch" the film. The clips also puncture the four corners of the film, which, when filed, can scratch other films in the same envelope. It is important to cut off the corners of films processed with clip hangers before filing to prevent scratches in the film emulsion of adjacent radiographs. When more than one film is processed at the same time in the tanks, the clips on the hangers can scratch neighboring films.

Wet Side

The wet side of the darkroom is where the actual chemical processing is performed. A darkroom where films are hand processed usually consists of three tanks, containing developer, water, and fix solutions. Different tank designs are available. The three tanks can be individually freestanding and warmed as required by means of an immersion heater (placed in the developer). Alternatively, the developer and fix tanks can be placed in one large tank filled with thermostatically controlled water. The latter is preferred and can be purchased as a complete package constructed with 3- or 5-gallon (9- or 22-L) individual tanks. The water tank is usually four times the size of the smaller developer and fix tanks. The central water tank should have a circulating water system to provide a means of regulating temperature and rinsing chemicals off the films during the processing procedure. A thermometer is an essential piece of equipment for the processing tanks because radiographic film is developed for a specified time based on the temperature of the chemicals.

The wet side should also have a film drying area consisting of either a drying rack or a drying cabinet. The drying rack should be placed in a dust-free area to prevent artifacts from sticking to the wet films. A drying cabinet is a heated forced-air unit that hastens the drying process. A viewing screen is also recommended on the wet side to evaluate radiographs. A "wet" film can be viewed, and, if a second radiograph is required, the radiographer can immediately evaluate the error. This evaluation is best achieved in the darkroom before too much time has elapsed.

Darkroom Lightproofing

As mentioned, one of the criteria of a good darkroom is that it be lightproof. Light leaks in a darkroom can cause significant film fog; therefore, taking appropriate measures to lightproof the darkroom is imperative. Lightproofing a room is more difficult than perhaps expected. The first step is locating the light leaks. Small light leaks may not be perceptible until the eyes have acclimated to the dark, and it may be necessary to

spend 5 minutes waiting for the eyes to adapt. To achieve a truly lightproof room, a number of tasks may be necessary.

The entrance to the darkroom is a common site for light leaks. A double-door system or revolving door is preferred but not always practical in a veterinary practice (Fig. 7.4). To lightproof a standard door, it should fit tightly into its frame against strips of felt or rubber molding. Weather stripping is also useful around doors to prevent the entrance of light. Light entering from underneath the door can be prevented by a vapor seal designed specifically for the bottom of a door. A sliding bolt lock or doorknob lock prevents someone from entering the darkroom at an inopportune time. A suspended ceiling can be a radiographer's nightmare. It may be necessary to lay a large black sheet of plastic above the ceiling tiles to prevent light in adjacent rooms from entering through the seams.

It is a common fallacy that the walls of a darkroom should be "dark." The opposite is true. The walls of the darkroom should be painted white or cream with a good quality, washable paint. By painting the walls a light color, more reflection of the safelight is produced, providing a more visible work environment. If the quality and intensity of the light are "safe," the illumination reflected from any surface also is "safe," regardless of the color of that surface.

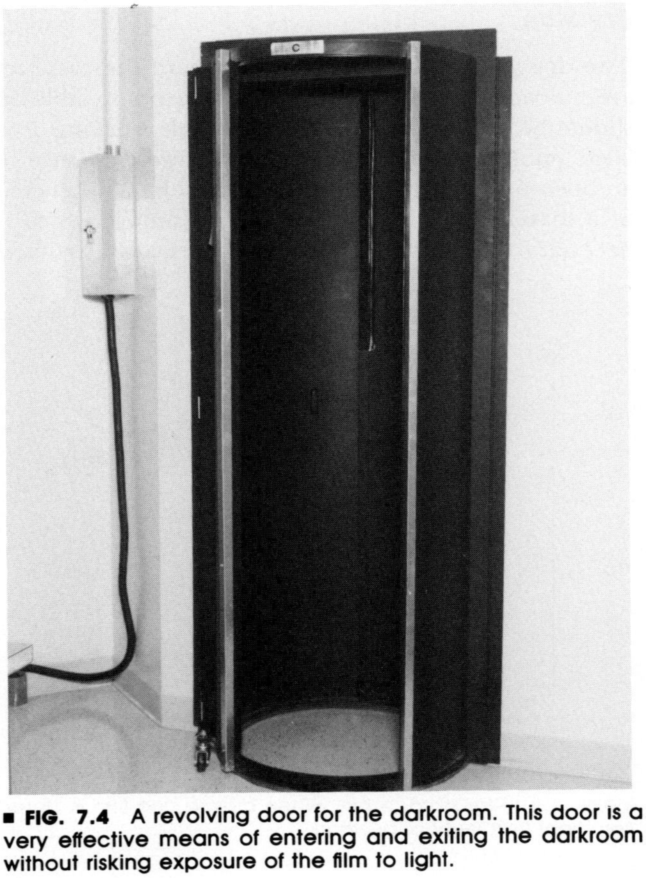

■ FIG. 7.4 A revolving door for the darkroom. This door is a very effective means of entering and exiting the darkroom without risking exposure of the film to light.

Darkroom Safelight

Correct safe lighting in the darkroom is crucial. A "safe" light means that the light produced will not affect the film. Radiographic film is sensitive to ultraviolet light. Safelights utilize a small-wattage bulb and a special filter to eliminate the light from the blue and green spectrum. The lightbulb should be 15 watt or less. The filter varies by manufacturer. The most common types are a brown filter (Wratten 6B, Kodak) for blue-light–sensitive film and a dark-red filter (Wratten 6BR or GS-1) for green-light–sensitive film. The dark-red filter is recommended because of its versatility: both green-light– and blue-light–sensitive film can be used in this lighting.

Safelights should be positioned so that work in the darkroom can be performed without fumbling. There are two types of safe lighting: direct and indirect (Fig. 7.5). Direct lighting is a diffused light shining directly over a work area, such as the dry or wet side of the darkroom. Indirect lighting is a filtered light directed toward the ceiling and reflected over the entire room. Indirect lighting is often combined with direct lighting. At no time should the safelight be closer than 4 feet to a work area. A safelight that is too close, has a too-high wattage bulb, or has incorrect filtration may cause film fog.

The efficiency of a safelight can be tested, which is discussed in Chapter 10. Remember, no light is "safe" if the film is exposed to it for a prolonged period. Therefore, the film bin should be open only when removing or replacing film. Fogging will result even with a safelight if the bin is left open or if film is left sitting on the counter.

FILM PROCESSING SOLUTIONS

Film processing, whether it is manual or automatic, comprises five basic steps: (1) developing, (2) rinsing or stop bath, (3) fixing, (4) washing, and (5) drying. The first step in learning how to process a film is having a basic understanding of the processing solutions. The chemical solutions can be purchased in a number of forms. Powders and liquid concentrates are the most

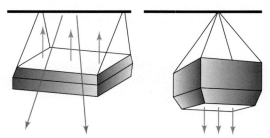

■ FIG. 7.5 Direct and indirect safe lighting for the darkroom.

commonly used in veterinary practice. Water is added to the concentrates according to the manufacturer's instructions to produce the proper amount of solutions for the processing tanks. It is important to prepare the chemicals correctly or the resulting solution may adversely affect the radiographic product.

Every effort should be made to keep the chemical solutions at a specified temperature—any variance may adversely affect the radiographic product. At temperatures below those recommended, some of the chemicals may become sluggish in action and may produce an underdeveloped or underfixed radiograph. At temperatures much above those recommended, the activity of the chemicals is too high for manual control.

Keep in mind also that all of the chemical solutions should be the *same* temperature. If the chemicals vary greatly in temperature, film reticulation can result. **Reticulation** appears as a mottled density on a finished radiograph due to irregular expansion and contraction of the film emulsion.

A quality assurance program should be established and maintained in the veterinary practice. This program not only allows reproducibility, it gives the radiographer confidence in the exposures used on each radiograph (see Chapter 10).

The Developer

The **developer** is a chemical solution that converts the latent image on a film to a visible image. The primary function of the developer is to convert the exposed silver halide crystals to black metallic silver.

The developing time is normally specified by the chemical manufacturer. Keep in mind that the temperature of the developer affects the developing time. Time-temperature developing is preferred over visual inspection when utilizing the manual processing technique. This manual inspection is called "sight developing." Sight developing consists of increasing or decreasing time according to visual inspection of film density while the film is still in the tank. This technique requires attention and skill and is often subject to error. Sight developing should be avoided if at all possible.

The developer consists of developing agents, accelerators, preservatives, restrainers, hardeners, and a solvent.

1. **Developing agents** are composed of chemical compounds, such as hydroquinone or phenidone, capable of converting exposed grains of silver halide to black metallic silver. The developing agent has little or no effect on the unexposed silver halide crystals.

2. **Accelerators** are chemicals that increase the activity of the developer. Substances such as potassium carbonate or sodium carbonate are used to increase the pH to an alkaline range of 9.8 to 11.4. The increase in pH causes the emulsion to swell and soften,

allowing the developing agent to work more effectively.

3. **Preservatives** prevent rapid oxidation that can occur with alkaline developing agents. They also help maintain a stable development rate and prevent staining of the emulsion layer.

4. **Restrainers** limit the action of the developing agent to the exposed silver bromide crystals in the film.

5. **Hardeners** are often added to developers in automatic processors. They harden the film during processing and prevent excessive swelling of the emulsion. If the gelatin emulsion were to swell extensively, it could be damaged by the rollers in the automatic processor.

6. The **solvent** consists of water to dissolve the chemicals.

The Rinse Bath

After a film has been in the developer, it retains a substantial amount of developer in the gelatin (approximately 60 cc on a 14×17 inch film). If the film were transferred directly into the fixer, the alkaline developer would neutralize the acid of the fixer. The **rinse bath** serves to stop the developing process, rinse the developer from the film, and prevent carryover contamination to the fixer.

Normally, the rinse bath consists of circulating water, and the film is rinsed for 30 seconds. A chemical solution such as acetic acid and water can be employed as another method of stopping the development procedure. This chemical solution is called a **stop bath.** In automatic processing, a rinse or stop bath is not necessary because the rollers tend to remove excess developer from the film before it reaches the fix tank.

The Fixer

After a film has been properly developed and the exposed silver halide crystals have been converted to metallic silver, one other step involving the silver crystals remains. The unexposed silver halide crystals remaining on the film are unaffected by the developer solution and must be removed. If the unexposed silver crystals were to remain on the film, they would discolor and darken with the exposure of light.

The **fixer** serves two basic purposes: (1) it clears the unexposed silver halide crystals from the film and (2) it hardens the gelatin coating so that it can be dried without damaging the film surface. This process is known as **fixation.** The general guideline is that the film should be fixed for twice the development time to ensure maximum hardening of the emulsion. (Note: A radiograph can be viewed briefly after it has been in the fix for 1 minute and then returned after evaluation.)

The fix solution consists of clearing or fixing agents, preservatives, hardeners, acidifiers, buffers, and a solvent.

1. **Clearing** or **fixing agents** dissolve and remove the unexposed silver halide crystals from the film emulsion. The two most common clearing agents are sodium thiosulfate and ammonium thiosulfate. The agent actually changes the appearance of the film from a milky white to a clear or transparent image. The black metallic silver portion of the film remains the same.

2. **Preservatives,** such as sodium sulfite, prevent decomposition of the fixing agent.

3. **Hardeners,** such as aluminum salt, prevent excessive swelling of the gelatinous emulsion during the fixation procedure and softening during the wash procedure. Hardeners shorten the drying time by essentially preventing the film from becoming "water-logged."

4. **Acidifiers** are compounds that accelerate the action of the other chemicals and neutralize any alkaline developer possibly carried over into the acidic fix solution.

5. **Buffers** are chemical compounds added to the solution to maintain the desired pH. Buffers stabilize the acidity against the addition of alkaline developer by carryover. Without the addition of a buffer, the alkaline developer would neutralize the acid of the fix solution, thus shortening the effective life of the fix. Some buffers also prevent sludge formation in the fix bath.

6. The **solvent** consists of water. The purpose of the solvent is to dissolve the other ingredients and assist the fixing agent to diffuse into the emulsion layer of the film. Once the fixing agent is in the emulsion layer, it can dissolve the unexposed silver halide crystals. The solvent then helps by carrying the silver halide away from the film.

The Wash Bath

The wash portion of the development procedure is vital to a quality radiograph. Unfortunately, the value of the wash procedure is often underestimated and inadequately performed. The purpose of the wash is to remove the processing chemicals from the film surface. If a film is not washed properly for a long enough period, the image will eventually discolor and fade.

Films should be washed in circulating water so that both surfaces of the film receive fresh water continuously. In manual processing, the average suggested wash time is 20 to 30 minutes with periodic agitation or water circulation. In automatic processing, the water system of the processor keeps a constant flow of temperate water through and around the wash rack and film.

Wetting Agent

A common problem of drip drying films is the possibility of water spots or other drying streaks. The drying process can be hastened and some artifacts avoided by using a wetting agent bath known as a surface-tension reducing agent (a detergent). These agents are commercially available.

Solution Replenisher

In manual processing, chemical depletion is a natural result of chemical carryover into adjacent tanks. As much as 60 cc of developer can be "carried" on a 14 × 17 inch piece of film into the rinse bath. Both the developer and the fixer need replenishment on a frequent basis to keep chemicals at a proper level to ensure that the entire film is covered.

Replenishment solutions are available in powder and liquid concentrate form. The liquids are easier to work with because they eliminate the problem of powder settling on the countertops of the darkroom. Generally, the replenisher has a higher concentration than the original solution to maintain chemical potency.

Solution Replacement

Exhausted processing chemicals (or, more likely, oxidation/deterioration of chemicals in limited-use situations) are a primary cause of poor quality radiographs. The developer and fixer solutions are often the last elements checked when a film has poor quality, yet exhausted chemicals are the most common cause. Chemicals that have lost their potency will produce radiographs that have increased film fog and decreased contrast and density.

Determining the need for developer and fixer replacement is based on a couple of clues. In general, the developer solution turns a brown to green color when it needs to be changed. The developer usually requires less changing than the fixer. Because each film brought into the fix tank brings with it a certain amount of water from the rinse tank, the fix tends to become diluted. The activity of the fix solution, however, cannot be determined by a change in color. The fixer needs to be changed when the "clearing time" is greater than 2 to 3 minutes. Clearing time refers to the amount of time it takes the fixer to clear the unexposed silver halide crystals off the film. If all of the silver complexes have not been removed, the film will fog or even turn black when exposed to light. In general, hand processing tank chemicals should be changed every 4 to 6 weeks.

Biologic Growth

A common problem encountered in hand processing tanks is the growth of bacteria and fungi, particularly during the warm seasons of the year. Bacterial and fungal growth can produce slime deposits that can build up in the tanks. The bacteria, fungi, and, at times, algae originate from the air, personnel, or incoming water supply. If not controlled, they can cause corrosion of the metal surfaces as well as artifacts on the films. The growth rate of the organisms is increased in stagnant water.

Biologic growth can be inhibited by good housekeeping. When the chemicals are changed and the processing tanks are drained, they should be scrubbed and quite possibly soaked with 1% chlorine bleach and water. The wash tank of automatic processors should be drained at the end of the day to reduce biologic growth. Organisms can be prevented from entering through the water line by a simple filtering system.

FILM PROCESSING TECHNIQUES

As mentioned, radiographic film can be processed in one of two ways: manually or with an automatic film processor. With the manual process, it takes approximately 1 hour to produce a finished product. With an automatic processor, a film can be processed and dried in as little as 90 seconds. Both methods produce a quality radiograph, and it is a matter of preference as to which method best suits the clinical situation.

Manual Processing Procedure

The manual (hand) processing procedure should be standardized as much as possible. By establishing a routine and following it, mistakes made in the darkroom are less likely to occur. Normally, the developing tanks are positioned so that the processing procedure starts at the left and ends at the right. In other words, the developing tank is on the left, the wash tank in the center, and the fix tank on the right (Fig. 7.6).

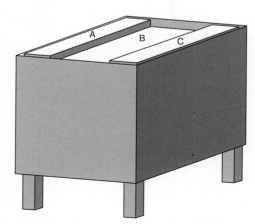

■ **FIG. 7.6** Bird's-eye view of hand processing tanks. The tank labeled A is the developer, B is the rinse and wash tank, and C is the fix tank.

Manual processing is not a difficult procedure, and the technique can be learned in a relatively short period.

Step 1—Preparation

Before the film is processed manually, the chemicals should be at the proper temperature (normally 20°C [68°F]) and should be stirred. Because the chemicals are suspensions, they tend to settle to the bottom of the tanks (Fig. 7.7). The paddles used to stir should not be shared between tanks: the developer paddle should never go into the fix tank and vice versa. (Note: Even slight fixer contamination in the developer can render it useless.) At this point, the white lights should be turned off and the safelight turned on.

Step 2—Unloading the Cassette

Care should be taken when taking the film out of the cassette. Fingernails should not be used as a tool to remove the film from the cassette corners. This technique can damage the sensitive intensifying screens. The proper method of removing the film is to open the backplate of the cassette and gently shake the top so that the film can be grasped by the corner between the thumb and the forefinger (Fig. 7.8). The x-ray film

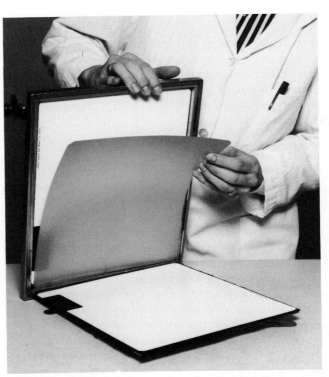

■ **FIG. 7.8** Proper method of removing a film from a cassette. The film should be "dumped" out of the cassette rather than "pried" out using fingers.

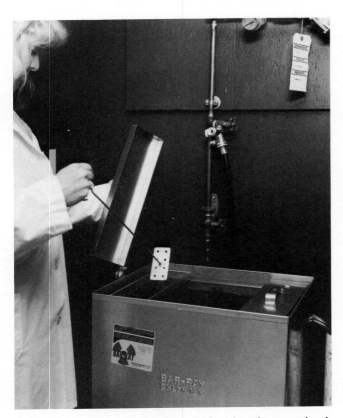

■ **FIG. 7.7** Stirring the chemicals before hand processing is very important. The chemicals tend to settle to the bottom of the tanks. Processing without stirring the chemicals could result in an unevenly developed film.

should be handled by the corners or edges only. The cassette should be closed while labeling the film and loading it onto the film hanger. Labeling film is discussed at the end of this chapter.

Step 3—Loading the Film on a Hanger

A tension clip hanger is loaded by inserting the film into the bottom, stationary clips first, then rotating the hanger right side up and inserting the film into the movable spring clips (Fig. 7.9). The film should be stretched so that it is taut enough to "bounce a coin on it." Mounting the film taut will prevent the film from touching adjacent films or walls in the processing tank.

If a channel hanger is used, it should be held in one hand while sliding the film into the channels with the other. All sides and corners of the film should be checked for correct placement in a channel. Once the film is in position, the top hinge can be closed.

Step 4—Developing the Film

The film is immersed into the developing tank, and the hanger is agitated two or three times to remove any air bubbles from the film surface (Fig. 7.10). The lid on the developer tank is replaced, and the timer is set for the appropriate development time. At this juncture, the hands should be dried and the cassette reloaded with film. Care should be taken in the re-

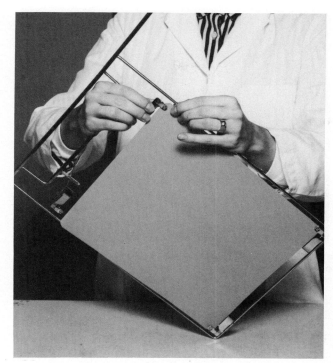

■ **FIG. 7.9** Loading a film on a clip film hanger.

loading process. The replacement film should meet all four corners of the cassette before closing so as not to compress any portion of the film in the cassette seams.

Step 5—Rinsing the Film

When the timer sounds, the film should be removed from the developer rapidly to avoid excessive dripping back into the developer tank (Fig. 7.11). For fast drainage, the hanger should be tilted so that the chemical carryover (spent developer) goes into the rinse or stop bath. Preventing the used developer from adding volume to the developer tank facilitates accurate tank replenishment. The film is immersed into the rinse bath and agitated for 30 seconds.

Step 6—Fixing the Film

After the film is in the rinse tank for 30 seconds, it should be drained of excess water and immersed into the fix tank (Fig. 7.12). The film is agitated two to three times to remove any air bubbles on the film surface, and the timer is set for the appropriate duration. The duration of the fixation process is usually twice the clearing time and after the film has lost its "milky" appearance. The milky appearance refers to the unexposed silver halide crystals remaining on the

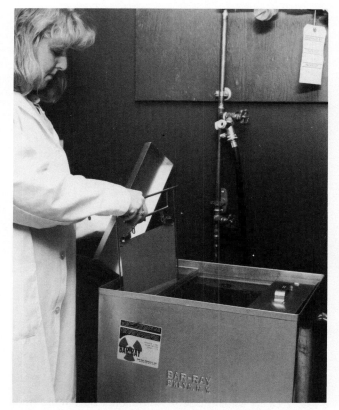

■ **FIG. 7.10** Immerse the film into the developing tank, and agitate two or three times to remove any air bubbles that may be attached to the side of the film. The developer temperature should be 68°F.

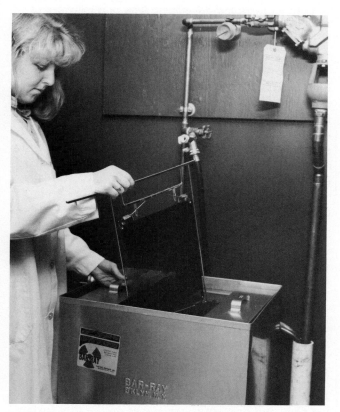

■ **FIG. 7.11** Rinse the film for 30 seconds. Before moving the film to the fix tank, tilt the hanger to allow for faster drainage of water off the hanger.

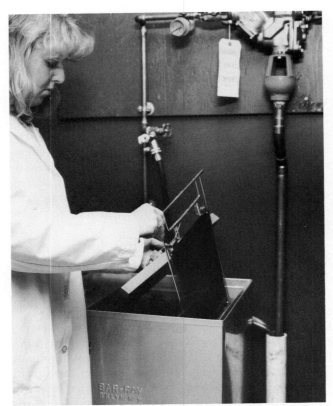

■ **FIG. 7.12** Immerse the film into the fix tank, and agitate the film a few times to remove any air bubbles. The film should be fixed for twice the developing time or a minimum of 10 minutes.

film. Once the silver is removed, the image will appear clear or transparent. After the film has been in the fix for a minute, it may be briefly viewed to evaluate the quality of exposure and positioning. It is important to put the film back into the fix tank after evaluation for a total of at least 10 minutes to allow maximum hardening of the film surface.

Step 7 — Washing the Film

The film is removed from the fix quickly so that chemical carryover (spent fixer) enters the wash tank. As with the developer, preventing carryover from entering the fix tank allows for accurate fix replenishment. The film should wash for 20 to 30 minutes (Fig. 7.13). The wash time depends on the water flow and exchange rate of the bath. The flow should have approximately eight complete changes per hour.

Step 8 — Optional Final Rinse

If facilities permit, a wetting agent can speed the drying time and prevent water marks on the film surface. The film is briefly dipped into the wetting agent prior to drying (Fig. 7.14).

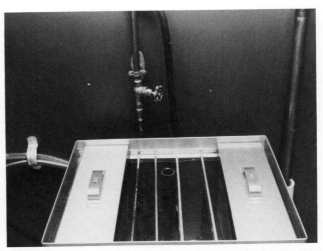

■ **FIG. 7.13** Wash the film for 20 to 30 minutes. If more than one film is being washed at once, allow enough space between each film to allow for adequate washing.

Step 9 — Drying the Film

The film should be dried in a dust-free area to prevent artifacts from sticking to the wet film surface. If channel hangers are utilized, the films should be removed from the hangers and hung with clips on a tension wire

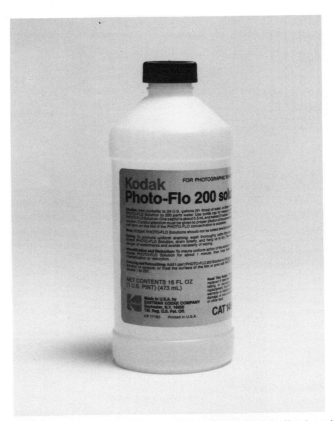

■ **FIG. 7.14** A wetting agent. An optional step in the hand processing procedure is to immerse the film briefly into a final rinse known as a wetting agent. The wetting agent decreases drying time and the chance of streaking while the film is drying.

(similar to a clothesline). Tension clip hangers can be hung on a drying rack (Fig. 7.15).

The films should be well separated and never allowed to touch each other while wet. When the films are dry, the sharp points on the corners of those processed with tension clip hangers need to be trimmed before filing. Trimming the sharp points prevents the emulsion of adjacent films from being scratched. The films can now be inserted into the appropriately labeled envelope.

Automatic Processing

Automatic processing involves the same basic principles as manual processing: the film is developed, fixed, washed, and dried. However, automatic processing has two major advantages over the manual method: (1) it is a highly standardized procedure with consistent quality and (2) it can produce a dry radiograph in a very short period. In a practice or clinic that has a high radiographic output, the amount of saved labor hours is remarkable. However, cost of an automatic processor is a primary factor that precludes many veterinary practices from having this convenience. For a low-volume veterinary practice, the expense of an automatic processor may not be justified.

A darkroom is still necessary for automatic processing, except a much smaller space is required. A counter is needed on the dry side to unload and load the cassettes, but the wet side consists of the processor only. Because the processor has its own drying mechanism utilizing heated forced air or infrared methods, an exhaust system or extractor fan must be in the darkroom to prevent excessive heat and fume accu-

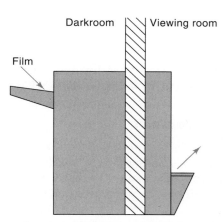

■ **FIG. 7.16** Cross section of an automatic processor that is designed to protrude through the darkroom wall. The film is loaded into the processor in the darkroom, and the finished product is delivered to the room adjacent.

mulation while in operation. Some automatic processors are designed to protrude through the darkroom wall so that a special exhaust system is not necessary (Fig. 7.16). In this case, the film is introduced into the processor in the darkroom and a finished, dry film exits in the room adjacent.

How Automatic Processors Work

Automatic processors involve roughly the same routine as manual processing, except they operate at much higher temperatures and have special formulated chemicals in order to speed development. The film is transported through the processor by a series of rollers similar to a conveyer belt in a factory. The rollers are driven by a motor moving the film at a constant speed (Fig. 7.17). The film must be transported at a controlled speed to ensure that the film is developed, fixed, and washed for the proper amount of time.

The exposed film is fed onto the tray of the machine and is then transported through the chemical

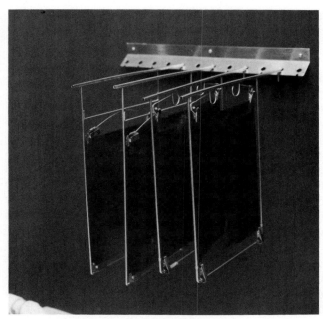

■ **FIG. 7.15** Films drying on a drying rack.

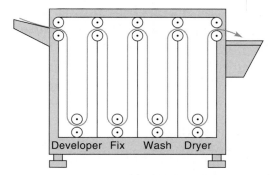

■ **FIG. 7.17** Cross section of an automatic processor showing its series of tanks and rollers. The rollers act as a conveyer belt, carrying the film from the developer, to the fix, to the wash, and finally to the drying racks.

baths and dryer by the roller assembly. In order to speed development, the rinse between the developer and fix is eliminated. The carryover chemicals are removed by compression as the film passes through squeegee rollers placed between the developer and the fix baths.

Processing Chemicals

The solutions are kept in peak condition because fresh chemicals are replenished at a predetermined rate based on machine usage. Without replenishment, chemical activity of the processing solutions would decrease with use as in manual processing. Accurate replenishment is essential to proper processing of film and to long life of the solutions. Generally, when the film is fed into the processor, pumps are activated to infuse replenisher from storage tanks to the baths inside the machine. The added replenisher is blended with the existing processing solutions by the recirculation pumps. Recirculation of the developer and fixer has two functions: to thoroughly mix the solutions and to help maintain the proper temperature and chemical activity. Excess processing solutions flow over the top of the tanks into the drain. Careful observation of the external replenishment tanks is necessary to maintain adequate chemical levels within the machine.

The temperature of the chemicals is constantly monitored and controlled within fine limits by a thermostatically operated water system. As in manual processing, the purpose of the water system is not limited to washing the films. Circulating water controls the temperature of the processing chemicals as well.

The method of water temperature control varies with the design of the processor. Hot and cold water may be blended to a proper temperature by a thermostatic mixing valve before the water enters the machine. Other processors are available that have cold incoming water that is electrically heated to the desired temperature.

Processor Maintenance

As with all mechanical devices, automatic processors can break down and need repair. In order to minimize the need for frequent repairs, proper maintenance is essential (Fig. 7.18). Recommendations for cleaning and maintenance procedures are furnished by the processor manufacturer and may include:

Solution level check
Replenishment rate check
Temperature check
Roller operation check
Rinsing and wiping of all roller racks
Regular cleaning of tanks

Although service engineers usually come as quickly as possible in the event of a processor break-

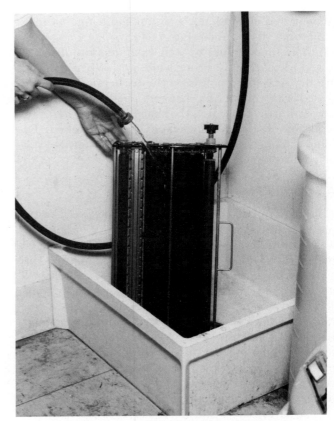

■ **FIG. 7.18** Processor maintenance is imperative to ensure proper film processing. The roller racks should be removed from the processor on a routine basis (at least monthly, depending on its use) and rinsed with warm water to remove any debris.

down, a back-up processing system is recommended. It is worthwhile to have the necessary chemicals and containers available so that emergency hand processing can be performed if required.

SILVER RECOVERY

In the present age of environmental awareness, recycling has become a national standard. Silver is a valuable natural resource and should be recycled whenever possible. In fact, most states in the United States require silver recovery as part of pollution control. All heavy metals are considered pollutants and cannot be disposed of in a septic system. Silver recovery not only is environmentally wise but is economically prudent as well.

During the processing procedure, the silver contained in the emulsion of the x-ray film either is transformed into black metallic silver in the developer solution or is removed by the fix solution. These two by-products, the fix solution and old radiographs, contain silver that can be recovered.

There are three methods of silver recovery from the fix solution: (1) metallic replacement, (2) electrolytic recovery, and (3) chemical precipitation.

Metallic Replacement

The metallic replacement method of recovery removes the silver from the exhausted fix by replacing the silver in the solution with another metal. The metal is normally iron in the form of steel wool. The steel wool dissolves in the acid fix solution and physically replaces the suspended silver, thus allowing the silver metal to precipitate to the bottom of the recovery unit.

A metallic replacer unit usually consists of a cartridge loaded with steel wool. The fix is poured into a top receptacle and allowed to "trickle" through the steel wool (Fig. 7.19). The fix containing no silver can then be discarded (according to local pollution control ordinances). Beware, the acid from the fix solution can harm pipes if water flow is low.

Up to 99% of the available silver can be recovered with the metallic replacement method, but the purity of recovered silver is low. This method is relatively inexpensive and is recommended for low-volume hand processing systems.

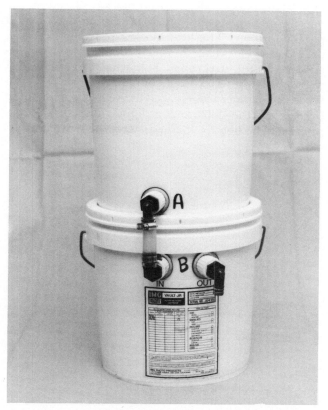

■ **FIG. 7.19** A Vault Junior trickle silver recovery system. The exhausted fix is poured into empty tank A and "trickled" through tank B. The fix containing no silver can then be discarded.

Electrolytic Recovery

Electrolytic recovery involves two electrodes (an anode and a cathode) placed either directly into the fix tank or into a separate holding container for the exhausted fix solution. As an electric current is passed between the two electrodes, the silver is attracted to the cathode. The silver is plated (collected) on the cathode. The advantage of electrolytic recovery is that the fix solution may be reused. Reusing fix solution, however, requires much chemical analysis. This method of reclamation recovers silver of high purity but is generally less efficient than metallic replacement.

Chemical Precipitation

The chemical precipitation technique of silver recovery involves additional chemical compounds to precipitate the silver from the fix solution. As the chemicals are added to the fix, the silver floats to the bottom of the receptacle and forms a sludge. The sludge is then filtered, dried, and packed to be sold to a refiner.

Gold and silver refiners/dealers often purchase exhausted fix solution and old radiographs for the reclamation of the silver that they contain. Companies that purchase fix solutions and discarded radiographs are normally listed in the telephone directory's yellow pages.

Before radiographs can be sold for reclamation, however, the veterinary practice is legally required to keep them for a specific length of time. The legal requirement for retaining radiographs is 7 years, but it is advisable to keep them until the patient is deceased.

FILM IDENTIFICATION

Every radiograph should be properly labeled with essential information so that the film can be identified at a later date. In many instances, additional radiographs need to be taken to evaluate healing or advancement of disease. Without proper labeling, progressive evaluation would be difficult. There is also the legal aspect to consider. If a medicolegal problem were to arise, a radiograph without proper labeling is of little value in a court of law. The only "legal" labeling of a radiograph is that which is in the film emulsion.

There are several methods of labeling a radiograph, and it is a matter of personal preference as to which method is adopted. All labeling systems should provide the same basic information: (1) name and address of the hospital/practice or veterinarian; (2) date the radiograph was taken; and (3) patient identification, including name of the owner and patient name, age, sex, and breed.

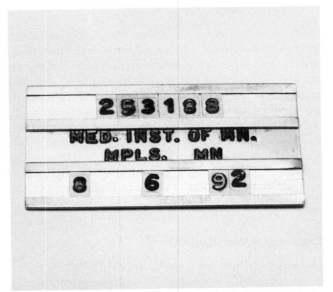

■ **FIG. 7.20** Lead letters placed in a holder designed to be placed on top of a cassette for film identification.

Lead Markers

One of the simplest methods of film labeling is with lead letters and numbers that are placed directly on the cassette before exposure. The lead digits can be placed in a holder or taped directly to the cassette (Fig. 7.20). The lead absorbs the primary radiation from the x-ray beam so that the film directly under the lead is left unexposed and appears transparent. It is possible to purchase prepared holders that include the name and address of the clinic spelled out permanently in lead letters. With a permanent prepared holder, it is necessary to change only the date and identification of the patient.

The disadvantages of this method of labeling are that it can be time-consuming and the small lead digits are easily lost. In addition, it limits tight collimation because the area outside the patient must be exposed to provide an image of the label.

Lead-Impregnated Tape

Another method of labeling a radiograph during exposure is with disposable lead-impregnated tape. By writing on the tape with a ballpoint pen or pencil, the soft lead is displaced, leaving indentations. Making indentations in the lead creates a difference in density that allows x-rays to penetrate to the film. The tape is then placed on a holder that has the name and address of the facility permanently attached (Fig. 7.21A,B). The lead tape can be used to label left or right, time intervals for a series of radiographs, and markers to indicate the direction of the x-ray beam for oblique views.

The lead-impregnated tape is available in 50- or 100-foot rolls or in precut 3-inch strips. The manufacturer of the tape will usually supply the lead-tape holder with the specified facility information.

Photoimprinting Label System

One label system utilizes a lead blocker placed on the outside of the cassette, an identification card, and a photoimprinter. The lead blocker prevents exposure to a 3 × 7 cm area, to which identification can be exposed in the darkroom. Following the removal of the film in the darkroom, but before processing, a typed or written card is placed between the unexposed portion of the film and a light source (photoimprinter). The light is "flashed," and the written infor-

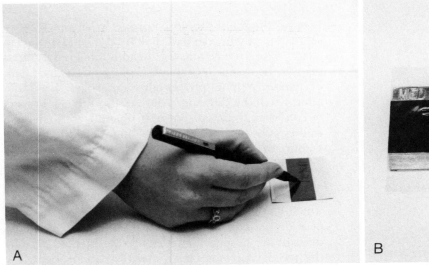

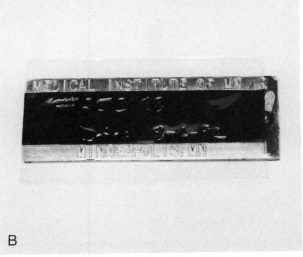

A   B

■ **FIG. 7.21** Lead-impregnated tape. The lead is displaced by means of a pointed writing instrument, leaving indentations (A). After the appropriate information is written, the tape is adhered to a specially designed holder (B).

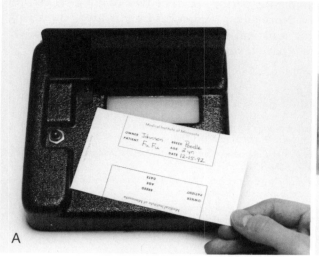

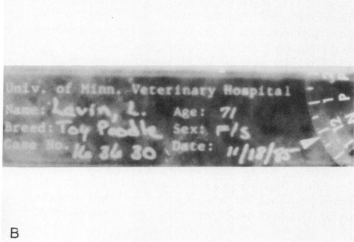

■ **FIG. 7.22** Film identification method known as photoimprinting. The identification card is placed on the photoimprinter with the film placed over the card (*A*). The imprinter is then closed, and a light is "flashed" under the card, which exposes the information onto the film. After the film is processed, the identification can be clearly seen in the corner of the film (*B*).

mation on the card is recorded on the previously unexposed area (Fig. 7.22A,B).

New cassettes can be purchased with the lead blocker already installed, or 3 × 7 cm pieces of lead can be purchased and installed on the face of the cassette. It is important that the lead blockers be placed in the same corner of all the cassettes. This consistency will prevent "flashing" the wrong corner in the darkroom. Caution should also be taken to ensure that no anatomic area of interest is positioned in the blocker area where no exposure will be made.

Miscellaneous Markers

Right (R) and left (L) markers are essential to identify a right or left limb or to identify the right or left side of the thorax or abdomen (Fig. 7.23). Markers may also be needed at times to identify a unique view, orientation, or beam direction. Labeling the front and rear limbs may be necessary, particularly in equine radiography because the anatomic structures of the

distal limbs of the horse are virtually identical. Time-sequence labels are also available for special procedures to indicate time elapse following the administration of radiopaque contrast media.

Other Identification Methods

In the event that identification was forgotten before exposure, it is possible to write on the film prior to development with a pencil or other pointed device. The pressure from the pointed device will distort the film emulsion and record the information, which will remain on the film throughout the processing procedure. It is also possible to scratch the information into the emulsion while it is still wet. Other methods include a permanent marker or a piece of adhesive tape on the dry film.

All of these identification techniques are considered temporary and are undesirable for routine film identification. They are not considered adequate markings should legal proceedings arise regarding the patient.

FILM FILING

An organized filing system is mandatory in any veterinary practice. It would be pointless to spend time correctly exposing the x-ray film and properly identifying and processing it only to place it in a pile of other radiographs taken in the past. In order to utilize x-rays for future referral or follow-up examinations, they must be placed in a suitable holder that is labeled appropriately.

Before filing x-rays, they must be completely dry. When x-ray film is hand processed with tension clip

■ **FIG. 7.23** Right (R) and left (L) markers for anatomic orientation.

hangers, very often the corners remain wet until the film is removed from the hanger and allowed to dry. Cutting the corners of the film where it was attached to the hanger clips may alleviate this problem.

The best method of filing radiographs is in a large, 14 × 17 inch (35 × 43 cm) file envelope regardless of the film size. Smaller-sized x-ray film could be filed in smaller envelopes, which would be a bit less expensive, but the smaller envelopes tend to get lost among the larger when filed together. Film filing envelopes can be purchased from any radiographic sales service.

Filing the films in a logical manner is crucial. The envelopes should be labeled with a description of the patient, name of owner, date, and type of radiographic examination performed. The type of filing system will vary. Normally, a numeric system is used, employing either a patient case number or a file number. Some clinics have a color-code system for easy retrieval.

BIBLIOGRAPHY

Eastman Kodak Company: *Kodak: The Fundamentals of Radiography,* 12th ed. Rochester, NY, 1980.

Gray JE, et al: *Quality Control in Diagnostic Imaging.* Aspen, Rockville, MD, 1983.

Morgan, JP, Silverman S: *Techniques in Veterinary Radiography.* Iowa State University Press, Ames, 1987.

Ticer, JW: *Radiographic Techniques in Small Animal Practice,* 2nd ed. WB Saunders, Philadelphia, 1984.

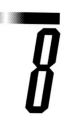

RADIOGRAPHIC
TECHNIQUE
EVALUATION

OBJECTIVES

Upon completion of this chapter, the reader should be able to:

- Describe briefly how radiography works
- Define density and contrast
- Describe the correct method of viewing a radiograph on a view box
- State the four questions of evaluation for a radiograph

- State the standard change made to kilovoltage to alter the penetreation of x-rays
- State the standard charge made to milliamperage to alter radiographic density
- List other error considerations that can cause a poor quality radiograph

I N T R O D U C T I O N

The production of a quality radiograph depends on many factors. Chapters 1 to 7 provide a detailed explanation of these factors, yet there is one element that remains to be discussed. This crucial factor involves the evaluation of a finished radiograph.

The ability of the technologist to evaluate a radiograph properly is imperative. Without this ability, the attempt to attain quality is futile. The need for a second radiograph at one time or another is unavoidable, no matter what your skill level. Assessing what is wrong with the radiograph and making the proper corrections are the skills that we seek. Radiographic quality depends on the technologist's understanding of the concepts and variables that produce a good radiograph.

Radiography can be an extremely difficult subject to grasp. The concepts of x-rays and how they are formed are complex. Mastering the physics of radiography is a challenge for every student. Quality radiographs are not attained by "luck" but by a conscious understanding of the variables. It is this understanding that can change a radiographic image into a piece of artwork.

PHYSICS OF RADIOGRAPHY: A REVIEW

X-rays are generated in an x-ray tube. The tube consists of a cathode side (with a negative electrical charge) and an anode side (with a positive electrical charge). In the tube, a stream of fast-moving electrons is attracted and directed from the cathode to the anode. As the electrons collide and interact with the atoms of the target on the anode, a great amount of energy is produced; 1% of this energy is in the form of x-rays.

The cathode consists of a wire filament that emits electrons when heated. The temperature of the filament is controlled by the milliamperage (mA) setting on the console of the machine. As the mA is increased, the temperature of the filament increases and the filament produces more electrons. The period of time

during which the electrons (x-rays) are permitted to leave the x-ray tube is measured in fractions of seconds (s). The number of electrons and the period set for their release determine how many x-rays are available. The **milliamperage-seconds (mA-s)** thus controls the total number of x-rays produced.

The anode, which attracts negatively charged electrons, is made of a metal (tungsten) that can withstand very high temperatures. This tolerance is necessary because of the great amount of heat produced during the collision of electrons. Ninety-nine percent of the energy produced at the impact of electrons is in the form of heat; only 1% is x-rays. The anode is constructed at an angle so that the electrons are directed downward (toward the cassette) through a window in the metal housing of the x-ray tube.

The electron speed necessary to create a high-energy impact is achieved by applying thousands of volts (kilovolts) across the anode and cathode. The available electrons thus travel at a tremendous speed toward the positive charge of the anode. High voltage produces x-rays with greater penetrating power and intensity. The **kilovoltage peak (kVp)** thus controls the penetrating power of the x-rays.

DENSITY AND CONTRAST: A REVIEW

The material covered in Chapter 5 gives a detailed explanation of density and contrast. In order to apply this knowledge in a practical manner, a review of the salient points is needed.

Radiographic density is defined as the degree of blackness on the radiograph. Density is primarily affected by mA-s. The higher the mA-s, the greater the density and the more blackness on the radiograph. The mA-s controls the total number of x-rays available. If x-rays make film black, more x-rays emitted by the machine cause more blackness on the film. The kVp may also influence density and increase blackness on the radiograph; mA-s and kVp can be differentiated because the latter also changes the contrast.

Radiographic contrast is defined as the density difference between two areas of a finished radiograph.

If the difference between two areas is great, the contrast is described as high. If there is a slight difference in density (an overall gray appearance), the contrast is low.

Radiographic contrast is primarily affected by the kVp. The higher the kVp, the lower the contrast. The kVp governs the penetrating power of the x-ray beam. If a high kVp setting is used, more x-rays reach the film because of the increased penetration (pushing power). The kVp also governs the energy spectrum of the x-ray beam. High kVp techniques not only have higher peak-energy photons in the beam, which enhance patient penetration, but also a wider variation of energies among all the photons in the beam, allowing for more variation in the degree of penetration among the photons. This broad photon energy spectrum contributes to the greater gray spectrum (long scale or low contrast), even with the high versus low kVp techniques. Scatter radiation, which is more prevalent with high kVp techniques, can influence image contrast as well, but the use of grids and the use of fast screens (i.e., rare-earth screens) minimizes this effect.

VIEWING A RADIOGRAPH

In order to evaluate a film accurately, a radiograph should be viewed on an evenly lit view box in a semi-darkened room. The view-box screen should be clean and all lightbulbs in working order.

The position of the film on the view screen is also important. Veterinary radiographers generally follow the medical protocol of viewing. Ventrodorsal or dorsoventral anatomy, such as an abdomen or a thorax, should be placed on the view screen so that the animal's head is at the top (or toward the top of the viewer) and the patient's right is on the viewer's left. In other words, the patient should be in the position to shake the hand of the viewer. All laterally positioned anatomy should face the viewer's left with the spine at the top.

EVALUATION OF RADIOGRAPHIC TECHNIQUE

In the technical evaluation of a radiograph, four basic questions should be asked:

1. Is the film too light or too dark?
2. Is there proper penetration?
3. Is the density suitable?
4. Is the contrast appropriate?

The answer to the first question is not always elementary. In examining a radiograph that seems too light, some personnel conclude that the film is overexposed. This misunderstanding stems from experience with photography. In taking a picture with a camera, increased exposure time increases the brightness of the picture. Radiography is the opposite of photography in this respect. The x-rays (more exposure) make the film black. If a radiograph is underexposed, the film seems too light; if the radiograph is too dark, it is overexposed.

When it has been established that a radiograph is too light or too dark, the next step is to determine why. This leads to the second question. Penetration is especially important if the film is too light. On a film with inadequate penetration, the anatomic parts (silhouettes) are indistinct or imperceptible. If, for example, kidney, liver, and bowel silhouettes are not visible on an abdominal radiograph, insufficient kVp was used. The standard change (increase or decrease) in kVp is 10 to 15%.

If the film is overpenetrated, it will be too dark. This problem of too much darkness is often confused with too much mA-s. Distinguishing between overpenetration and too much density due to mA-s depends on the consideration of the contrast.

The third question to be addressed concerns film density. Insufficient film density is usually indicated if the film is too light and the anatomic silhouettes of interest are visible but not aesthetically sound; that is, the image is visible but not dark enough to be seen well. The film does not have enough blackness, and more x-rays are needed to increase the density. If a film is too dark because of excessive density, the image is too dark but the contrast is not significantly affected. To improve a radiograph by altering the density, the mA-s is increased or decreased by 30 to 50%.

The fourth question involves radiographic contrast. There is much confusion concerning contrast and its relationship to poor quality radiographs. The kVp controls the scale of contrast on a finished film. High kVp is responsible for low contrast and gives a radiograph an overall gray appearance.

Low kVp is used to establish high contrast and generates many blacks and whites on the radiograph. Contrast is a primary factor in evaluating an overexposed radiograph and determining whether it is overpenetrated or has too much density due to the mA-s. If a radiograph is too dark because of overpenetration, the bones are gray. Too much density caused by excessive mA-s has very little effect on the contrast. The soft tissue is dark, but the bones remain relatively white. The flow chart in Figure 8.1 can be used as a reference for quick evaluation.

A quality radiograph has adequate penetration, sufficient density, and good contrast. These requirements differ for bone and soft tissue. To be of diagnostic value, a radiograph must have the correct scale of contrast. For soft tissue, low contrast is desirable. An abdominal radiograph, for example, should have many soft grays to facilitate differentiation of the intra-abdominal organs (Fig. 8.2). High contrast is necessary for bone radiography. The image should be well defined, and the bone should be distinct from the surrounding tissue.

PRACTICAL APPLICATION

In the four scenarios that follow, evaluate the specified radiographs by answering the four basic questions.

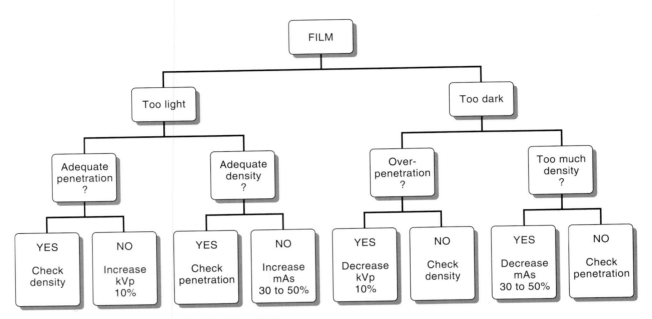

■ **FIG. 8.1** Exposure technique evaluation flow chart.

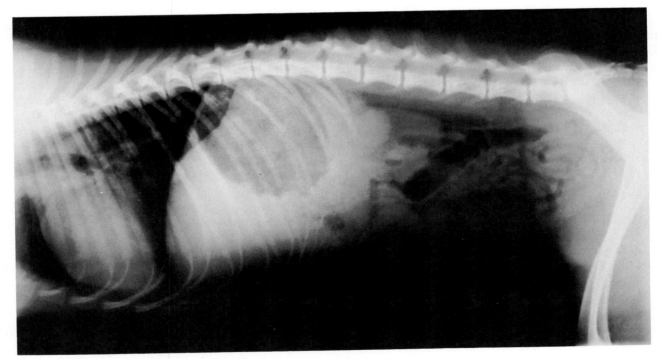

■ **FIG. 8.2** A properly exposed abdominal radiograph (lateral view).

SCENARIO I

Examine the Radiograph in Figure 8.3

The film is too light. This indicates insufficient kVp or mA-s. A close examination demonstrates that the anatomic parts are not clearly visible, especially in the cranial portion behind the diaphragm. This information answers the second question: there is insufficient penetration. The kVp should be increased 10 to 15% to improve the penetration and density and to achieve a suitable scale of contrast for an abdominal radiograph.

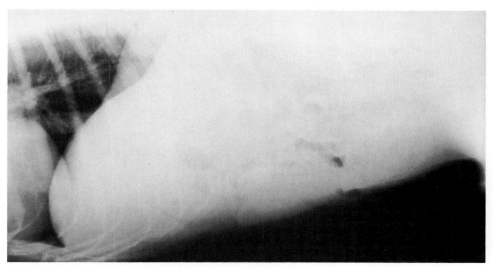

■ **FIG. 8.3** Scenario I for evaluating radiographic technique.

SCENARIO II

Examine the Radiograph in Figure 8.4

Initial examination indicates that the radiograph is too light. On further inspection, the anatomy is visible but lacks density. Penetration is suitable, but the contrast is inappropriate. By increasing the mA-s by 50%, the image will be improved by the creation of more blackness on the radiograph. This correction will enhance the overall density and appearance of the film.

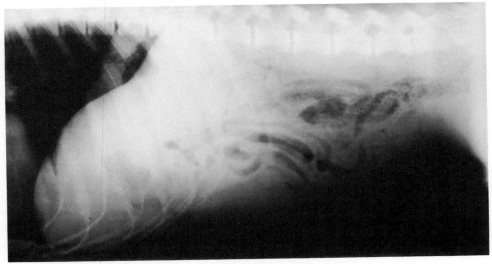

■ **FIG. 8.4**   Scenario II for evaluating radiographic technique.

SCENARIO III

Examine the Radiograph in Figure 8.5

It is evident that the radiograph is too dark. The film has too much density. The problem is difficult to assess until the contrast (which is inappropriate) is examined. Examination of the bone tissue in the radiograph demonstrates that the spine and pelvis are gray, an indication of overpenetration. Overpenetration of the patient has affected the density and leads to confusion as to the cause of the dark image. The radiograph will be of greater diagnostic value if the kVp is decreased by 10 to 15%.

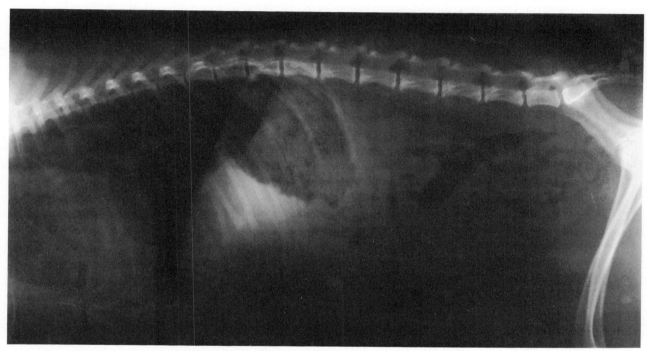

■ **FIG. 8.5** Scenario III for evaluating radiographic technique.

SCENARIO IV

Examine the Radiograph in Figure 8.6

This radiograph is also too dark. Initial examination to determine the cause does not conclusively demonstrate overpenetration. There is an overabundance of density, but overpenetration and excessive density due to mA-s cannot be distinguished until the contrast (which is appropriate) is evaluated. The spine and pelvis remain relatively white despite the excessive density. Based on this observation, it can be concluded that the kVp level is appropriate but that the mA-s should be decreased by 50%.

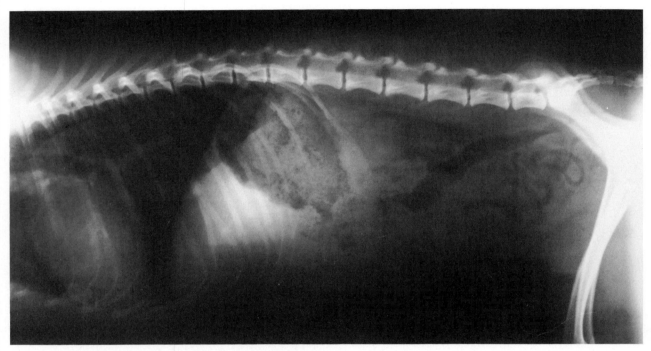

■ **FIG. 8.6** Scenario IV for evaluating radiographic technique.

OTHER ERROR CONSIDERATIONS

In evaluating a quality radiograph, the technologist should be aware of other pitfalls that can generate a poor quality film. Certain standards must be maintained in the darkroom as well as with the radiographic equipment. A radiograph that has been processed with exhausted chemicals or exposed with a poor film-screen combination, for example, will mimic a film that has been underexposed. In order to eliminate all possible pitfalls, proper quality control should be maintained. Chapter 10 covers this topic in detail.

BIBLIOGRAPHY

Cunliffe-Lavin LM: Radiographic technique: A ray of hope. Vet Technician J 444–451:12, 1991.

DEVELOPING A TECHNIQUE CHART

OBJECTIVES

Upon completion of this chapter, the reader should be able to:

- State the purpose of a technique chart
- List the factors that influence a technique chart
- List the recommended screen variable kVp technique charts based on anatomy for a small animal practice
- List the equipment necessary for variable kVp technique chart formulation
- Describe how the exposure factors— kVp, milliamperage, and exposure time(s)—are calculated
- List the base mA-s factors for the three speeds of screens
- Describe the modifications necessary for the exposure technique when using a grid

- State in chronological order the steps essential for variable kVp technique chart formulation
- Describe how the appropriate mA-s setting is chosen for all of the anatomical areas of small animals
- Describe the method of formulating a variable mA-s technique chart
- Describe the modifications necessary when a technique chart fails to produce adequate radiographic density because of patient size, condition, or pathology

G L O S S A R Y

SANTES' RULE: Calculation for determining an approximate amount of kilovoltage (kVp) necessary for a given anatomic area based on measurement and the grid being used: (2 × tissue thickness in cm) + 40 + grid factor = kVp.

TECHNIQUE CHART: A chart that is based on tissue thickness and anatomic part that can be consulted for predetermined machine settings.

I N T R O D U C T I O N

The **technique chart** is an invaluable resource for a radiographer. The purpose of the technique chart is to provide a consistent method of choosing the proper exposure factors to create a diagnostic radiograph. Based on the thickness of tissue and anatomic area of the body, the technique chart can be consulted by the radiographer for a predetermined machine setting. Without this resource, one would have to calculate a new technique each time a radiograph is taken or use a questionable technique performed previously. A technique chart prevents the need for second radiographs due to inappropriate exposure factors.

Every x-ray machine should have its own formulated technique chart. It is often thought that a successful exposure technique used on x-ray machine A will also work on x-ray machine B. This is not true. Even x-ray machines of the same make and model vary in both quantity and quality of output because of variations in input voltage and calibration. Several other factors influence the chart:

Speed of screens
Age of screens
Speed of film
Source-image distance (SID)
Amount of beam filtration
Temperature and time of film processing
Type of grid

The factors affecting a technique chart should be standardized as much as possible. The SID, amount of beam filtration, film processing, and type of grid should remain constant. The success of a technique chart depends on the radiographer's willingness to maintain continuity of the variables.

The only variables that will change are the types of film and screens used. The film type and speed should be preselected and limited. The screen speed chosen should fit the needs of the practice and be limited to one or two speeds. A veterinary practice that has a number of screen types will have to formulate many technique charts. Working with a number of film and screen types with coinciding technique charts

can be confusing and may increase the incidence of errors.

SUGGESTED CHARTS

Another misconception is that just one technique chart is needed for an x-ray machine. On the contrary, anatomic and technical differences call for more than one chart. Several charts may be needed and may include:

Screen and nonscreen
Grid and nongrid
Various film-screen combinations
Species specific
Anatomy specific

In general, five (screen) variable kVp technique charts based on species and anatomy are recommended for a small animal veterinary practice:

1. Extremity and skull (canine/feline), no grid.
2. Abdomen (canine/feline), with grid.
3. Thorax (canine/feline), with grid.
4. Pelvis and spine (canine/feline), with grid.
5. Avian and exotics, no grid.

TECHNIQUE CHART FORMULATION

Several methods are used in veterinary practice to formulate a technique chart; all are effective and vary slightly. The method presented here is different from others because of a few short cuts that the technologist may find helpful. The principles of technique chart formulation can be applied to any species and anatomic area. The method presented here applies to x-ray machines that have variable kVp and exposure time settings.

To create a workable technique chart, a series of trial exposures need to be made using a cooperative, average-sized patient. Theoretically, by exposing one radiograph, all five suggested technique charts can be formulated by this means.

Equipment needed for this procedure should be gathered before proceeding. A mature dog with average conformation (neither obese nor emaciated), weighing approximately 50 pounds, is an ideal patient for this procedure. With this size dog, a 14 × 17 inch cassette should be employed. The x-ray film used should be medium speed because of its versatility in veterinary practice.

Exposure Factors

To formulate a variable kVpp technique chart, a test radiograph will be made of the canine abdomen in lateral recumbency. The measurement will be in the range of 11 to 16 cm, and the exposure factors will be based on the screen type and grid ratio used. Remember, any measurement exceeding 10 cm necessitates the use of a grid to reduce fog-producing scatter radiation.

- *Kilovoltage*: Use **Santes' rule**: (2 × tissue thickness in cm) + SID (40 inches) + grid factor = kVp.
- *Milliamperage*: Highest setting possible.
- *Exposure time*: Selection based on milliamperage-seconds (mA-s) needed for screen type (discussed next).

Base mA-s Factors (Table 9.1)

The following base mA-s requirements for the intensifying screens are merely starting points for the radiographer. Each individual radiographic system may require slightly different exposures.

SCREEN TYPE	M A - s RANGE
Fast (high speed)	2.5 to 10
Medium (par speed)	5 to 12.5
Slow (ultradetail)	30 to 40

Exposure Modification for Grid Use

When using a grid, increased exposure is needed to maintain adequate radiographic density. Addition of a grid usually requires doubling the exposure time. For example, if the exposure technique needed for a table-top (nongrid) exposure is 2.5 mAs (1/120 [s] at 300 mA), the new exposure for grid use would be at least 5.0 mA-s (1/60 [s] at 300 mA).

The kVp will also need to be modified. The amount of modification will vary according to the grid ratio being used.

GRID RATIO	ADDED KVP TO SUM OF SANTES' RULE
5:1	6 to 8
8:1	8 to 10
12:1	10 to 15
16:1	15 to 20

T A B L E 9 . 1

Milliamperage-Seconds (mA-s) Chart

TIME (s)	25 mA	50 mA	100 mA	150 mA	200 mA	300 mA
1/120	.2	.4	.8	1.3	1.7	2.5
1/60	.4	.8	1.7	2.5	3.3	5
1/40	.6	1.3	2.5	3.8	5.0	7.5
1/30	.8	1.7	3.3	5	6.7	10
1/24	1	2.1	4.2	6.2	8.3	12.5
1/20	1.25	2.5	5	7.5	10	15
1/10	2.5	5	10	15	20	30
2/10	5	10	20	30	40	60
1/4	6.3	12.5	25	37.5	50	75
3/10	7.5	15.0	30	45	60	90
4/10	10	20	40	60	80	120
1/2	12.5	25	50	75	100	150
6/10	15	30	60	90	120	180
3/4	18.8	37.5	75	112.5	150	225
1	25	50	100	150	200	300
1 1/4	31.3	62.5	125	187.5	250	375
1 1/2	37.5	75	150	225	300	450
2	50	100	200	300	400	600
2 1/2	62.5	125	250	375	500	750
3	75	150	300	450	600	900

PROCEDURE FLOW CHART: VARIABLE kVp TECHNIQUE CHART

I. Canine abdomen with the use of a grid
- A. Select a dog
    1. Cooperative adult
    2. Moderate muscling
    3. Average weight (approximately 50 pounds)
    4. Haircoat clean/medium to short length
- B. X-ray machine
    1. Evaluate line voltage
    2. Set SID (constant)
- C. Exposure technique
    1. Kilovoltage: Use Santes' rule from lateral measurement plus additional kVp for grid use
    2. Milliamperage: Highest setting possible (to achieve shortest exposure time)
    3. Exposure time: Chosen according to required mA-s for selected intensifying screen
- D. Film-screen system
    1. Select the intensifying screen that best represents an average age of other screens (fast screens recommended)
    2. Select film that is not expired or damaged (medium-speed film recommended)
    3. A 400- to 600-speed film-screen system is suggested
- E. Grid
    1. Ensure grid position
    a. Placed on cassette centered with central x-ray
    b. Under tabletop with Bucky tray centered to central x-ray
- F. Test exposure
    1. Use calculated exposure technique
- G. Process in standardized darkroom
    1. Solutions adequate strength (hand processing)
    2. Replenisher at recommended rate (automatic processing)
- H. Evaluate radiograph
    1. Too dark: Decrease mA-s 30 to 50% or kVp 10 to 15%
    2. Too light: Increase mA-s 30 to 50% or kVp 10 to 15%
- I. Repeat test exposure
    1. Repeat step H
- J. Formulate and plot technique chart
    1. 0 to 80 kVp: Increase or decrease kVp by increments of 2
    2. 80 kVp and above: Increase or decrease kVp by increments of three

TRIAL EXPOSURE—EXAMPLE 1

Known Information

Lateral abdomen measurement = 13 cm
Film speed = medium
Screen speed = fast

TABLE 9.2

Trial Exposure: Example 1

AREA: ABDOMEN   GRID: 8:1   SID (INCHES): 40

THICKNESS (cm)	kVp	mA	TIME (s)	mA-s
5	58	300	1/40	7.5
6	60	300	1/40	7.5
7	62	300	1/40	7.5
8	64	300	1/40	7.5
9	66	300	1/40	7.5
10	68	300	1/40	7.5
11	70	300	1/40	7.5
12	72	300	1/40	7.5
13	74	300	1/40	7.5
14	76	300	1/40	7.5
15	78	300	1/40	7.5
16	80	300	1/40	7.5
17	83	300	1/40	7.5
18	86	300	1/40	7.5
19	89	300	1/40	7.5
20	92	300	1/40	7.5
21	95	300	1/40	7.5
22	98	300	1/40	7.5
23	101	300	1/40	7.5
24	104	300	1/40	7.5
25	107	300	1/40	7.5

Grid ratio = 8 : 1
SID = 40 inches
Milliamperage capability = 300
kVp = 120

Calculation for Kilovoltage

(2 × 13 [cm]) + 40 (SID) + 8 (grid factor) = 74 kVp

Calculations for mA-s

300 × $\frac{1}{120}$ =   2.5 mA-s ⎤

300 × $\frac{1}{60}$ =   5.0 mA-s ⎥ mA-s range based

300 × $\frac{1}{40}$ =   7.5 mA-s ⎥

300 × $\frac{1}{30}$ = 10.0 mA-s ⎦ on fast screen speed

300 × $\frac{1}{24}$ = 12.5 mA-s

In order to choose the appropriate mA-s for an abdominal radiograph, it is necessary to consider the tissue density being exposed and the grid being used. As stated earlier, the suggested technique charts for the canine are (1) extremity/skull, (2) abdomen, (3) thorax, and (4) pelvis/spine. All of the anatomic areas listed need to be assigned a suitable mA-s setting. The thorax, for example, possesses less x-ray–absorbing tissues than other parts of the anatomy, and therefore fewer x-rays are needed to produce a proper radiographic density. The thorax requires 50 to 75% less mA-s than the abdomen. The pelvis, in comparison, requires 50 to 75% more mA-s due to its increased tissue density. The lowest mA-s of the base settings is normally sufficient for tabletop extremity/skull use.

The following is a suggested distribution based on the tissue density of each of the anatomic areas and whether or not a grid is needed.

S U G G E S T E D   D I S T R I B U T I O N

2.5 mA-s ▪ Extremity/skull (no grid used)
5.0 mA-s ▪ Thorax (8 : 1 grid used)
7.5 mA-s ▪ Abdomen (8 : 1 grid used)
10.0 mA-s ▪ Pelvis/spine (8 : 1 grid used)

Based on the machine milliamperage capability of 300, the following calculation can be made to attain the proper time setting:

300 mA × _____ = 7.5 mA-s

where

time (s) = $\frac{1}{40}$.

Trial Exposure 1

The following is the exposure setting for a 13-cm canine abdomen (see Table 9.2 for plotted technique chart):

- kVp = 74
- Milliamperage = 300
- Time in seconds = $\frac{1}{40}$

Notice that a grid is used for the abdomen even with a measurement thickness less than 10 cm. It is possible to use a grid with measurements under 10 cm as long as the proper kVp settings are used. Using a grid for *all* measurements of an abdomen, thorax, and pelvis eliminates the confusion created when grid and nongrid techniques are used on the same chart. The use of a grid for measurements under 10 cm will not decrease radiographic quality. On the contrary, radiographic quality is increased whenever a grid is used. For all technique charts, except the extremity/skull chart, a grid can be used for all centimeter thickness increments.

TRIAL EXPOSURE — EXAMPLE 2

Oftentimes, the x-ray machine used in veterinary radiography does not have a 300 milliamperage capability. In this second example, a 100 milliamperage/100 kVp capacity machine is used.

Known Information

Lateral abdomen measurement = 14 cm
Film speed = medium
Screen speed = fast
Grid ratio = 8 : 1
SID = 40 inches
Milliamperage capability = 100
kVp capability = 100

Calculation for kVp

(2 × 14 [cm]) + 40 (SID) + 8 (grid factor) = 76 kVp

Calculations for mA-s

100 × $\frac{1}{120}$ =   0.8 mA-s

100 × $\frac{1}{60}$ =   1.6 mA-s

$100 \times \frac{1}{40} = 2.5$ mA-s

$100 \times \frac{1}{30} = 3.3$ mA-s

$100 \times \frac{1}{24} = 4.2$ mA-s   mA-s range based

$100 \times \frac{1}{20} = 5.0$ mA-s   on fast screen speed

$100 \times \frac{1}{15} = 6.6$ mA-s

$100 \times \frac{1}{12} = 8.3$ mA-s

$100 \times \frac{1}{10} = 10.0$ mA-s

$100 \times \frac{1}{8} = 12.5$ mA-s

SUGGESTED DISTRIBUTION

2.5 mA-s ▪ Extremity/skull (no grid)
5.0 mA-s ▪ Thorax (8:1 grid)
8.3 mA-s ▪ Abdomen (8:1 grid)
10.0 mA-s ▪ Pelvis/spine (8:1 grid)

Trial Exposure 2

The following is the exposure setting for a 14-cm canine abdomen (see Table 9.3 for plotted technique chart):

- kVp = 76
- Milliamperage = 100
- Time in seconds = $\frac{1}{12}$

OTHER FORMULATION METHODS

Some x-ray machines will limit the alterations made in kilovoltage and milliamperage. Certain older or smaller x-ray machines do not allow for kilovoltage variations in steps of 1 or 2 kVp. A compromise between kVp and mA-s will need to be made for this type of machine. For example, if the kVp settings can be altered in 10-kVp intervals only, increased radiographic density may be attained by increasing the mA-s. For each centimeter of increased patient thickness, a small amount of mA-s is added to the exposure technique. This is called a variable mA-s technique chart.

Table 9.4 is an example of a variable mA-s technique chart. For the tissue thickness of 1 to 5 cm, the same kilovoltage (50) was used. The mA-s, on the other hand, was increased approximately 20 to 30% for each centimeter increase. When the chart reaches the centimeter thickness of 6, the kVp is increased to 60 and the mA-s is decreased to its original value and the mA-s cycle begins again.

MODIFICATION RECOMMENDATIONS

In some instances, a technique chart may fail to produce a quality radiograph because of excessive patient thickness or pathology. It may be necessary to increase the mA-s at a particular centimeter measurement to maintain adequate radiographic density. For example,

---

T A B L E 9 . 3

Trial Exposure: Example 2

AREA: ABDOMEN   GRID: 8:1   SID (INCHES): 40

THICKNESS (cm)	kVp	mA	TIME (s)	mA-s
5	58	100	$\frac{1}{12}$	8.3
6	60	100	$\frac{1}{12}$	8.3
7	62	100	$\frac{1}{12}$	8.3
8	64	100	$\frac{1}{12}$	8.3
9	66	100	$\frac{1}{12}$	8.3
10	68	100	$\frac{1}{12}$	8.3
11	70	100	$\frac{1}{12}$	8.3
12	72	100	$\frac{1}{12}$	8.3
13	74	100	$\frac{1}{12}$	8.3
14	76	100	$\frac{1}{12}$	8.3
15	78	100	$\frac{1}{12}$	8.3
16	80	100	$\frac{1}{12}$	8.3
17	83	100	$\frac{1}{12}$	8.3
18	86	100	$\frac{1}{12}$	8.3
19	89	100	$\frac{1}{12}$	8.3
20	92	100	$\frac{1}{12}$	8.3
21	95	100	$\frac{1}{12}$	8.3
22	98	100	$\frac{1}{12}$	8.3
23	100	100	$\frac{1}{12}$	8.3

TABLE 9.4

Variable Milliamperage-seconds (mA-s) Technique Chart

THICKNESS (cm)	kVp	mA	TIME (s)	mA-s	SID	GRID
1	50	100	1/20	5	40	No
2	50	100	1/15	6.7	40	No
3	50	75	1/10	7.5	40	No
4	50	100	1/12	8.3	40	No
5	50	100	1/10	10	40	No
6	60	100	1/20	5	40	No
7	60	100	1/15	6.7	40	No
8	60	75	1/10	7.5	40	No
9	60	100	1/12	8.3	40	No
10	60	100	1/10	10	40	No

at the centimeter measurement thickness of 15 on an abdominal technique chart, the increase in tissue density may demand more milliamperage. At this juncture, the time setting should be increased for the rest of the centimeter intervals (Table 9.5).

In veterinary radiography, radiographs of patients that are unhealthy are often needed. Pathologic conditions may require a variation from the standard exposure technique. For patients that are obese or those that have pathologic conditions, such as pleural effusion, massive cardiomegaly, or ascites, an increase in exposure factors is needed to produce adequate radiographic density. Pathologic conditions can decrease radiographic quality by decreasing density and image clarity. Under most circumstances, if an increase of radiographic density is needed because of fluid-filled lungs or abdomen, the mA-s should be increased. Increasing the mA-s improves the density without causing excessive scatter radiation that can fog a radiograph further. If circumstances call for a

TABLE 9.5

Technique Chart Exhibiting Milliamperage-seconds (mA-s) Change

AREA: ABDOMEN   GRID: 8 : 1   SID (INCHES): 40

THICKNESS (cm)	kVp	mA	TIME (s)	mA-s
5	58	300	1/40	7.5
6	60	300	1/40	7.5
7	62	300	1/40	7.5
8	64	300	1/40	7.5
9	66	300	1/40	7.5
10	68	300	1/40	7.5
11	70	300	1/40	7.5
12	72	300	1/40	7.5
13	74	300	1/40	7.5
14	76	300	1/40	7.5
15	78	300	1/30	10
16	80	300	1/30	10
17	83	300	1/30	10
18	86	300	1/30	10
19	89	300	1/30	10
20	92	300	1/30	10
21	95	300	1/30	10
22	98	300	1/30	10
23	101	300	1/30	10
24	104	300	1/30	10
25	107	300	1/30	10

shorter exposure time, the kilovoltage can be increased 10 to 15% instead of increasing the mA-s. The following is a list of suggested modifications:

1. Pleural fluid/massive cardiomegaly: Increase mA-s 50%.
2. Ascites: Increase mA-s 50%.
3. Obesity or heavy muscling: Increase mA-s 50%.
4. Plaster cast: Increase mA-s 50%.
5. Neonatal dog or cat: Decrease mA-s 50%.
6. Special procedures using radiographic contrast media: Increase mA-s 50%.

BIBLIOGRAPHY

Eastman Kodak Company: *Kodak: The Fundamentals of Radiography*, 12th ed. Rochester, NY, 1980.

Johns HE, Cunningham JR: *The Physics of Radiology*, 3rd ed. Charles C Thomas, Springfield, Ill, 1974.

Morgan JP, Silverman S: *Techniques in Veterinary Radiography*, 4th ed. Iowa State University Press, Ames, 1987.

Ticer JW: *Radiographic Technique in Small Animal Practice*, 2nd ed. WB Saunders, Philadelphia, 1984.

Watters JW: Development of a technique chart for the veterinarian. Compend Cont Educ 2:568–571, 1980.

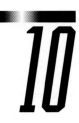

QUALITY ASSURANCE/ QUALITY CONTROL

Susan L. McClanahan

OBJECTIVES

Upon completion of this chapter, the reader should be able to:

- Define quality assurance
- Define quality control
- Understand the reasons for quality assurance/quality control
- Describe the various quality control tests
- List the equipment necessary to complete the quality control tests
- Describe how to interpret the results of the quality control tests
- Describe how to keep the records necessary to track the results of the quality control tests
- Understand when to call for service personnel to correct a problem

GLOSSARY

QUALITY ASSURANCE: A system of activities whose purpose is to provide assurance that the overall quality control is in fact being done effectively. The system involves a continuing education of the adequacy and effectiveness of the overall quality control program with a view to having corrective measures initiated where necessary.

QUALITY CONTROL: The overall system of activities whose purpose is to provide a quality product or service that meets the needs of the users. The aim of quality control is to provide quality that is satisfactory, adequate, dependable, and economic.

INTRODUCTION

Quality assurance is an area that has become more recognized by the medical industry as a necessary tool for overall control of diagnostic radiographs. **Quality assurance** is defined as:

> *A system of activities whose purpose is to provide assurance that the overall quality control job is in fact being done effectively. The system involves a continuing evaluation of the adequacy and effectiveness of the overall quality control program with a view to having corrective measures initiated where necessary. (Thomas, 1973)*

The activities of a quality assurance program are numerous. They include (1) preventive maintenance, (2) quality control, (3) equipment calibration, (4) inservice education of the personnel responsible for radiography, and (5) other items such as the evaluation of new products.

Quality control, being just one aspect of the quality assurance program, is defined as:

> *The overall system of activities whose purpose is to provide a quality of product or service that meets the needs of the users; also the use of such a system. The aim of quality control is to provide quality that is satisfactory, adequate, dependable and economic. (Thomas, 1973)*

If the quality assurance program is the "umbrella" or management portion, then the quality control segment of this program covers the integrity and function of the equipment and the measurement of image quality (Fig. 10.1).

The purpose of having a quality assurance/quality control (QA/QC) program is threefold. First, it provides a way to minimize the dose of radiation not only to the patient but also to the individuals who are assisting with the radiograph. Second, it allows production of a quality radiograph that will provide information for an accurate diagnosis. Third, its use leads to a decreased number of repeated films and thereby reduced overall cost per examination.

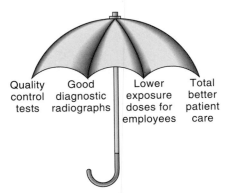

■ **FIG. 10.1** Umbrella of quality assurance/quality control.

Quality control tests | Good diagnostic radiographs | Lower exposure doses for employees | Total better patient care

QUALITY ASSURANCE/QUALITY CONTROL IN VETERINARY RADIOGRAPHY

Questions have been raised as to the validity of a quality assurance program and the quality control tests in a veterinary practice. The basis for these questions has been that the patients being radiographed are not human and therefore the question of repeated radiographs and unnecessary radiation becomes mute. However, the consideration should be for the persons assisting in positioning the animal or otherwise involved with the procedure during the radiographic exposure. Therefore, whether the patient is human or not is certainly not the issue, but rather it is the protection of any involved individuals from unnecessary ionizing radiation.

A veterinary technician is an important part of any quality assurance program as it is the technician's job to do most of the quality control tests, interpret the data, and keep the records. Therefore, the remainder of this chapter addresses these tests, their interpretation, and the records that should be kept.

To understand the quality control tests, the data gathered will be objective. We will not deal with opinions or personal preferences as to contrast and image quality. The technician will measure, plot, and analyze the data. This information will be gathered at a point where it is not yet visible to the eye on the radiograph.

Equipment

The actual equipment that one must have to perform quality control testing depends on the size of the facility or practice. For a small facility, the following equipment will allow you to accomplish a very informative quality control testing protocol:

> Sensitometer
> Densitometer
> Thermometer
> Nine pennies
> Tape measure
> Carpenter's level
> Screen-film contact mesh
> Simple instructions for use and interpretation

Storage of these items should be kept within easy access and together. This will eliminate confusion and delay when it is time to conduct the tests. Most of these tests are done only annually; when this is not the case it will be noted.

Tracking Charts

The purpose of tracking charts is to provide a means to record the data for ease in interpretation and tracking of results. There is no right or wrong way to keep this information except for the sensitometry/densitometry tests. The charts that the technician makes and relies on for the tracking of the equipment parameters are the mainstay of the quality assurance program. By charting the information, it is easy to inspect the data from the measurements and assess any changes. Changes that do occur can be brought to the attention of the veterinarian prior to it becoming a problem that necessitates a second radiograph. When the charts indicate to the technician that the control limits have been reached or exceeded, action should be taken immediately.

Equipment Needed:
Graph paper or commercially prepared tracking charts

Pencil and ruler
Notebook/folder for retention of tracking charts

Procedures

The procedures for the use of the test equipment are described in detail at the appropriate tests. The following tests can be conducted frequently as they are easy to do and provide the practice with a quick look at the physical nature of the radiographic equipment and the environment.

QA / QC TESTS FOR THE X-RAY APPARATUS

SID (Source-Image Distance) Marks:

EQUIPMENT NEEDED:
Tape measure
Carpenter's level

OBJECTIVE:
To ensure the accuracy of the SID.

PROCEDURE:
1. Using a steel measuring tape, measure from the focal spot mark on the tube housing to the table top. If there is no mark on the tube housing, simply divide the tube housing end cap into fourths. Using the bottom fourth as the focal spot, mark this on the end cap with a permanent marker, and proceed with the measurement.

2. Measure from the tabletop to the top of the cassette in the Bucky tray.

3. Add these two numbers together. They should equal the SID that is marked (Fig. 10.2A,B).

4. Measure the marks on the tube stand for accuracy as well. Replace any "missing" marks with permanent marker, nail polish, or paint. If the collimator has a tape measure on it, check this for accuracy with the external tape measure. This information should be recorded for comparison and included in the quality control tests notebook or file.

Perpendicularity

EQUIPMENT NEEDED:
Carpenter's level

OBJECTIVE:
To ensure that thex-ray beam is properly centered, we must be sure that the tube stand, collimator, and x-ray tube are perpendicular and properly aligned.

PROCEDURE:
1. When the x-ray tube is positioned in the normal position, use the level to confirm that the tube is level and parallel with the table (Fig. 10.3). Stand at

continued

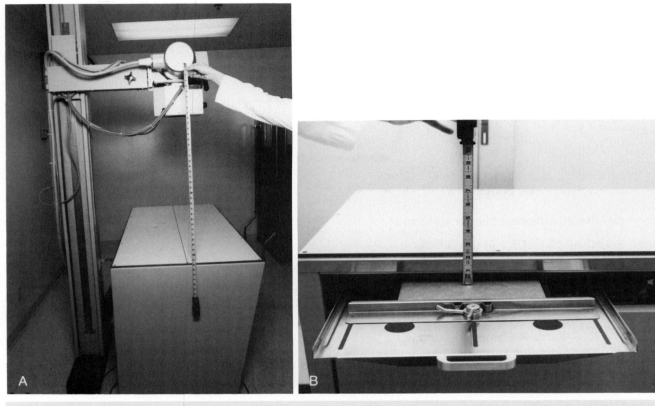

■ **FIG. 10.2** With a tape measure, the source-image distance (SID) from the focal spot of the x-ray tube to the table is measured and recorded (*A*). With the same tape measure, the distance from the tabletop to the top of a cassette placed in the Bucky tray is measured (*B*). The two measurements are added together and should match the SID marked on the tube stand.

the end of the table and look at the tube, collimator, and tube stand. Visually verify that they appear to be perpendicular.

2.   Stand alongside the table and verify the same information as to the perpendicularity of the collimator, x-ray tube, and tube stand.

3.   If the tube, the collimator, or the tube stand look crooked or canted, adjust it or have it repaired before attempting any alignment tests or taking any radiographs. This information should be recorded and whether the test was negative or what was canted and how it was corrected. If the problem was serviced, the repair report should be kept for future reference. The information should be recorded for comparison.

QA / QC TESTS FOR THE X-RAY APPARATUS *Continued*

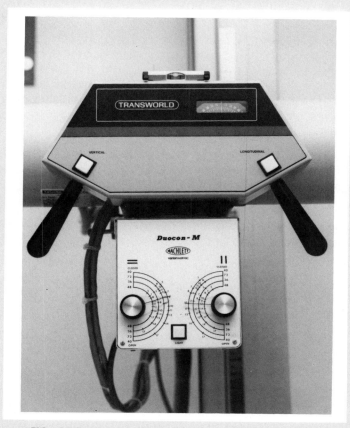

■ **FIG. 10.3** Perpendicularity. A level is used to determine that the x-ray tube is level and parallel to the tabletop.

Tube/Table/Crane Locks

EQUIPMENT NEEDED:
None

OBJECTIVE:
To check the function of the locks to eliminate any unnecessary motion from the x-ray tube, table, or crane.

PROCEDURE:
1. Physically place locks on and off to see whether they lock securely and unlock properly.

2. Check to make sure that the lock switch itself is not broken and that it functions properly. This should be recorded for future reference.

X-Ray Field Light

EQUIPMENT NEEDED:
Water and cloth

OBJECTIVE:
To ensure that the field light can be seen properly with the normal lights on in the radiographic room.

continued

QA / QC TESTS FOR THE X-RAY APPARATUS *Continued*

PROCEDURE:
1.   Turn off the power to the machine. Wash the plastic covering of the x-ray collimator with warm water and mild soap. The plastic covering over the tube output area should be clean and free of debris and dirt. If not, artifacts can show up on the radiograph. (Note: On some older equipment, the plastic covering may be part of the filtering of the x-ray beam. If this is the case, do not damage or remove this without having a service person correct the filtration on the equipment.)

2.   Turn on the power to the machine. To check the brightness of the light, leave room lights on and turn on the collimator light. If there is no difficulty in seeing the edges of the field, there is no problem.

3.   If the dimensions of the light field are difficult to see, there is a problem, and a service person will need to be called to increase the light intensity. This should be recorded for future comparison and reference.

Light Field Size

EQUIPMENT NEEDED:
Steel tape measure

OBJECTIVE:
To ensure that the light field that is determined by the collimator dials is accurate.

PROCEDURE:
1.   Using the tape measure, verify the SID to the tabletop.

2.   Set the collimator size indicators at some field size. Remember to use the scare for the SID you use routinely. (An example of a field size to use is 8 × 10 inches) (Fig. 10.4 A,B).

3.   Turn on the collimator light.

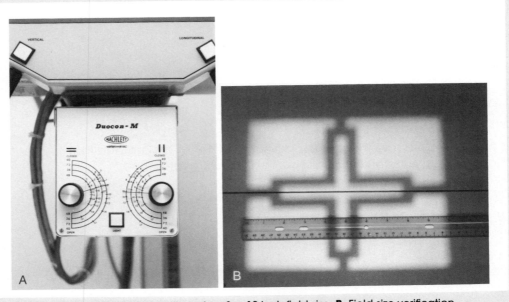

■ **FIG. 10.4**   **A,** Collimator setting of an 8 × 10 inch field size. **B,** Field size verification.

QA / QC TESTS FOR
THE X-RAY APPARATUS *Continued*

4.   Using the tape measure, measure the light field on the tabletop. This measurement should be within 2% of the SID for light field accuracy. This should be recorded for future comparison and reference.

Collimator/Cones/Diaphragms

If the x-ray equipment does not have a lighted collimator but uses slide-in diaphragms to collimate to the cassette sizes, this is the test that should be conducted.

EQUIPMENT NEEDED:
One cassette to match each of the cone/diaphragm sizes or diameters

OBJECTIVE:
To ensure that the cones or diaphragms used are the correct size for the cassettes available for use within the practice.

PROCEDURE:
1.   Slide the different cones/diaphragms into or onto the x-ray tube one at a time.

2.   Place the appropriate size cassette in the Bucky tray (be sure to recheck the SID).

3.   Make an exposure. Use a technique for this exposure that is approximately that for a fetlock or carpus.

4.   Develop this film. The corners of the developed film will be clear (as if cut off) if the cone/diaphragm used matched the size of the cassette used in the Bucky tray. If there is no Bucky tray and all the radiographs are done tabletop, then do this test tabletop making sure that the SID is accurate. Record this information in the QA/QC file for future reference.

Locks/Cables/Overhead Crane Movement

EQUIPMENT NEEDED:
None, except the x-ray equipment

OBJECTIVE:
To ensure adequate locking and movement so that the x-ray tube does not drift during the exposure.

PROCEDURE:
1.   Lock and unlock the locks. When each of the locks is in the locked position, the item that you are testing should not be able to move. For example, if you are testing the Bucky tray lock, then, in the locked position, you should not be able to move it. If you are testing x-ray tube motion, then, in the locked position, you should be unable to move the x-ray tube.

2.   To assess the overhead crane movement, the x-ray tube must be moved around its known limitations. The tube should move easily and without obstruction. Record this information for future reference.

continued

QA / QC TESTS FOR THE X-RAY APPARATUS *Continued*

Angulation Indicator

EQUIPMENT NEEDED:
Carpenter's level
Protractor

OBJECTIVE:
To ensure that the angle indicator is correct when using any angulation on the x-ray tube for a radiographic exposure.

PROCEDURE:

1. Place the carpenter's level on the tabletop—it should be level.

2. Place the carpenter's level on the bottom of the collimator—this also should be level.

3. Note that at both of these places, the appropriate indicators should be zero.

4. Rotate the x-ray tube to 15 degrees, and, using the protractor, measure the degree of angulation. This should also be 15 degrees.

5. Repeat this rotation of the x-ray tube to 30 and 45 degrees, reading the angle indicator and measuring each degree change with the protractor (Fig. 10.5). Record this information for future reference.

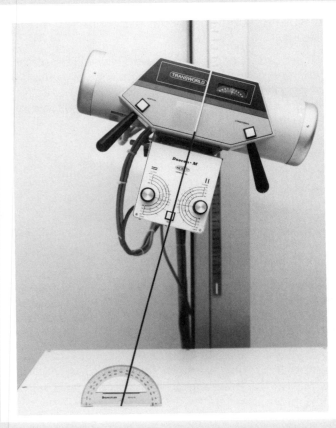

■ **FIG. 10.5** Angulation verification. With the use of a protractor, a rotation of the x-ray tube of 15 degrees is verified.

QA / QC TESTS FOR THE X-RAY APPARATUS *Continued*

View-box Uniformity

EQUIPMENT NEEDED:
Light meter
You can use a photographic light meter if it has a measurement scale. When using certain types of photographic light meters, the denominator of the shutter-speed light intensity is in foot-candles.

OBJECTIVE:
To ensure uniform bulb intensity and color for even light transmittance for radiographic evaluation.

PROCEDURE:
1.   Unplug the view box from the electrical outlet. Clean the view box, inside and out. Use soft cloth and warm water with mild soap. Do not use nail polish remover or other harsh abrasives as these will scratch the view-box surface.

2.   When you are cleaning inside, ensure that the bulbs are the same brand and the same color (e.g., daylight or soft white).

3.   To measure the intensity of the lights, turn on the view box for 2 minutes before doing the test. This will allow the bulbs to stabilize.

4.   Turn off all the room lights.

5.   Measure the intensity using the light meter in three different areas on the viewer.

6.   Calculate the average of the intensity of the viewer. An average or normal range would be within 400 to 580 foot-candles. Record this average information to monitor the life of the bulbs and their intensity as they age.

Light Field/X-ray Field Alignment

EQUIPMENT NEEDED:
Nine pennies
10 × 12 inch cassette loaded with film

OBJECTIVE:
To ensure that the x-ray field is actually going where the light field indicates.

PROCEDURE:
1.   Center the x-ray tube over the table.

2.   Set the SID to 40 inches or your normal SID, and verify that the collimator is level.

3.   Put a cassette in the Bucky tray.

4.   Center to the tray under the table.

5.   Set the collimator field indicators at a field that is approximately 6 × 8 inches.

6.   Turn the collimator light on, and place one penny in the middle of each edge of the light field inside the light and one penny in the middle of each edge of the light field outside the light. The edges of the pennies should have the light field running between them, but the pennies should be touching (Fig. 10.6).

continued

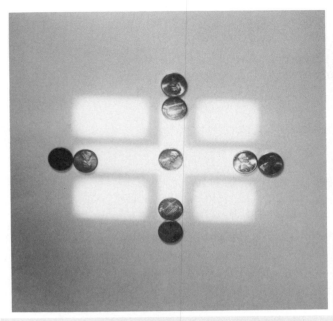

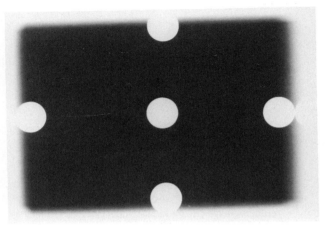

■ **FIG. 10.7** Radiograph of a nine pennty test. This test result is within normal limits.

■ **FIG. 10.6** Light field-x-ray field alignment verification. Nine pennies are laced on the edges of the collimator light field, as shown, and an exposure is taken.

7. Make an exposure. The technique should be approximately the same as for a carpus or a stifle.

8. Develop the film. When developed, the radiograph should show the pennies just as they were placed on the table, on either side of the light field. If they are not, the collimator is in need of adjustment (Fig. 10.7). The width of a penny is 0.75 inch, and 2% of a 40-inch SID is 0.8 inch. Therefore, if the x-ray field is off the width of one penny, it is time to call service personnel.

To ensure that the center of the light and the x-ray field are aligned, draw diagonally from corner to corner on the film itself (all four corners). Make the same drawing from corner to corner on the exposed part. These two pairs of "X's" also should not be more than 2% of the SID apart. If they are, realignment by service personnel is needed. Record this information in the QA/QC file for future reference.

Screen-Film Contact

E Q U I P M E N T   N E E D E D :
Copper wire mesh contact tool with ⅛ inch spacing of the wires
Densitometer

O B J E C T I V E :
To ensure that the adhesive on the back of the screens within the cassettes is still holding the screen tightly.

P R O C E D U R E :
1. Each cassette that is to be tested should be allowed to sit for about 10 minutes before this test is performed. This will allow any trapped air (from loading the film into it) to dissipate.

QA / QC TESTS FOR THE X-RAY APPARATUS *Continued*

2.   Place the cassette on the tabletop.

3.   Place the cassette so that the long axis is perpendicular to the anode-cathode axis of the x-ray tube. This is to minimize the anode heel effect.

4.   Place the wire mesh over the cassette.

5.   Use at least a 40-inch SID.

6.   Cone down to the size of the cassette.

7.   Make an exposure using approximately a carpus or a stifle technique for tabletop.

8.   Process the film.

9.   When viewing the film, place on view box in a dimly lit room.

10.   Stand approximately 6 to 8 feet back from viewer. You will be looking for areas of darkness or unsharpness on the film. Areas of poor contact appear as dark areas on the film (Fig. 10.8A,B). If this area is in the middle of the cassette or in an area where you are likely to have a patient's area of interest, this screen should be attended to. This may be as simple as regluing the edges of the screen to the felt. Any household white glue (e.g., Elmer's) can be used or you can use double-backed tape (e.g., carpet tape). It may be possible that the screens in the cassette need to be replaced. This test must be done on all cassettes.

Uniformity of Screen Speed

EQUIPMENT NEEDED:

Control cassette, for each speed within the practice (this cassette is usually one that is the newest or most consistent for exposure)
Densitometer
One box of film, to be used with each screen size within the practice

OBJECTIVE:

To determine periodically whether screens have lost speed through wear and tear

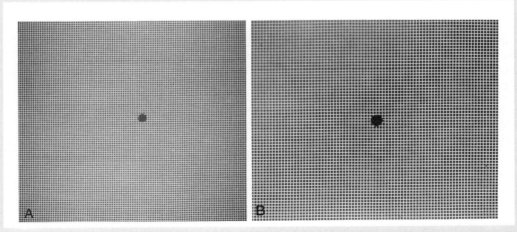

■ **FIG. 10.8 A,** Radiograph of a screen contact test. Note that the grid on the radiograph is well defined: this cassette has good screen-to-film contact. **B,** Radiograph of a screen contact test. Note the dark, blurred area in the corner: this is an example of poor screen-to-film contact.

QA / QC TESTS FOR THE X-RAY APPARATUS *Continued*

PROCEDURE:

Prior to starting, visually inspect each cassette for properly functioning locks, intact hinges, and screen-felt contact. The screens should be checked for scratches, worn spots, or chips and should be clean.

1. Sort all the cassettes by screen type or speed group (high speed, par, detail, rare earth). Test each speed group separately.

2. Select one cassette from a sorted speed group as the control cassette.

3. Record the number of this cassette so that you will be able to repeat this test when needed.

4. Load the cassettes from the film box designated for this procedure. Cutting a 14 × 17 inch film into fourths and placing one fourth into one corner of each cassette will help to limit the cost of this procedure. Just remember which corner of the cassette has the film in it.

5. SID should be at least 50 inches if possible. You may have to put the cassettes on the floor to get this distance.

6. Place the corners of the cassettes together.

7. Center the x-ray tube over the area where the cassettes meet.

8. Cone down to approximately 8 × 8 inch field size.

9. Mark the cassette that is the control, place this cassette into the upper right quadrant position of the four cassettes (Fig. 10.9).

10. Make an exposure, using approximately a carpus or a stifle technique. A technique that could be used for a medium-speed system is 10 mA-s at 50 to 60 kVp. For a faster speed system, 5 mA-s at the same range of kVp would be acceptable.

11. Process these films.

12. Read the densities of each film in the center on the densitometer.

13. Record the density for each of the screens.

14. Repeat this procedure until all the screens within the same speed group have been done.

15. Determine the average density of the films for each speed group. Divide the measured density of each film by the control's density to determine each screen's ratio.

16. If there is more than one speed in the practice, this procedure must be repeated for the other speed groups starting from the choice of a control cassette to the recording of the densities. The range of acceptable ratios between screens is between 0.85 and 1.15. Any screen that falls outside of the ratio range should be removed from service. Record this information for future reference.

QA / QC TESTS FOR THE X-RAY APPARATUS

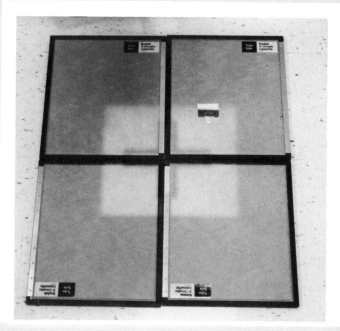

■ **FIG. 10.9** Screen match setup with an "X" on the standard cassette.

Machine Parameters for Calibration (kVp, mA, Timer, and Filtration)

Calibration should be conducted at least annually. The rationale for having the x-ray equipment calibrated is to ensure that when 80 kVp is chosen, 80 kVp is delivered. Likewise, it is done to ensure that the mA stations and the timer are correct. Calibration involves a series of tests that a service person must perform.

An example of a parameter that can change is kilovoltage. As an x-ray machine ages, kilovoltage can fluctuate. This can be a problem with incoming line voltage. Many veterinary clinics do not have a dedicated line for the radiographic equipment, and the voltage can change dramatically with an increase or a decrease in the incoming line voltage. This, of course, will effect the penetration on the radiographs. Another possibility of kilovoltage fluctuation is that of bad internal workings, whether it is a computer chip, board, or drive that is not functioning correctly. These will be apparent in radiographs that are incorrectly penetrated and need to be repeated.

Darkroom Quality Control

Darkroom cleanliness is so important for good film processing that it is addressed separately. Just wiping up the counter is not enough, but it is a start. There must be no eating and no smoking in the darkroom. Crumbs in the cassettes can cause artifacts that could be interpreted as part of the diagnosis for the patient. Remember that the lit end of a cigarette is not a "safe" light and can fog your radiographs. This type of fog is called darkroom fog. Darkroom fog, no matter what the cause, is unacceptable. Fog can be caused from white light leaks from around a door, cracked safelights, improper-wattage bulb in the safelight, improper safelight filter, safelight too close to the counter with a too-high wattage bulb, improper chemical temperature, improper chemical balance.

Fog Test

EQUIPMENT NEEDED:
Lightly exposed radiograph
Watch or timer
Densitometer

OBJECTIVE:
To assess any fog in the darkroom that might be adding unwanted density to the radiograph during processing.

PROCEDURE:
1. Expose a cassette with a film in it, using a small extremity technique.

2. Take cassette into the darkroom.

3. Remove the film from the cassette, place film on counter, cover half of film with cassette.

4. All the safelights should be on as in routine processing of a radiograph.

5. Leave the film and cassette in this position for 2 minutes by the watch or timer (Fig. 10.10).

6. Process the film normally.

7. When the film has been processed, notice the difference.

8. Measure each side of the radiograph with the densitometer. The difference should be no greater than 0.08 optical density (OD) for routine film-screen combination and routine darkroom processing. If the difference is greater than 0.8 OD, location of the source of the radiographic fog problem must be found (Fig. 10.11). This test should be done quarterly as it will provide a good follow-up on fog. Record this information for future reference.

Sensitometry and Densitometry

EQUIPMENT NEEDED:
Film, one box designated for sensitometry (this should be the same type/speed used every day but of the smallest size, that is, 8 × 10 inch)
Sensitometer
Densitometer
Sensitometry graph paper
Thermometer

OBJECTIVE:
To ensure that the processing of the radiographs is optimized, thereby providing the best quality radiograph. This is done by testing the processing procedure using a nonradiographic light source that is constant.

PROCEDURE:
1. In the darkroom, before doing anything else in this procedure, take the temperature of the developer in the processor or hand tank.
2. Using the sensitometer, expose one edge of a piece of radiographic film from the box of film dedicated for sensitometry (Fig. 10.12A,B).
3. Process the film normally.

QA / QC TESTS FOR THE X-RAY APPARATUS *Continued*

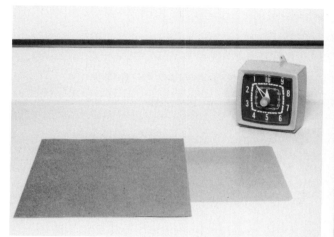

■ **FIG. 10.10** Fog test setup in the darkroom. A piece of unexposed film is placed on the counter in the darkroom, and one half of the film is covered. After 1 minute, the film is processed and examined.

■ **FIG. 10.11** Radiograph of a darkroom fog test. Note that the two halves of the film have different densities. This is an example of film fog.

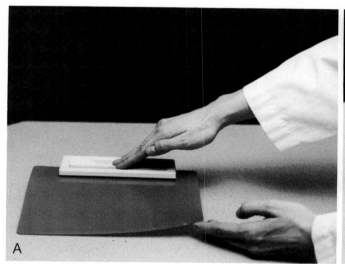

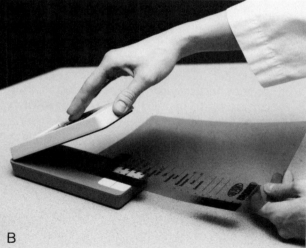

■ **FIG. 10.12** **A,** Exposing a test strip with the sensitometer. **B,** Reading the test strip with the densitometer.

QA / QC TESTS FOR
THE X-RAY APPARATUS *Continued*

4. After the film has been processed, the optical density of the steps will be read using the densitometer and recorded on the graph paper (Fig. 10.13) according to the procedure in 5 to 14.

5. Measure the density in the center area of the film without any exposure.

6. Plot this densitometer reading number in the base + fog area on the graph.

7. The base + fog should not increase more than +0.05 from the original or normal reading.

8. Next, read the steps of the sensitometry exposure and record numbers on the film or a piece of scratch paper. These numbers will be used to determine which step will be used for contrast strip and the speed strip.

9. From these numbers, determine which step is within a density range of 1.0 to 1.3. This is known as the speed step.

10. Plot the density reading for the speed step in the area on the graph. This step will be used for the speed step for the entire box of sensitometry film. Variations should not be greater than ±0.15 of the initial reading. If they are beyond this parameter, corrective action must be taken.

11. Using the numbers for the steps off the scratch paper, determine the density of the steps above and below the speed step.

12. Subtract these two densities for the reading for the contrast strip. These two steps will be used for the contrast strip for the entire box of sensitometry film.

13. Plot this number on the graph portion for contrast. The variations should not be greater than ±0.20. If they are beyond this parameter, corrective action must be taken (Fig. 10.14).

14. These densities from the same steps on the sensitometry strip will be read and plotted daily on the graph paper.

It is imperative that this sensitometry and densitometry test be done each day prior to processing any radiographs to determine the processing environment before films are taken to reduce the need for retaking films. (Note: All sensitometers and densitometers come with detailed instructions on how to do the procedures and the corrective actions to be taken when test results are outside of the designated parameters.)

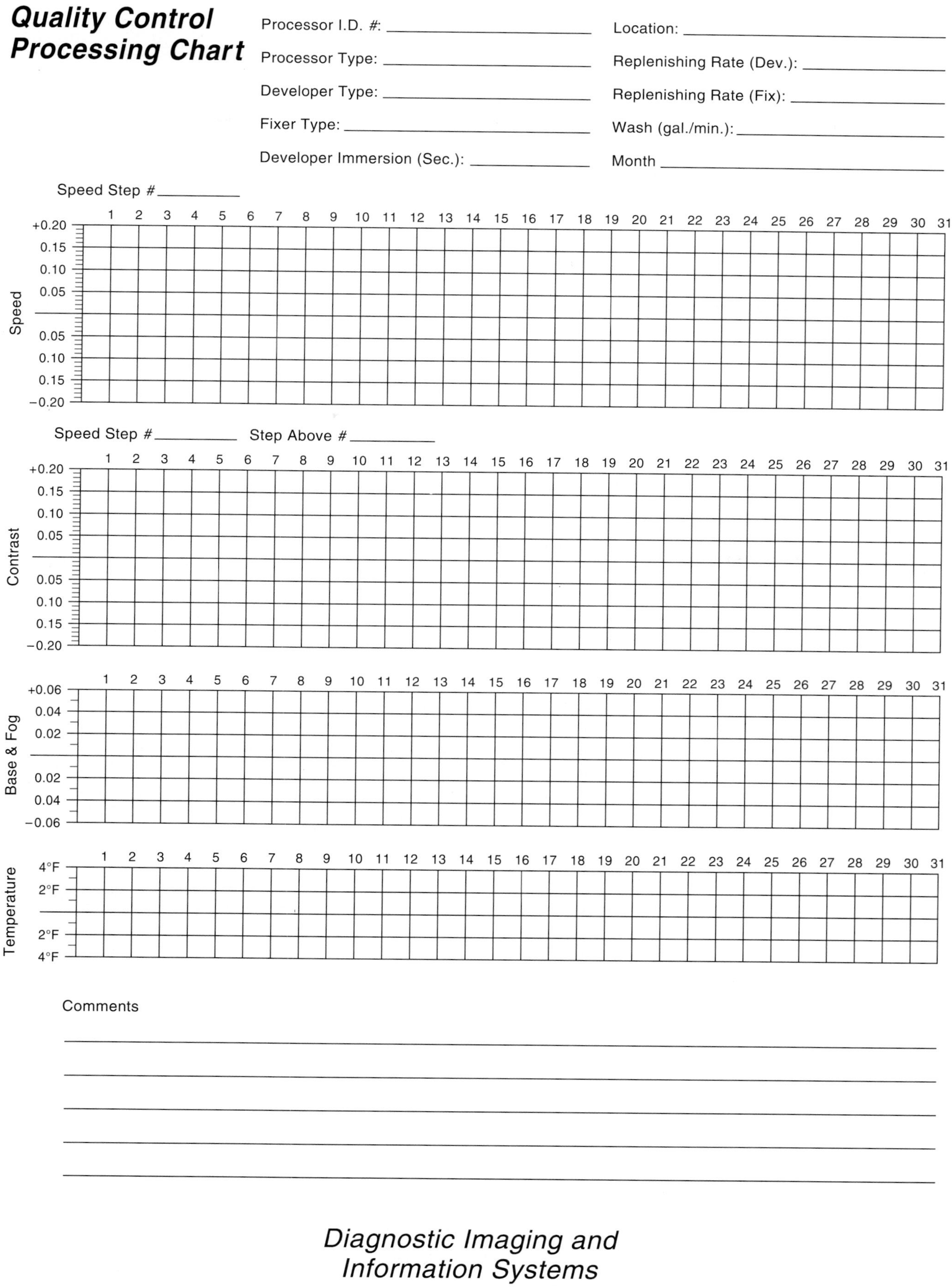
Quality Control Processing Chart
Processor I.D. #:
Location:
Processor Type:
Replenishing Rate (Dev.):
Developer Type:
Replenishing Rate (Fix):
Fixer Type:
Wash (gal./min.):
Developer Immersion (Sec.):
Month
Speed Step #
Speed
+0.20
0.15
0.10
0.05
0.05
0.10
0.15
−0.20
Speed Step #
Step Above #
Contrast
+0.20
0.15
0.10
0.05
0.05
0.10
0.15
−0.20
Base & Fog
+0.06
0.04
0.02
0.02
0.04
−0.06
Temperature
4°F
2°F
2°F
4°F
1 2 3 4 5 6 7 8 9 10 11 12 13 14 15 16 17 18 19 20 21 22 23 24 25 26 27 28 29 30 31
Comments
Diagnostic Imaging and Information Systems

■ **FIG. 10.13** Example of a graph used to plot information received from the sensitometer/densitometer test strip.

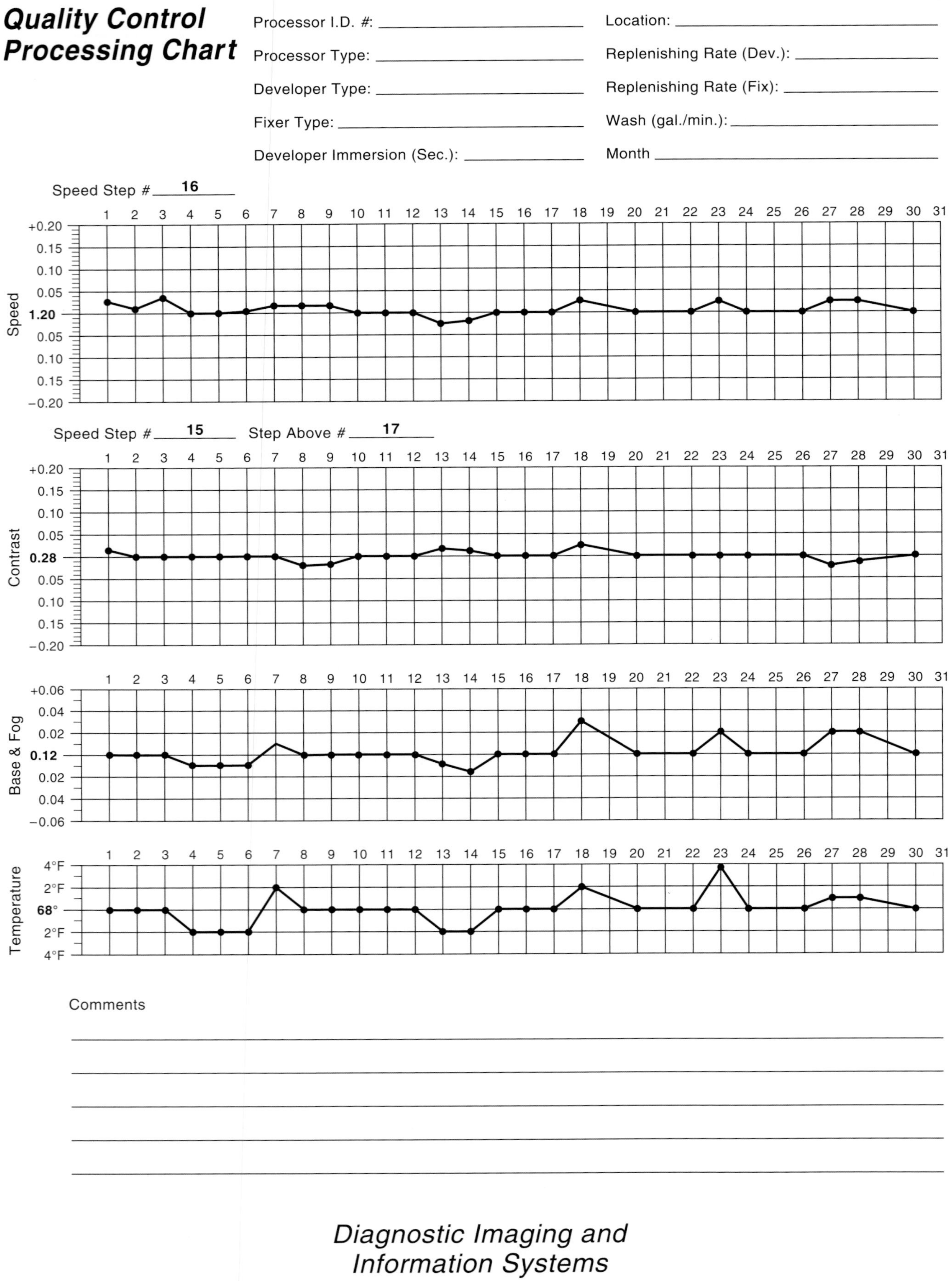

Quality Control Processing Chart

Processor I.D. #: _____ Location: _____

Processor Type: _____ Replenishing Rate (Dev.): _____

Developer Type: _____ Replenishing Rate (Fix): _____

Fixer Type: _____ Wash (gal./min.): _____

Developer Immersion (Sec.): _____ Month _____

FIG. 10.14 A completed sensitometry/densitometry graph for a month.

B I B L I O G R A P H Y

Gray JE, et al: *Quality Control in Diagnostic Imaging.* Aspen, Rockville, Md, 1983.

T E C H N I C A L
A R T I F A C T S
A N D   E R R O R S :
C A S E   S T U D I E S

O B J E C T I V E S
Upon completion of this chapter, the reader should be able to:

- State the importance of minimizing radiographic artifacts
- List and describe the common artifacts that occur in veterinary radiography
- State the preventive measures used to eliminate the occurrence of radiographic artifacts
- Identify the artifacts exhibited in each case study and their prevention

G L O S S A R Y

ARTIFACT: Anything that decreases the quality of the radiograph resulting in difficult evaluation and interpretation.

I N T R O D U C T I O N
Radiographic **artifacts** are a menace to any radiographer. A radiograph is often marred by various artifacts resulting from a number of causes. An artifact not only decreases the quality of the radiograph, it may lead to a misdiagnosis. It is the responsibility of the radiographer to be able to recognize the error and to be able to correct it. This chapter is designed to expose the reader to many possible artifacts and to challenge the reader's ability to identify common film faults. Table 11.1 is a list of common artifacts and their causes. It is important that the radiographer be-

come familiar with this list and understand how to prevent these artifacts from occurring.

If an artifact consistently appears on radiographs, the cassette should be isolated and the screens cleaned and examined for damage. If the fault is persistent, the cassette should be labeled "faulty screens." However, if the damage could lead to a misdiagnosis, the screens should be discarded and replaced.

After examining the list of artifacts in Table 11.1, read through the following case studies and try to determine the cause and correction of the artifacts before looking at the answers.

T A B L E 11 . 1

Common Artifacts and Their Causes

Artifact	Cause	Artifact	Cause
Film too dark	Overexposure due to too much kVp or mA-s	Heavy lines on radiograph (generalized)	Grid lines due to:
	Overdevelopment due to too much time in developer or increased developer temperature		Grid out of focal range
			Grid out of alignment to x-ray central beam
			Grid upside-down
	Overmeasurement of part under examination		Damaged grid
	Machine (meters or timer) out of calibration		Roller marks as result of film jammed in automatic processor
	SID not correct for grid use	Inconsistent film density	Collimation of primary beam
Film too light	Underexposure due to insufficient kVp or mA-s		Bucky tray not positioned directly under primary x-ray beam
	Underdevelopment due to decreased temperature or time of development, developer exhausted or diluted		Cassette not locked into Bucky tray correctly
			Light leak into cassette
			Quantum mottle
	X-ray tube failure		Target damage (pitted anode)
	Incorrect film-screen combination		Variable screen-film contact
	Machine timer out of calibration	Black marks (not generalized)	Crimping or folding of film
	Drop in incoming line voltage		Two films sticking together during development
Film gray/lack of contrast	Too much kVp		Static electricity
	Radiation fog due to exposure of film to radiation other than desired exposure		Developer on film before processing
			Fingerprints as a result of developer on hands while loading or unloading cassette
	Light leak in darkroom		
	Storage fog due to conditions that are too hot or too humid	Clear areas on film (white marks; not generalized)	Hair in cassette
			Scratch in film emulsion
	Chemical fog due to old chemicals, increased chemical temperature, or increased time of development		Line due to scratch on screen surface
			Contrast media on cassette or table
			Air bubble on film during developing procedure
	Film out of date		Film touching side of the tanks during manual processing
	Lack of a grid with use of high kVp		
	Double exposure		Fingerprints due to film handling with contaminated hands
	Incorrect bulb wattage or filter for safelight in darkroom		Fixer splashes on film before developing
Lack of detail	Increased object-film distance	Yellow radiograph	Premature age due to improper fixation
	Blurring due to poor screen-film contact		Film sticking together during fixing process
	Blurring due to patient motion		Incomplete washing so residual fixer oxidizes to yellow powder while destroying the image.
	Blurring due to x-ray tube motion		
	Distorted image due to central x-ray not directed at center of film		
	Double exposure		

1

C A S E   S T U D Y   1

Examine the Radiograph in Figure 11.1

This radiograph exhibits a blurred image that lacks detail and definition—a classic example of motion. This artifact can be the result of a number of causes. The most common cause is patient movement during exposure. Patient motion is the most common artifact in veterinary radiography.

To minimize the occurrence of patient motion, a number of preventive measures can be taken. For example, motion can be limited by physical and chemical restraint. Sedation may be necessary for uncooperative patients or for views that are difficult to position without patient compliance. In instances when the patient is panting, holding the muzzle closed or a short, quick blow on the nose while simultaneously making the exposure can be an effective method of temporarily stopping rapid respiration. Another method to decrease the chance of motion is to utilize a short exposure time. This can be achieved by using the highest milliamperage setting possible on the x-ray machine and fast intensifying screens.

Another cause of a blurred radiographic image is x-ray tube or cassette motion. This problem primarily occurs in equine radiography, in which a standard x-ray table is not applicable. The cassette must be manually held next to the anatomic area of interest and the x-ray tube positioned on a portable stand. A sturdy tube stand and cassette holder (discussed in Part II of this text) can minimize this type of motion.

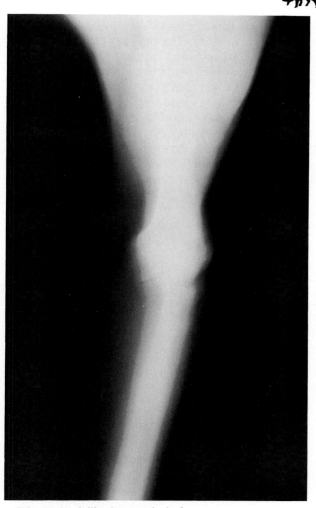

■ **FIG. 11.1** Artifact case study 1.

CASE STUDY 2

2

Examine the Radiograph in Figure 11.2

This radiograph exhibits a general lack of density. This artifact can be attributed to many causes. On first glance, the radiographer may believe that the radiograph lacks sufficient kilovoltage (kVp) or milliamperage-seconds (mA-s). Insufficient exposure factors can certainly cause a radiograph to be too light. However, more than the image is light: the background (area surrounding the patient anatomy) is also light. This type of insufficient film density can be the result of faulty film processing incorrect film-screen matching, or an x-ray machine out of calibration.

If the processing solutions are expired or are too cold or if the film is developed for an insufficient length of time, a radiograph such as the one in Figure 11.2 can result. Strictly adhering to the standard processing procedure designated for the radiographic film being used and changing the solutions on a regular basis will prevent poor quality radiographs.

An incorrect film-screen combination can result in a radiograph that is too light or too dark. The intensifying screens must match the film being used. If there is any question, the manufacturer should be consulted.

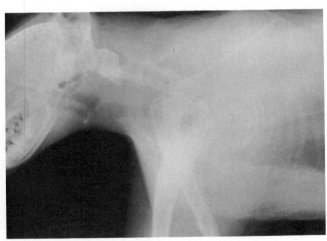

■ **FIG. 11.2** Artifact case study 2.

3

CASE STUDY 3

Examine the Radiograph in Figure 11.3

Improper film handling is the cause of this radiographic artifact. A black "tree" pattern or a linear dot pattern is the result of static electrical charge released on the film. Static electricity is most common in dry winter months, when the darkroom has relatively low humidity. To avoid static, the film should be handled carefully to avoid friction. X-ray film should be removed from the storage box slowly and placed in the cassette without being dragged across any surface.

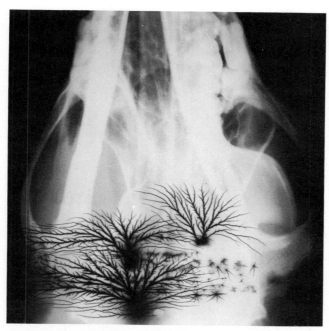

■ **FIG. 11.3** Artifact case study 3.

4

CASE STUDY 4

Examine the Radiograph in Figure 11.4

This radiograph, similar to the radiograph in Case Study 1, exhibits a blurred image. Under close examination, one can see that two identical images are actually superimposed. This radiograph is an example of a double exposure. Under stressful circumstances, it is possible to inadvertently push the exposure button twice. It is also possible that the audible exposure indicator (''beep'' or ''ding'' during exposure) malfunctioned and a second exposure was taken. If there is any question of the machine function, a service representative should be summoned.

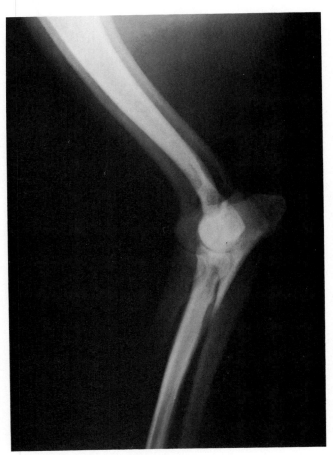

■ **FIG. 11.4** Artifact case study 4.

5

CASE STUDY 5

Examine the Radiograph in Figure 11.5

The artifact on this radiograph is a classic example of a finger pressure mark due to incorrect film handling. This artifact is called a finger crescent and commonly occurs when the radiographer is in a hurry to remove the x-ray film from the cassette. When two fingers are placed on the film a small distance apart and pinched together to remove the film from the cassette, a black crease mark can result from the pressure placed on the film by the fingertips (Fig. 11.6). To avoid this artifact and others that are similar, x-ray film should be handled by the edges only.

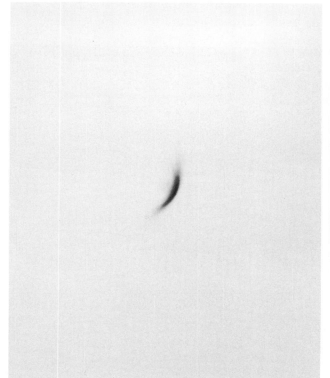

■ **FIG. 11.5** Artifact case study 5.

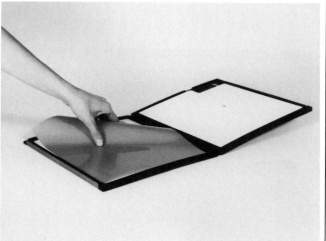

■ **FIG. 11.6** Improper method of film removal from a cassette.

CASE STUDY 6

6

Examine the Radiograph in Figure 11.7

The artifact on this radiograph exemplifies the importance of proper animal preparation before radiography. The gray streaks are the result of a wet haircoat. These streaks can potentially inhibit a proper diagnosis or even mimic a pathologic lesion. Radiopaque contrast media, urine, blood, or water can create this artifact.

Before any animal is exposed, debris should be removed and the haircoat should be dry. When radiographing a large animal, such as a horse, the area of interest should be clean, dry, and debris-free. In equine pedal radiography, the frog of the hoof should be picked and washed, ensuring the removal of dirt, manure, and rocks. Sheep and llama radiography can be a challenge if the wool is long and full of debris. In some instances, sheering may be necessary to alleviate excessive artifacts.

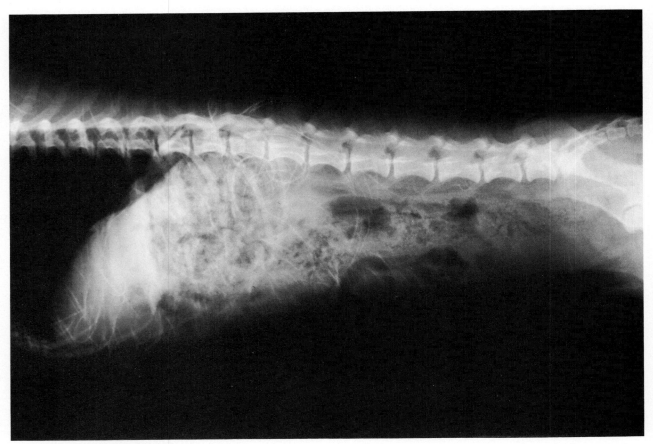

■ **FIG. 11.7** Artifact case study 6.

CASE STUDY 7

Examine the Radiograph in Figure 11.8

This radiographic artifact is one example of what can happen when a technologist is in a hurry to reload a cassette. Care was not taken to ensure that all corners of the film were placed correctly in the corners of the cassette. The film was folded onto itself as the cassette was closed. The fold in the film creates a dark line across the radiograph and a mirror image on either side of the crease. Although this artifact is not common, it is an example of what can occur if the film is not properly loaded into a cassette.

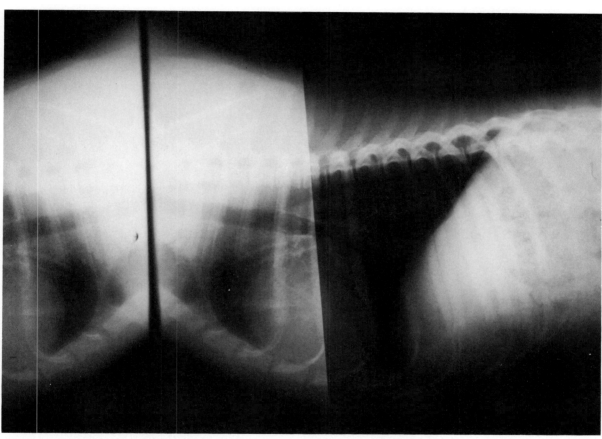

■ **FIG. 11.8** Artifact case study 7.

8

C A S E   S T U D Y   8

Examine the Radiograph in Figure 11.9

The artifact on this radiograph is the result of a foreign object in the cassette. Unwanted foreign matter in the cassette is not uncommon. This artifact happens to be a piece of paper that was inadvertently placed in the cassette during the film loading process. A number of radiographic manufacturers supply x-ray film with a sheet of thin paper between each piece of film. If a radiographer is not careful during the cassette loading process, it is easy for a sheet of the paper to slip into the cassette with the film.

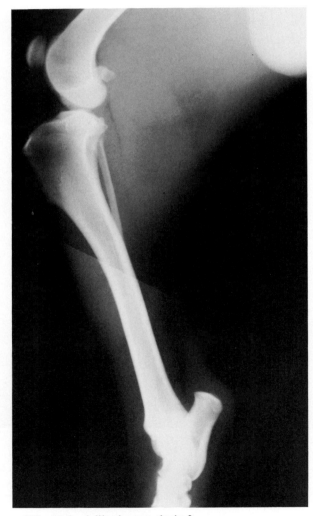

■ **FIG. 11.9**   Artifact case study 8.

9

CASE STUDY 9

Examine the Radiograph in Figure 11.10

The emulsion of the x-ray film is very sensitive to damage, especially when wet. This radiograph exhibits a common artifact that occurs during hand processing: a scratch in the emulsion. Unless proper care is taken, the emulsion can become marred as a result of contact with adjacent hangers or other projections. Scratched emulsion is a common occurrence when a number of films are developed at one time. This is especially true with the use of tension clip hangers as opposed to channel hangers. When processing more than one film at a time, care must be taken to ensure sufficient space between each film within the tank. It is important to remember that even when a radiograph is completely dry, the emulsion can be damaged. Proper film handling is imperative at all times—before, during, and after processing.

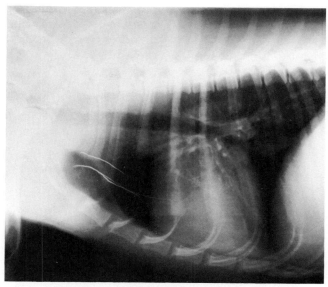

■ **FIG. 11.10** Artifact case study 9.

10

CASE STUDY 10

Examine the Radiograph in Figure 11.11

The artifact on this radiograph is a classic example of film fog. At some point, either before or after the exposure was made, light exposed a portion of the film. Unwanted light can reach the film in three common ways: (1) the film bin door is ajar, (2) a film box lid is loose or damaged, and (3) the cassette is not closed properly or is damaged.

The film bin in which x-ray film is stored should be light-tight when the door is completely closed. If the technologist is in a hurry and the door is left open or has a faulty seal, light can leak in. In the same respect, if the film boxes are not kept in a film bin and the lid of the box is not secure, film fog is inevitable. In each case, more than one film could be fogged. In fact, an entire box of film could be ruined, which would be quite costly to the clinic.

Not latching the cassette completely will allow light to leak in and expose a portion or all of the film. Improper loading of the cassette can also lead to film fog resulting from a portion of the film sticking out of the closed cassette. Light can also enter a cassette if it is damaged by being dropped or not handled carefully, preventing a latch from locking. By using care when loading and handling a cassette, these problems can be prevented.

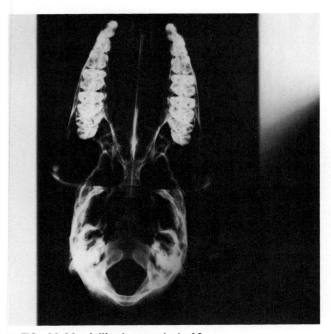

■ **FIG. 11.11** Artifact case study 10.

CASE STUDY 11

11

Examine the Radiograph in Figure 11.12

This radiographic artifact is uncommon and is a challenging mystery to solve. Notice that the radiograph has a number of superimposed exposures, all of which are too light. The artifact was the result of accidentally leaving an unexposed cassette in the cassette tray while various extremities were exposed with a cassette on the tabletop. Later, when the cassette was found in the tray, it was subsequently processed and found to be exposed numerous times. If a film is suspected of being exposed, it is best to discard or process the film to prevent the need for additional radiographs.

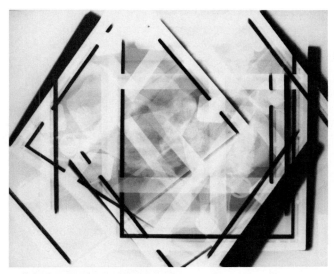

■ **FIG. 11.12** Artifact case study 11.

12

CASE STUDY 12

Examine the Radiograph in Figure 11.13

This radiographic artifact is a common occurrence during or after the use of radiopaque contrast media. Contrast media are used for special radiographic procedures such as an upper gastrointestinal study or cystogram (discussed in Part II). Whenever radiopaque contrast media are used in veterinary radiography, the possibility of spillage exists. If a contrast medium is present on the cassette or on the x-ray table, it will prevent the x-rays from reaching the film properly. To minimize the occurrence of this artifact, the tabletop and cassettes should be monitored and cleaned frequently if necessary.

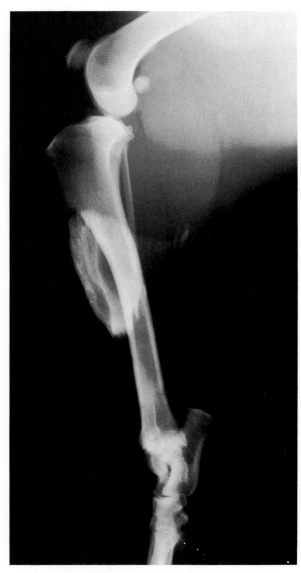

■ **FIG. 11.13** Artifact case study 12.

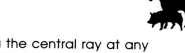

13 CASE STUDY 13

Examine the Radiograph in Figure 11.14

The artifact on this radiograph is due to a portion of the film being unexposed. On one side of the radiograph, there is a definite line where the x-rays are not reaching the film. Collimation can reduce the primary beam field size, but in this case the clear areas on the radiograph would be symmetric (on both sides of the film). There are two primary causes for the type of artifact shown here: (1) the central x-ray is not perpendicular to the cassette and (2) the cassette was not directly under the entire primary x-ray beam.

The importance of having the central ray perpendicular (forming a 90-degree angle) to the x-ray film is discussed in Chapter 5. Aiming the central ray at any angle other than 90 degrees will not only prevent the entire film from being exposed, it will cause geometric distortion.

The cause of the artifact in this case study was not the tube angle (no distortion is noted), but that the cassette was not directly under the entire primary x-ray beam. If the cassette is placed into the cassette tray incorrectly, a portion of the primary beam will not reach the film. To ensure proper exposure, the cassette must be locked into the tray with the cassette locks, the tray must be pushed under the tabletop completely, and the center of the cassette tray must be in line with the central x-ray.

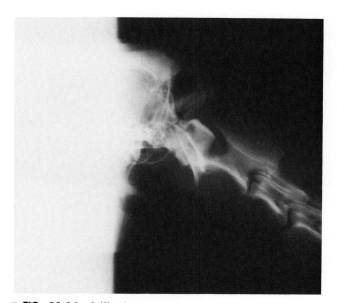

■ **FIG. 11.14** Artifact case study 13.

CASE STUDY 14

14

Examine the Radiograph in Figure 11.15

The artifact in this radiograph appears as small clear (white) areas. Close examination reveals that the white blotches are actually fingerprints. This artifact is most likely the result of having fix solution on the hands while handling the film before processing. It is imperative that the hands be clean and dry before handling any film. (Remember, fingerprints are a dead giveaway to the culprit of artifactual crime!)

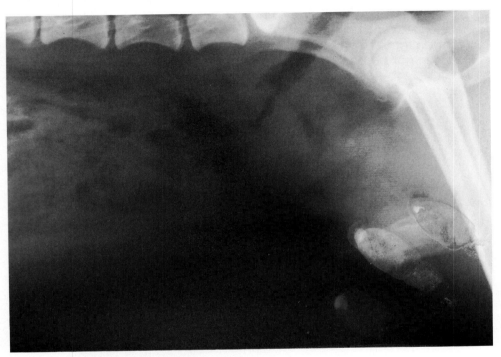

■ **FIG. 11.15** Artifact case study 14.

CASE STUDY 15

Examine the Radiograph in Figure 11.16

This radiograph exhibits numerous white dots. There is no pattern to the position of the dots, but they are primarily located near the caudal portion of the patient. A second view would confirm that this artifact is located inside the body of the patient and not a problem with the cassette, film, or processing. The white dots are buckshot from a shotgun shell. This patient is most likely a hunting dog that was too close to the hunter's aim of fire (or was running away from an unhappy neighbor). This artifact is a common occurrence in field dogs and should not be a cause for alarm. Under most circumstances, the pellets are located in the muscle tissue and will remain there or work themselves out of the body with time.

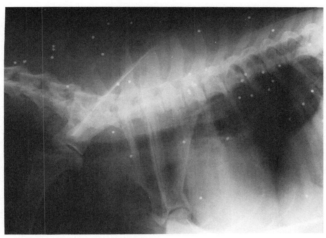

■ **FIG. 11.16** Artifact case study 15.

BIBLIOGRAPHY

Douglas SW, Herrtage ME, Williamson HD: *Principles of Veterinary Radiography,* 4th ed. Bailliere Tindall, Philadelphia, 1987.

Eastman Kodak Company: *Kodak: The Fundamentals of Radiography,* 12th ed. Rochester, NY, 1980.

Gray JE, et al: *Quality Control in Diagnostic Imaging.* Aspen, Rockville, Md, 1983.

Morgan JP, Silverman S: *Techniques in Veterinary Radiography,* 4th ed. Iowa State University Press, Ames, 1987.

Sweeney RJ: *Radiographic Artifacts: Their Cause and Control.* JB Lippincott, New York, 1983.

Ticer JW: *Radiographic Techniques in Small Animal Practice,* 2nd ed. WB Saunders, Philadelphia, 1984.

RADIOGRAPHIC
POSITIONING

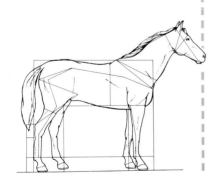

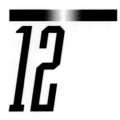

12

GENERAL
PRINCIPLES
OF POSITIONING

CHAPTER OUTLINE

- POSITIONAL TERMINOLOGY
- PATIENT POSITIONING:
  BASIC CRITERIA
- FILM IDENTIFICATION

OBJECTIVES
Upon completion of Part II of this text, the reader should be able to:

- List and define the proper anatomic positional terminology used in veterinary radiography
- State the four factors that need to be considered for an accurate reproduction of an anatomic area
- Describe the proper handling of the patient for radiography
- List the basic guidelines for veterinary radiographic positioning
- State the technical preparation necessary before positioning the patient
- Describe how a measurement of the anatomic area of interest is taken
- List the required views of each anatomic part
- State the advantage of "splitting" a cassette

- Explain the importance of collimation
- List and describe the appropriate patient preparation necessary to minimize radiographic inhibitory artifacts
- List and describe the patient restraint and positioning aids available
- State the proper labeling of various anatomic positions
- State the importance of label placement
- Describe the proper radiographic positioning techniques for all anatomic areas of small, large, and exotic animals
- List and describe the common special procedures involving contrast medium utilized in small animal radiography

POSITIONAL TERMINOLOGY

Understanding the correct terminology for the various anatomic views is essential to a radiographer. The directional terms cited in this text are based on the revised terminology system advocated by the American Committee of Veterinary Radiologists and Anatomists. This relatively new system exactly defines the position and direction of the primary x-ray beam. The correct veterinary anatomic directional terms and abbreviations for radiographic projections follow (Figs. 12.1 and 12.2).

Left (Le)	Dorsal (D)
Right (Rt)	Ventral (V)
Medial (M)	Lateral (L)
Cranial (Cr)	Rostral (R)
Caudal (Cd)	Palmar (Pa)
Oblique (O)	Plantar (Pl)

on the dorsal side. Directional terms can also be combined for oblique views. For example, DMPaLO of the carpus indicates that the carpus is rotated to a selected degree angle and the central x-ray enters the dorsal/medial surface and exits out of the palmar/lateral surface. It is necessary for the radiographer to become familiar with these directional terms in order to label and expose anatomic areas appropriately.

PATIENT POSITIONING: BASIC CRITERIA

Part II of this text is dedicated to the instruction of correct anatomic positioning. Positioning small animal patients for radiographic examinations may require the use of sedation or general anesthesia and positional devices. Overt manual restraint should be minimized

---

D E F I N I T I O N S
The meanings of the directional terms are as follows:

DORSAL: Upper aspect of the head, neck, trunk, and tail. The term also means toward the upper aspect of the animal. Dorsal also describes those aspects of the legs from the carpus and tarsus joints distally that face toward the head.

VENTRAL: Lower aspects of the head, neck, trunk, and tail. The term also means toward the lower aspect of the animal.

CRANIAL: Describes parts of the neck, trunk, and tail positioned toward the head from any given point. Cranial also describes those aspects of the limb above the carpal and tarsal joints that face toward the head.

ROSTRAL: Parts of the head positioned toward the nares from any given point on the head.

CAUDAL: Describes parts of the head, neck, and trunk, positioned toward the tail from any given point. Caudal also describes those aspects of the limbs above the carpal and tarsal joints that face toward the tail.

PALMAR: Used instead of caudal when describing the forelimb from the carpal joint distally

PLANTAR: Used instead of caudal when describing the hind limb from the tarsal joint distally.

PROXIMAL: Nearness to the point of origin of a structure

DISTAL: Farther away from the point of origin of a structure.

SUPERIOR AND INFERIOR: Used to describe the upper and lower dental arcades, respectively.

LATERAL: The x-ray beam enters through either the left or the right side of the body and emerges on the opposite side, where the cassette is positioned.

MEDIOLATERAL: The x-ray beam enters a limb through the medial side and exits on the lateral side. Most lateral radiographs of the limbs are taken in mediolateral projection in small animal radiography.

LATEROMEDIAL: The x-ray beam enters a limb through the lateral side and exits on the medial side. Most lateral radiographs of the limbs are taken in lateromedial projection in large animal radiography.

RECUMBENT: The animal is lying down when the radiograph is made. Most radiographs of the dog and cat are made with the animal in the recumbent position, and this position should be presumed unless otherwise stated on the radiograph.

Beam Direction

The abbreviated term used for the position designates the direction of the x-ray beam. The first letter states where the x-ray beam enters the body, and the second designates where it exits. For example, the abbreviation VD (ventrodorsal) indicates that the x-ray beam enters through the ventral side of the animal and exits

as much as possible and should be used only when chemical restraint is contraindicated.

Care must be taken to include all essential anatomic regions in the primary beam when positioning patients. The primary goal of positioning for radiography is devising the most suitable posture for the animal patient from which an accurate reproduction of the anatomic area can be produced. Several important

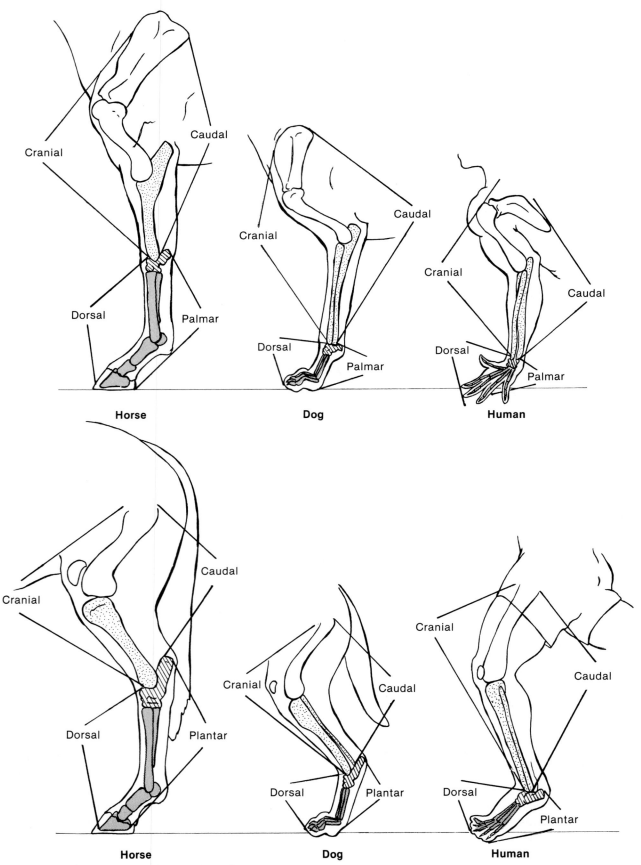

Horse   **Dog**   **Human**

Horse   **Dog**   **Human**

■ **FIG. 12.1** Correct anatomic directional terms.

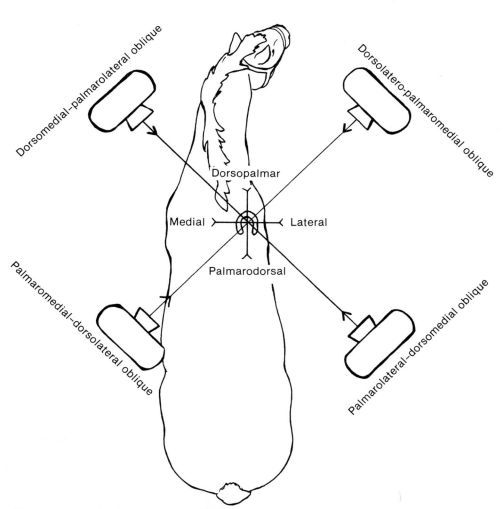

■ FIG. 12.2   Correct anatomic directional terms for oblique views.

factors must be considered if an accurate reproduction is to be made:

1. Welfare of the patient.
2. Restraint and immobilization of the patient.
3. Minimal trauma to the area of interest.
4. The least risk of exposing those assisting with the examination to radiation.

The Patient

The comfort and welfare of the patient should be considered at all times. Patience is vital, especially with animals that cannot be sedated. Remember, radiography can be a frightening experience to an animal. The animal is unsure what is happening and, from its perspective, is certain the procedure will be painful. To minimize anxiety, animals should be handled in a slow, quiet manner. Most animals respond to a calm, soft voice and gentle stroking. Quick, loud movements and severe restraint usually result in a frightened, tense, and even aggressive patient.

The rotor noise (spinning of the rotating anode) of the x-ray tube often startles animals. It is a good idea to start and release the rotor switch when working with patients that exhibit signs of anxiety. The rotor will continue to spin for several minutes, allowing the animal to become accustomed to the noise.

As much technical preparation for the exposure as possible should be done prior to positioning the animal on the table. That is, the patient should be measured, the exposure technique set on the machine console, the cassette placed on the table or Bucky tray, and the label made before positioning the patient. Most animals tolerate being restrained in a particular position for a short time.

Measurement

To measure the anatomic area of interest, a caliper is used. A caliper is an inexpensive device used to measure part thickness in centimeter increments (Fig. 12.3). (The site where the measurement should be taken is given for every anatomic area in the positioning series, Chapters 13 to 20.) If the radiographer is unsure of where to measure a particular part, the measurement should be made over the part's thickest area. When there is a large difference in thickness in a particular area, it is advisable to make two separate radiographs with different exposures. If only a small difference in tissue density exists, a compromise should be made.

Required Views

Because a radiograph is a two-dimensional picture of a three-dimensional structure, two views of each anatomic area taken at right angles to each other are the minimum recommended. The importance of two

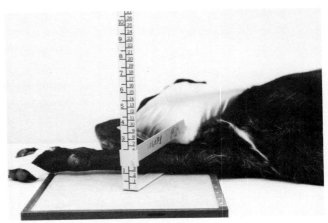

■ **FIG. 12.3** Proper use of a caliper.

views is exemplified when radiographing a fractured bone. For example, one view of a nondisplaced oblique fracture of a long bone may appear normal. A lateral and craniocaudal view would be necessary to visualize the fracture line.

Another guideline is to have the area of interest closest to the film. This reduces distortion and magnification of the area under examination. In addition, if a limb is being radiographed, it may be helpful to radiograph the opposite corresponding limb. This would allow the pathologic structure of one leg to be compared with the normal anatomy of the other.

In order to radiograph more than one view on the same piece of film to minimize the number of films used per patient, the cassette can be "split" by placing a sheet of lead over one half to prevent its exposure (Fig. 12.4). Once one side has been exposed, the lead

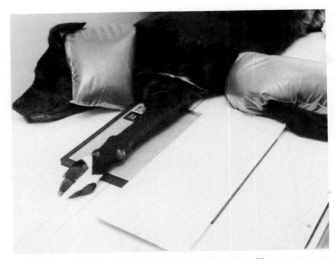

■ **FIG. 12.4** Example of splitting a cassette with a commercially available lead sheet. One view can be exposed on one side of the cassette, and the opposite view can be exposed on the other.

sheet can be moved to the already exposed area and the other side can be exposed. Lead sheets can be purchased from most x-ray supply companies. The sheets are usually supplied in preselected sizes, or larger sheets can be purchased and cut to the desired size. The lead should be at least 2 mm thick. If a lead sheet is unavailable, a lead glove can be placed over the area to be shielded.

Splitting a cassette is possible only when the cassette is used on the tabletop, without the use of the film (Bucky) tray and/or grid. The cassette can be split into any number of areas as long as there is enough space for each anatomic view. When splitting a cassette, it is important to position the animal so that all views of the area are facing the same direction on the film. For example, if a lateral view of the tarsus was exposed with the toes of the patient facing the right side of the cassette, the craniocaudal view should have the toes facing the same side of the cassette (Fig. 12.5).

Collimation

Collimation of the primary x-ray beam is very important whether the technician is splitting a cassette or not. The smallest field size possible should be used for any given area of the body. For example, when radiographing the carpus of a cat, the collimator light should include the carpus and a small portion of the long bones distal and proximal to the carpus (Fig. 12.6). It is not necessary to expose a large area surrounding the carpus. In fact, exposing a large area will increase the amount of scatter radiation, which will decrease radiographic contrast.

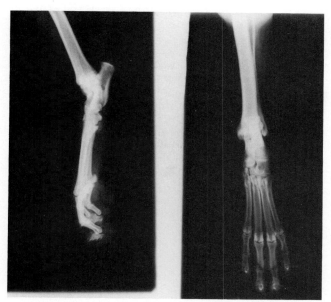

■ **FIG. 12.5** Radiograph of a canine tarsus, lateral and dorsoplantar views. Note that the toes of the patient are facing the same direction on the film.

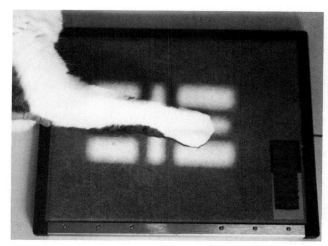

■ **FIG. 12.6** Example of proper collimation ("coning down") for a radiograph of the carpus of a cat.

Positioning Guidelines

In general, the central x-ray beam should be centered directly over the area of interest. For example, the x-ray beam is centered over the caudal border of the 13th rib for an abdomen. By centering here, the entire abdomen is included (assuming the proper size cassette is used).

The measurement for any anatomic region should be taken over the thickest area. This ensures that all regions of the part of interest will be penetrated with sufficient exposure factors.

Specific anatomy must be included for each anatomic area. For example, all radiographs of long bones (humerus and femur) should include the shaft of the bone as well as the joints distal and proximal to the bone. For joint radiography, the x-ray beam must be centered over the joint space and the beam should include a portion of the long bones distal and proximal.

Patient Preparation

The patient should be clean and free of any debris. If the haircoat of the animal is wet or full of debris, confusing artifacts can appear on the radiograph. Collars, harnesses, and leashes of any sort, especially those made of metal, should be removed. In addition, bandages, splints, and casts should be removed prior to radiography unless there is a definite medical reason for leaving them in place. Pedal radiography of the horse may require removing the shoes and cleaning the frog of the foot to alleviate any artifacts that may impinge over an area of interest. For radiography of the small animal abdomen, the gastrointestinal tract must be free of ingesta and fecal material. A cathartic such as an enema or a laxative may be indicated to remove the obstructive material. A more detailed discussion concerning animal preparation for abdominal study is in Chapter 17, in the section on abdominal radiography.

Restraint

As mentioned, chemical restraint is preferred. If manual restraint is required, however, all personnel in the radiographic suite during exposure must be shielded properly with the appropriate lead apparel. (See Chapter 3 for proper manual restraint and shielding.) With manual restraint, the canine patient usually responds to a calm, authoritative approach, whereas a feline patient will resist too much restraint.

Positioning Aids

To assist in the positioning of the animal patient, devices such as sandbags, foam blocks and wedges, wood blocks, and a radiolucent trough can be used (see Fig. 12.2). Tape, gauze, rope, and compression bands are also useful as positioning aids. With these devices, and sedation if necessary, very little manual restraint is needed. Positioning devices are commercially available or can easily be made by hand. Most fabric stores sell foam that can be cut into the desired shape with a scalpel blade or electric knife. Sandbags can easily be sewn and filled with sand for a fraction of the cost of those commercially available. Positioning aids should not be placed under or over the area of interest because none are completely nonradiopaque. Foam tends to produce an air density shadow and has the tendency to absorb and retain liquids that might be radiopaque when dry.

FILM IDENTIFICATION

Proper labeling of a radiograph is mandatory for legal and practical reasons. The film identification should include the appropriate patient information and/or access number as described in Chapter 7. A marker must also be used to identify the right or left (R or L) side of the patient, the limb being radiographed (front or rear), as well as the view, if necessary.

Placement of the label is also important. Anatomic areas that are symmetric (e.g., dorsoventral view of a dog skull) or anatomically identical to another area (e.g., an equine limb distal to the carpus and tarsus) are difficult to distinguish without proper labeling. For example, a lateral view of the front fetlock joint of a horse must be labeled "Left (L) Front."

When a marker is placed on a cassette for craniocaudal or caudocranial views, it should be placed on the lateral aspect of the extremity, as shown in Figure 12.4. In dorsoventral or ventrodorsal views, the marker should be placed on the cassette to identify one side or the other. That is, the lead "R" or "L" should be placed on the appropriate side of the animal. When a lateral projection of the abdomen or thorax is taken, the marker should indicate the side that is down on the table or cassette. For example, if a dog is in left lateral recumbency, the cassette should be labeled "L." When a lateral projection of an extremity is taken, the marker should be placed cranially to (in front of) the leg.

It is also important to mark sequential radiographs with the appropriate numbers that identify time elapsed or order taken. For example, special procedures such as a gastrointestinal contrast study require sequential radiographs over a period of time. In such an instance, each set of radiographs should be labeled with the appropriate time elapsed (hours and minutes).

BIBLIOGRAPHY

Douglas SW, Herrtage ME, Williamson HD: *Principles of Veterinary Radiography*, 4th ed. Bailliere Tindall, Philadelphia, 1987.

Habel RE: *Applied Veterinary Anatomy*, 2nd ed. RE Habel, Ithaca, NY, 1978.

Kleine LJ, Warren RG: *Small Animal Radiography*. CV Mosby, St. Louis, 1982.

Ryan GD: *Radiographic Positioning of Small Animals*. Lea & Febiger, Philadelphia, 1981.

Schebitz H, Wilkins H: *Atlas of Radiographic Anatomy of the Dog and Cat*. WB Saunders, Philadelphia, 1986.

Smallwood JE, et al: A standardized nomenclature for radiographic projections used in veterinary medicine. Vet Radiol J 26:2–9, 1985.

Smallwood JE, Shively MJ: Nomenclature for radiographic views of limbs. Equine Pract 1:41–45, 1979.

Ticer JW: *Radiographic Technique in Small Animal Practice*, 2nd ed. WB Saunders, Philadelphia, 1984.

SMALL ANIMAL FORELIMB

CHAPTER OUTLINE

- SCAPULA
- SHOULDER
- HUMERUS
- ELBOW

- RADIUS AND ULNA
- CARPUS
- METACARPUS-PHALANGES

SCAPULA

Lateral View

There are two methods for radiographing a lateral view of the scapula: (1) with the scapula placed dorsal to the vertebral column and (2) with the scapula superimposed over the lung field.

Dorsal to Vertebral Column

The best unobstructed view of the scapula is achieved by pushing the leg of interest dorsally so that the scapula is positioned dorsal to the vertebral column.

The patient is placed in lateral recumbency with the affected limb closest to the cassette. The affected leg is held perpendicular to the spine. The limb is then pushed dorsally by grasping it firmly below the elbow and extending the elbow joint. With the elbow in extension, the joint cannot flex, allowing the scapula to be pushed dorsally. As the affected leg is pushed dorsally, the opposite leg is pulled ventrally. By pulling the opposite leg, the thorax becomes slightly rotated, which isolates the scapula dorsal to the body. At this point, the scapula should be seen bulging above the dorsal spinous processes of the thoracic vertebrae. Sedation is usually indicated for this view because of the firm manipulation necessary.

BEAM CENTER: Middle of scapula
MEASUREMENT: Thickest area of scapula

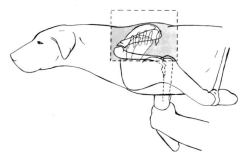

■ **FIG. 13.1** Correct positioning for the lateral view of the scapula positioned dorsal to the vertebral column.

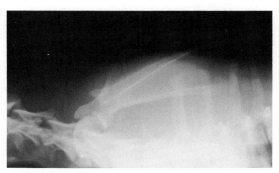

■ **FIG. 13.2** Radiograph of the lateral view of the scapula dorsal to the vertebral column.

Superimposed over Cranial Thorax

The view of the scapula superimposed over the cranial thorax is indicated for a patient that is in pain and when excessive manipulation may induce further injury. The body of the scapula is placed over the radiolucent lung fields, allowing visualization of the majority of the bone. Although the entire scapula is not visible, this view is valuable for the evaluation of the neck and body.

The patient is placed in lateral recumbency with the affected limb next to the cassette. The affected limb is pulled caudally and ventrally. The upper limb should be extended cranially, out of the area of interest. The sternum can be rotated away from the table slightly to visualize the dorsal border of the scapula better.

BEAM CENTER: Middle of scapula
MEASUREMENT: Cranioventral thorax where scapula is positioned

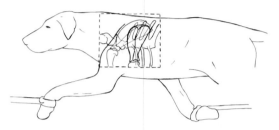

■ **FIG. 13.3** Correct positioning for the lateral view of the scapula superimposed over the cranial thorax.

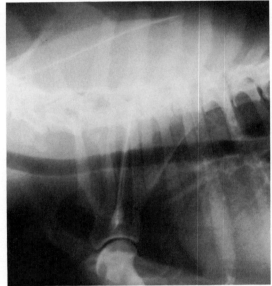

■ **FIG. 13.4** Radiograph of the lateral view of the scapula superimposed over the cranial thorax.

Caudocranial View

The patient is placed in dorsal recumbency (on its back) with both forelegs extended cranially. The patient's sternum should be rotated away from the scapula approximately 10 to 12 degrees. This rotation alleviates any superimposition of the ribs of the thoracic cavity over the scapula and gives a clear, unobstructed view of the structure.

BEAM CENTER: Middle of scapula
MEASUREMENT: Thickest area (scapulohumeral joint)

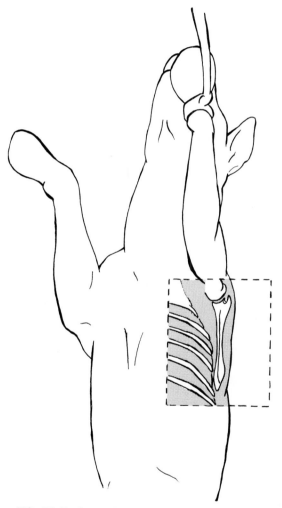

■ **FIG. 13.5** Correct positioning for the caudocranial view of the scapula.

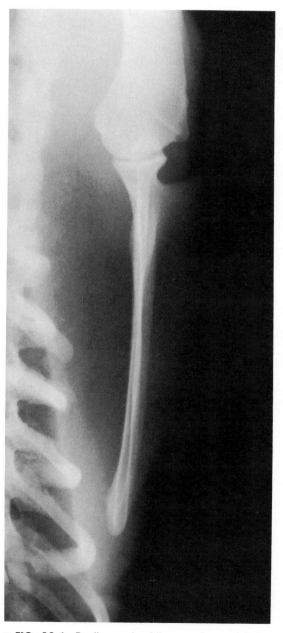

■ **FIG. 13.6** Radiograph of the caudocranial view of the scapula.

SHOULDER

Lateral View

The patient is placed in lateral recumbency with the shoulder of interest closest to the cassette. In order to alleviate any superimposition of structures over the shoulder, the leg must be extended cranial and ventral to the sternum. The opposite limb is pulled in a caudodorsal direction, and the neck is extended dorsally. This gesture will rotate the sternum slightly away from the shoulder joint. Care should be taken not to over-rotate the thorax as the shoulder may be lifted up off of the cassette.

BEAM CENTER: To shoulder joint
MEASUREMENT: Thickest area over shoulder joint

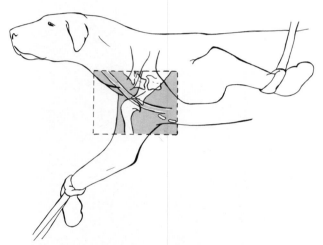

■ **FIG. 13.7** Correct positioning for the lateral view of the shoulder.

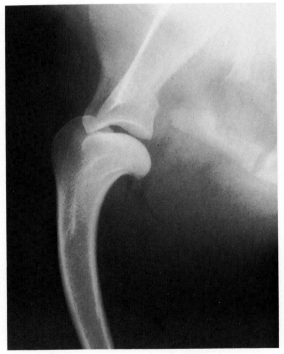

■ **FIG. 13.8** Radiograph of the lateral view of the shoulder.

Caudocranial View

The position for the caudocranial shoulder is very similar to the corresponding view of the scapula. The patient is placed in dorsal recumbency with both fore-limbs extended cranially. The limb should be extended so that the humerus is close to parallel to the cassette. Sedation may be necessary to allow such extension. As the forelimb is extended, care must be taken not to rotate the humerus. Any rotation would create an oblique view of the shoulder joint.

In some cases, it may be advantageous to expose both shoulders simultaneously. This would allow the veterinarian to examine and compare both joints. The only disadvantage to the simultaneous exposure is that the x-ray beam cannot be centered directly over one joint but is centered in the middle of the two.

BEAM CENTER: To shoulder joint
MEASUREMENT: Over shoulder joint (armpit)

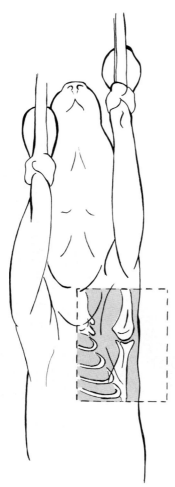

■ **FIG. 13.9** Correct positioning for the caudo-cranial view of the shoulder.

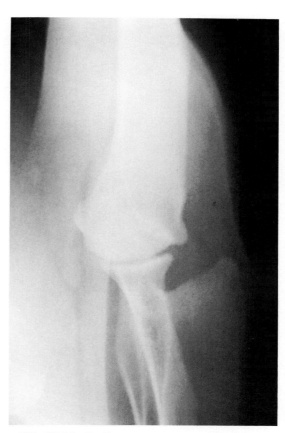

■ **FIG. 13.10** Radiograph of the caudocranial view of the shoulder.

HUMERUS

Lateral View

The patient is in lateral recumbency with the affected limb placed on the cassette. The leg is extended in a cranioventral direction with the opposite limb drawn in a caudodorsal direction. The head and neck should be extended dorsally. The field of view should include both the shoulder and the elbow joint with the humerus centered to the cassette.

BEAM CENTER: Center of humerus
MEASUREMENT: Thickest area over shoulder joint

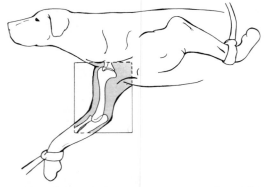

■ **FIG. 13.11** Correct positioning for the lateral view of the humerus.

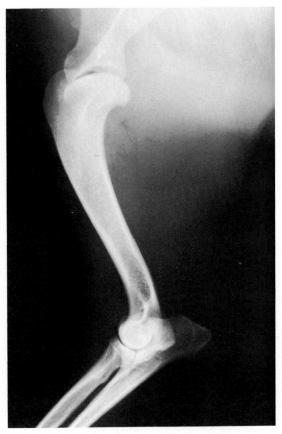

■ **FIG. 13.12** Radiograph of the lateral view of the humerus.

Caudocranial View

The patient is placed in dorsal recumbency with the forelimbs extended cranially. The leg of interest should remain as parallel to the cassette as possible to minimize distortion. The head and neck should remain between the forelimbs to eliminate superimposition and rotation of the body. The humerus should be centered to the cassette, and both the shoulder and the elbow should be included in the field of view.

BEAM CENTER: Middle of humerus
MEASUREMENT: Thickest area over shoulder region

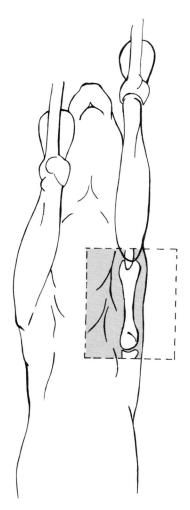

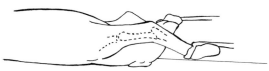

■ **FIG. 13.13** Correct positioning for the caudo-cranial view of the humerus.

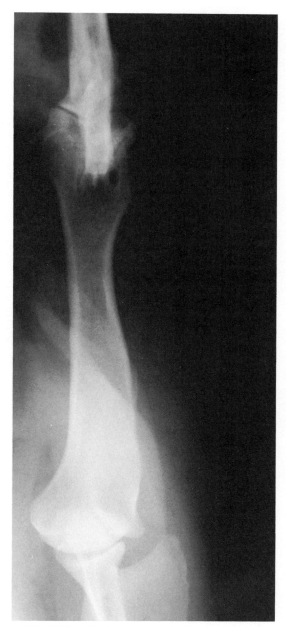

■ **FIG. 13.14** Radiograph of the caudocranial view of the humerus.

Craniocaudal View

The patient is placed in dorsal recumbency with the affected limb pulled caudally until the line of the humerus is parallel to the cassette. The limb should be abducted slightly from the thorax to alleviate any superimposition of ribs over the area of interest. The field of view should include the shoulder, humerus, and elbow. This view of the humerus has a relatively long object-film distance and will usually exhibit some magnification.

BEAM CENTER: Middle of humerus
MEASUREMENT: Thickest area over shoulder region

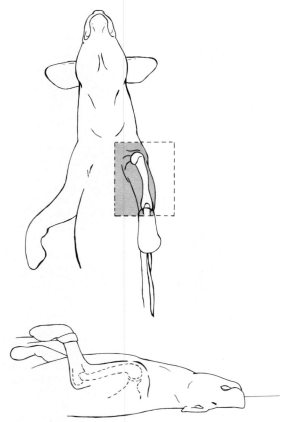

■ **FIG. 13.15** Correct positioning for the craniocaudal view of the humerus.

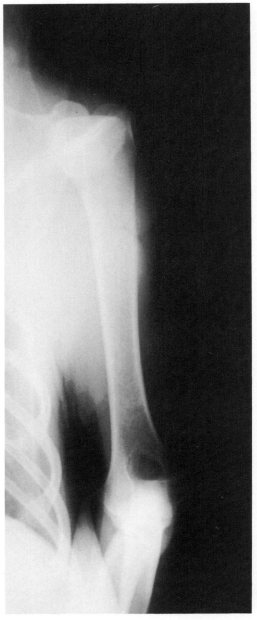

■ **FIG. 13.16** Radiograph of the craniocaudal view of the humerus.

ELBOW

Craniocaudal View

The patient is placed in sternal recumbency with the affected limb extended cranially. The patient's head should be elevated and positioned away from the affected side. Care should be taken to prevent the elbow from displacing laterally or medially when pulling the head to one side. To maintain a true craniocaudal position, the olecranon should be placed between the medial and the lateral humeral epicondyles. Placing a foam pad under the point of the elbow may alleviate rolling and prevent rotation.

BEAM CENTER: Over elbow joint
MEASUREMENT: Thickest area (distal humerus)

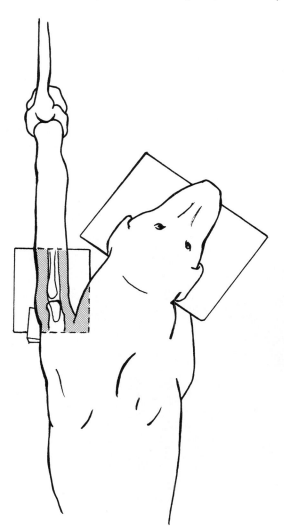

■ **FIG. 13.17** Correct positioning for the craniocaudal view of the elbow.

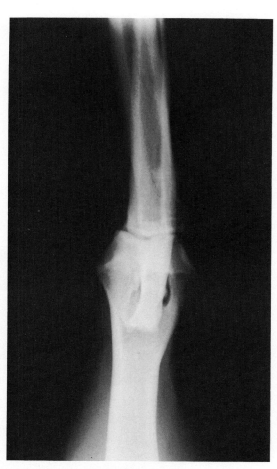

■ **FIG. 13.18** Radiograph of the craniocaudal view of the elbow.

Lateral View

The patient is placed in lateral recumbency with the affected limb positioned on the cassette. The head and neck should be extended slightly in a dorsal direction and the unaffected limb pulled in a caudodorsal direction. A foam wedge can be placed under the metacarpal region to maintain a true lateral view of the elbow.

BEAM CENTER: Over elbow joint
MEASUREMENT: Distal humerus

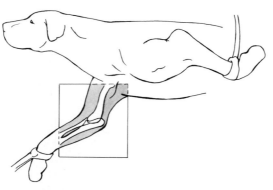

■ **FIG. 13.19** Correct positioning for the lateral view of the elbow.

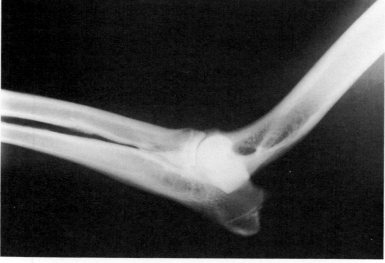

■ **FIG. 13.20** Radiograph of the lateral view of the elbow.

Flexed Lateral View

The patient is placed in the same position as for the routine lateral projection. The carpus is pulled toward the neck region, flexing the elbow. Care should be taken to keep the elbow in a true lateral position during flexion. By keeping the carpus lateral, the elbow should also remain in a true lateral position.

BEAM CENTER: Middle of elbow
MEASUREMENT: Distal humerus

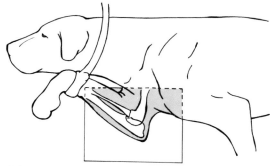

■ **FIG. 13.21** Correct positioning for the flexed lateral view of the elbow.

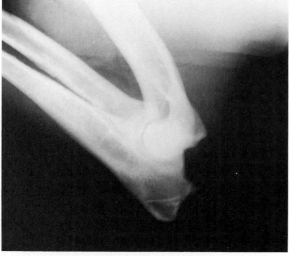

■ **FIG. 13.22** Radiograph of the flexed lateral view of the elbow.

RADIUS AND ULNA

Lateral View

The patient is placed in lateral recumbency with the affected limb centered on the cassette. The opposite limb is drawn caudally out of the way. The primary x-ray beam should include the elbow and carpal joints.

BEAM CENTER: Middle of radius and ulna
MEASUREMENT: Over elbow

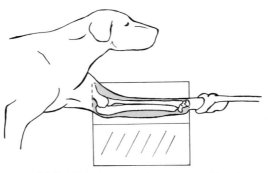

■ **FIG. 13.23** Correct positioning for the lateral view of the radius and ulna.

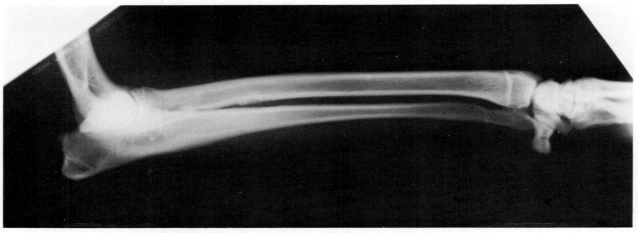

■ **FIG. 13.24** Radiograph of the lateral view of the radius and ulna.

Craniocaudal View

The patient is placed in sternal recumbency. The affected limb is extended cranially with the radius and ulna centered on the cassette. The head should be elevated and positioned away from the affected side. A true craniocaudal position should be ensured by confirming the placement of the olecrenon between the humeral condyles. The collimated x-ray beam should include the elbow and the carpus.

BEAM CENTER: Middle of radius and ulna
MEASUREMENT: Over distal humerus

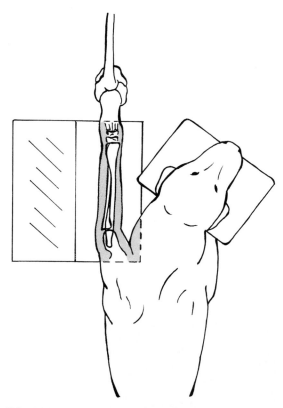

■ **FIG. 13.25** Correct positioning for the craniocaudal view of the radius and ulna.

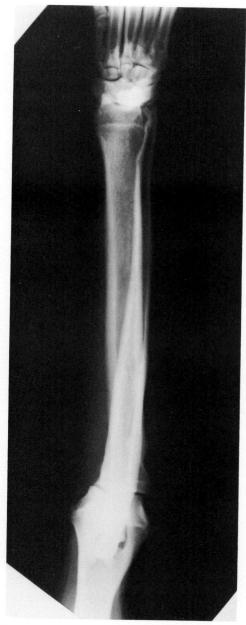

■ **FIG. 13.26** Radiograph of the craniocaudal view of the radius and ulna.

CARPUS

Lateral View

The patient is placed in lateral recumbency with the affected limb on the center of the cassette. A foam wedge pad can be placed under the elbow to prevent the carpus from moving away from the cassette. The opposite limb is pulled caudally out of the field of view. A flexed lateral view of the carpus can be taken in this position as well, if necessary.

BEAM CENTER: Over distal row of carpal bones
MEASUREMENT: Middle of carpus

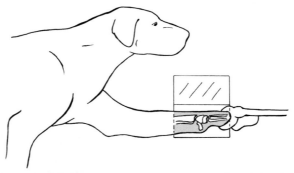

■ **FIG. 13.27** Correct positioning for the lateral view of the carpus.

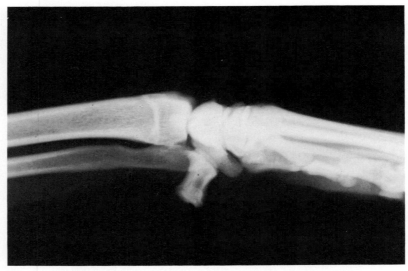

■ **FIG. 13.28** Radiograph of the lateral view of the carpus.

Dorsopalmar View

The patient is placed in sternal recumbency with the affected limb extended cranially. The carpus is placed flat on the cassette. A foam pad may be placed under the elbow to prevent rotation.

Because some injuries are difficult to detect radiologically on the standard dorsopalmar and lateral views, it may be helpful to take oblique views. Dorsopalmar mediolateral and dorsopalmar lateromedial oblique views are taken at 45 degrees off of the dorsopalmar view.

Other views that may be useful to detect joint instability of the carpus are dorsopalmar stressed views. With the affected carpus placed in dorsopalmar position, the radius and ulna are held firmly in place. The paw is pushed medially or laterally with a ruler or wooden paddle. Care should be taken not to apply too much force on the joint to avoid further injury.

BEAM CENTER: Middle of distal row of carpal bones
MEASUREMENT: At beam center site

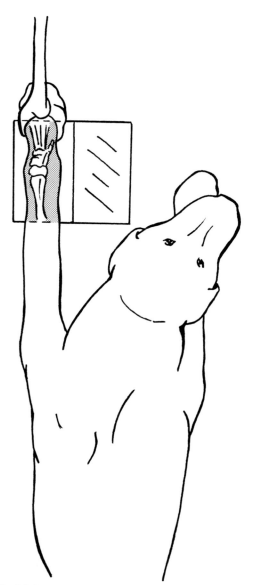

■ **FIG. 13.29** Correct positioning for the dorsopalmar view of the carpus.

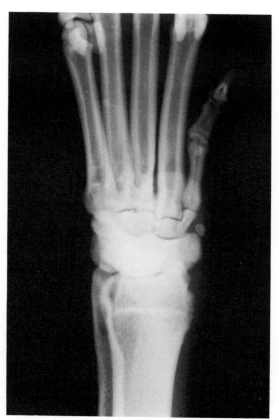

■ **FIG. 13.30** Radiograph of the dorsopalmar view of the carpus.

METACARPUS-PHALANGES

Dorsopalmar View

The patient is placed in sternal recumbency with the limb of interest extended. The paw is placed flat on the cassette. A piece of adhesive tape can be used to flatten the digits, if necessary. The field size should be large enough to include the carpal joint and the tips of the digits.

BEAM CENTER: Middle of metacarpal bones
MEASUREMENT: Middle of metacarpal bones

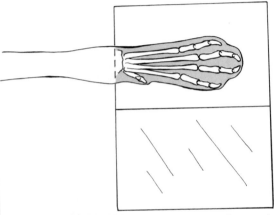

■ **FIG. 13.31** Correct positioning for the dorsopalmar view of the metacarpus-phalanges.

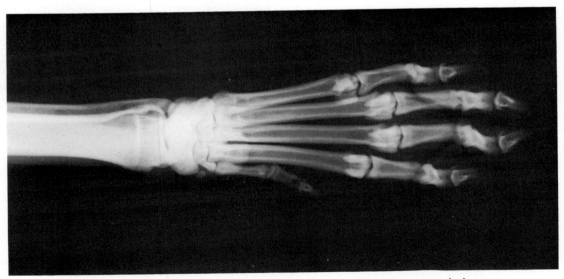

■ **FIG. 13.32** Radiograph of the dorsopalmar view of the metacarpus-phalanges.

Lateral View

The patient is placed in lateral recumbency with the affected side down. The limb of interest is placed on the cassette. A foam pad can be placed under the elbow to alleviate any rotation and any separation of the paw from the cassette. The beam center and measurement are the same as for the dorsopalmar view.

Some difficulty may be experienced viewing the digits as a result of superimposition. If it is necessary to examine one digit, it will be necessary to isolate the affected digit from the others. The specific digit to be examined is pulled cranially and fixed in position with tape. The other digits can be pulled in a caudal direction with another band of tape. The field of view should include the carpal joint and the tips of the digits.

BEAM CENTER: Center of digit
MEASUREMENT: Level of middle phalanx

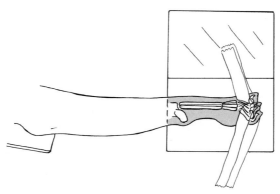

■ **FIG. 13.33** Correct positioning for the lateral view of phalangeal isolation.

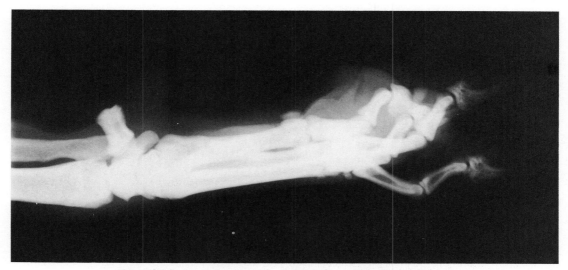

■ **FIG. 13.34** Radiograph of the lateral view of phalangeal isolation.

BIBLIOGRAPHY

Douglas SW, Herrtage ME, Williamson HD: *Principles of Veterinary Radiography,* 4th ed. Bailliere Tindall, Philadelphia, 1987.

Habel RE: *Applied Veterinary Anatomy,* 2nd ed. RE Habel, Ithaca, NY, 1978.

Kleine LJ, Warren RG: *Small Animal Radiography.* CV Mosby, St. Louis, 1982.

Miyabayashi T, den Toom OI, Morgan JP: Application of positional radiographic techniques in the dog and cat. Part III — Skeleton. Cal Vet 7:11.5, 1983.

Morgan JP, Silverman S: *Techniques of Veterinary Radiography,* 4th ed. Iowa State University Press, Ames, 1987.

Ryan GD: *Radiographic Positioning of Small Animals.* Lea & Febiger, Philadelphia, 1981.

Schebitz H, Wilkins H: *Atlas of Radiographic Anatomy of the Dog and Cat.* WB Saunders, Philadelphia, 1986.

Smallwood JE, Shively MJ: Nomenclature for radiographic views of limbs. Equine Pract 1:41–45, 1979.

Ticer JW: *Radiographic Technique in Small Animal Practice,* 2nd ed. WB Saunders, Philadelphia, 1984.

S M A L L   A N I M A L
P E L V I S   A N D
H I N D   L I M B

CHAPTER OUTLINE

- PELVIS
- FEMUR
- STIFLE JOINT

- TIBIA AND FIBULA
- TARSUS
- METATARSUS-PHALANGES

PELVIS

Lateral View

The patient is placed in lateral recumbency with the side of interest closest to the cassette. A foam wedge should be placed between the patient's stifle joints to keep the femurs parallel to the cassette. A foam wedge will also alleviate rotation and ensure that the two sides of the pelvis are superimposed. In order to distinguish the right femur from the left on the finished radiograph, the limb closest to the cassette should be pulled slightly cranial and the top leg caudal. This staggering of the femurs is especially important if the patient has a hip luxation and one femur needs to be differentiated from the other. The field of view should include the entire pelvis and a portion of the lumbar spine and the femurs. The pelvis should be centered in the middle of the cassette.

BEAM CENTER: Over greater femoral trochanter
MEASUREMENT: At level of trochanter

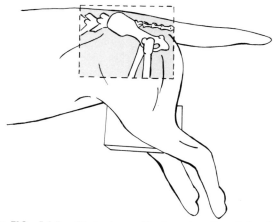

■ **FIG. 14.1** Correct positioning for the lateral view of the pelvis.

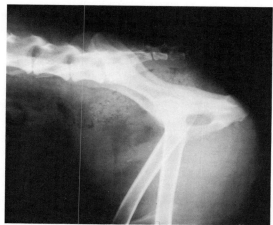

■ **FIG. 14.2** Radiograph of the lateral view of the pelvis.

Ventrodorsal View

Frog Leg Projection

The frog leg view of the pelvis is suitable when pelvic trauma is suspected. Minimal stress and tension are placed on the pelvis and hip joints in this projection.

The patient is placed in dorsal recumbency. A V trough is a useful positioning device to maintain bilateral symmetry. The pelvic limbs can assume a normal flexed position. The femurs should be at a 45-degree angle to the spine and can be secured in position by placing sandbags over the tarsal joints. It is important that the limbs be positioned identically to maintain symmetry.

BEAM CENTER: Over level of pubis and acetabulum
MEASUREMENT: Over acetabulum (groin)

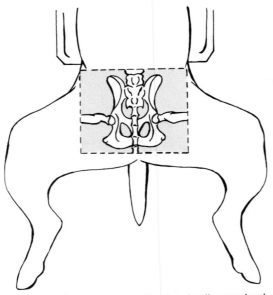

■ **FIG. 14.3** Correct positioning for the ventrodorsal frog view of the pelvis.

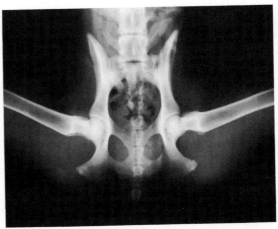

■ **FIG. 14.4** Radiograph of the ventrodorsal frog view of the pelvis.

Extended Projection

The extended view of the pelvis is standard for the evaluation of the hip joints for hip dysplasia. Symmetry and precision are vital for this view. Sedation is usually required.

A number of steps are necessary to achieve proper positioning of the pelvis. The patient is placed in dorsal recumbency with its back in a V trough or maintained with the aid of sandbags. The pelvic limbs are flexed into a frog position, and the tarsal joints are firmly grasped. At this point, the stifle joints are rotated medially toward each other. When the stifles are within 1 or 2 inches of each other, the limbs are extended caudally until the femurs are parallel to the cassette or until resistance is encountered. The hind legs can be secured with adhesive tape or hand held with the use of lead gloves (Figs. 14.5 to 14.8).

For correct positioning, the following criteria must be met:

1. Femurs are parallel to each other.
2. Both patellae are centered between the femoral condyles.
3. Pelvis is without rotation; obturator foramens, hip joints, hemipelvis, and sacroiliac joints appear as a mirror image.
4. The tail is secured with tape (if necessary) between the femurs.
5. Field of view includes the pelvis, femurs, and stifle joints.

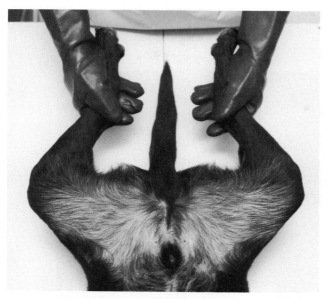

■ **FIG. 14.5** Ventrodorsal extended view of the pelvis: place the patient in the ventrodorsal frog position.

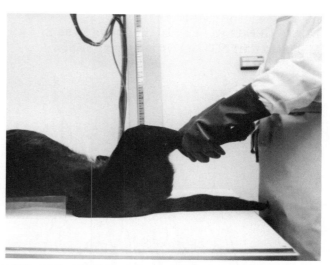

■ **FIG. 14.6** Ventrodorsal extended view of the pelvis: rotate the stifle joints medially so that they are an inch or two apart.

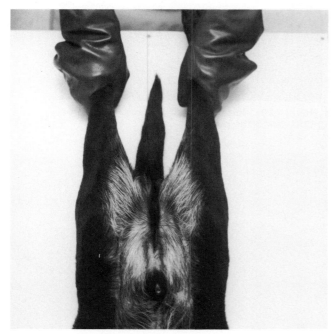

■ **FIG. 14.7** Ventrodorsal extended view of the pelvis: extend the femurs in a caudal direction while keeping them parallel to the table.

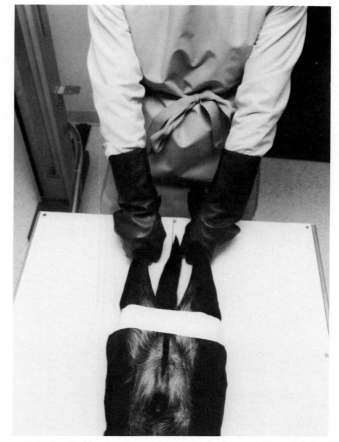

■ **FIG. 14.8** Ventrodorsal extended view of the pelvis: if manual restraint is unwarranted or insufficient, gauze or tape can be used around the distal femurs to secure the pelvis in the position.

BEAM CENTER: Caudal portion of ischium
MEASUREMENT: Over midfemur region

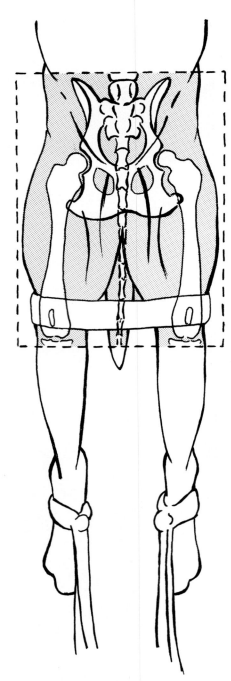

■ **FIG. 14.9**   Correct positioning for the ventrodorsal extended view of the pelvis.

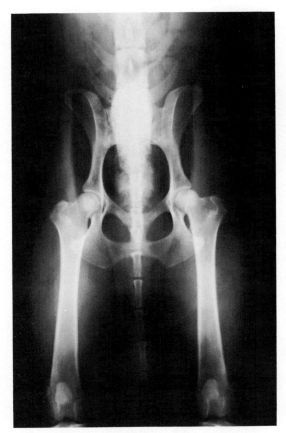

■ **FIG. 14.10**   Radiograph of the ventrodorsal extended view of the pelvis.

FEMUR

Lateral View

The patient is placed in lateral recumbency with the affected limb closest to the cassette. The opposite limb is abducted and rotated out of the line of the x-ray beam. A foam pad can be placed under the proximal tibia to alleviate any rotation of the femur. The field of view should include the hip joint, femur, and stifle joint.

BEAM CENTER: Middle of femur
MEASUREMENT: Middle of femur

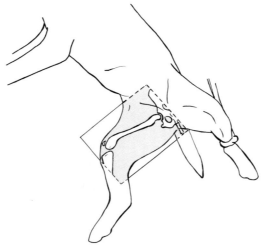

■ **FIG. 14.11** Correct positioning for the lateral view of the femur.

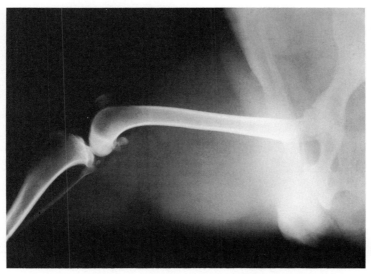

■ **FIG. 14.12** Radiograph of the lateral view of the femur.

Craniocaudal View

The patient is placed in dorsal recumbency with the limb of interest extended caudally. Slight abduction of the affected limb will eliminate superimposition of the proximal femur over the tuber ischium. The opposite limb can be flexed and rotated laterally to facilitate the abduction. Proper alignment is essential so that the femur is in a true craniocaudal position; the patella should be between the two femoral condyles. The field of view should include the hip joint, femur, and stifle joint.

BEAM CENTER: Middle of femur
MEASUREMENT: Middle of femur

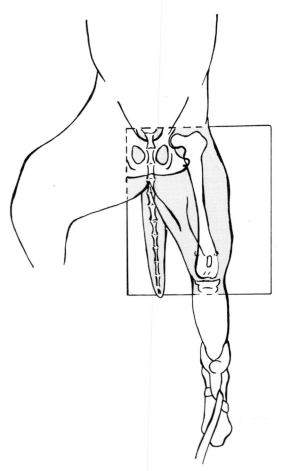

■ **FIG. 14.13** Correct positioning for the craniocaudal view of the femur.

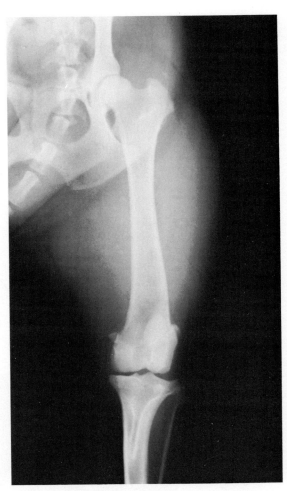

■ **FIG. 14.14** Radiograph of the craniocaudal view of the femur.

STIFLE JOINT

Caudocranial View

The patient is positioned in sternal recumbency with the affected limb pulled into a position of maximum extension. The opposite limb is flexed and elevated with a sponge or sandbag. Elevation of the opposite limb will control the lateral rotation of the stifle joint under examination. Determining the proper degree of rotation is critical to achieve a true caudocranial view; the patella should be centered between the femoral condyles. Palpation of the femoral condyles and the tibial tuberosity may be helpful to ensure symmetry.

A craniocaudal view of the stifle joint is also possible. The patient is positioned in dorsal recumbency with the limb under investigation extended as for the craniocaudal view of the femur. Although this view may be easier to position, it has the disadvantage of some magnification and distortion of the image due to increased object-film distance.

BEAM CENTER: Over stifle joint
MEASUREMENT: Distal end of femur

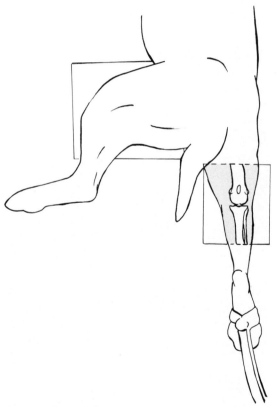

■ FIG. 14.15 Correct positioning for the caudocranial view of the stifle joint.

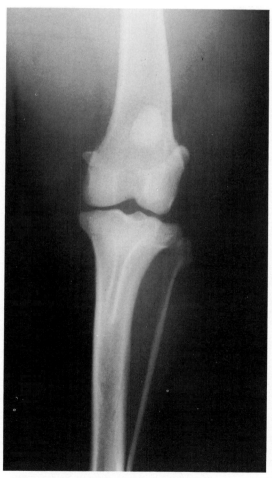

■ FIG. 14.16 Radiograph of the caudocranial view of the stifle joint.

Lateral View

The patient is placed in lateral recumbency with the affected joint placed on and centered to the cassette. The opposite limb is flexed and abducted from the line of the x-ray beam. The stifle joint should be in a natural, slightly flexed position. A sponge pad can be placed under the tarsus so that the tibia is parallel to the cassette surface. Elevation of the tibia will ensure superimposition of the two femoral condyles and facilitate a true lateral projection.

BEAM CENTER: Over stifle joint
MEASUREMENT: Over femoral condyles

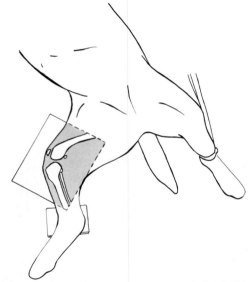

■ **FIG. 14.17** Correct positioning for the lateral view of the stifle joint.

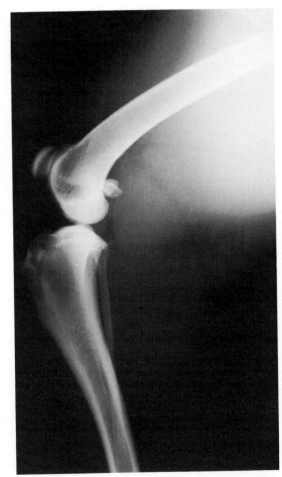

■ **FIG. 14.18** Radiograph of the lateral view of the stifle joint.

Skyline Projection of Patella (Sunrise View)

The skyline projection demonstrates changes that can occur to the patella and the femoral trochlear groove.

The patient is placed in lateral recumbency with the opposite limb down on the table. The affected limb should be in a fully flexed position. Tape or roll gauze can be placed around the midtibia and femur to hold the stifle joint in this flexed position. The stifle should remain horizontal and can be supported on a foam pad. The cassette is placed behind the stifle joint vertically, and a horizontal x-ray beam is centered to the patella.

BEAM CENTER: Over patella
MEASUREMENT: Site of patellar articulation

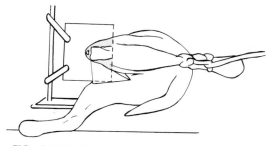

■ **FIG. 14.19** Correct positioning for the skyline view of the patella.

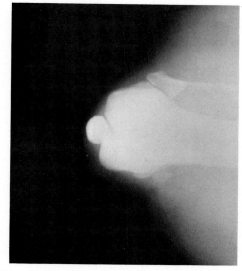

■ **FIG. 14.20** Radiograph of the skyline view of the patella.

TIBIA AND FIBULA

Lateral View

The patient is placed in lateral recumbency with the affected limb placed on the cassette. The stifle should be slightly flexed and maintained in a true lateral position. A sponge wedge can be placed under the metatarsus to eliminate any rotation of the tibia. The opposite limb is pulled cranially or caudally so that it is out of the line of the x-ray beam. The field of view should include the stifle joint, tibia and fibula, and tarsal joint.

BEAM CENTER: Middle of tibia and fibula
MEASUREMENT: Over stifle joint

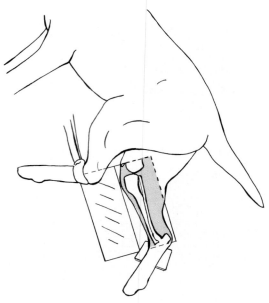

■ **FIG. 14.21** Correct positioning for the lateral view of the tibia and fibula.

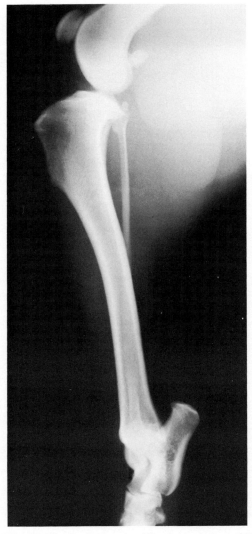

■ **FIG. 14.22** Radiograph of the lateral view of the tibia and fibula.

Caudocranial View

The patient is placed in sternal recumbency with the affected limb extended caudally. The tibia and fibula are centered to the cassette. The body can be supported in position with foam blocks placed beneath the caudal abdomen and pelvic region. Elevating the hind end will minimize the weight placed on the stifle joint extended caudally and will facilitate positioning. The tibia and fibula should be in a true caudocranial position so that the patella is placed between the two femoral condyles. The opposite limb should be flexed and placed on a sponge pad to control rotation of the limb of interest. If the patient has a long tail, it should be secured with tape out of the field of view. The field of view should include the stifle joint, tibia and fibula, and tarsal joint.

BEAM CENTER: Middle of tibia and fibula
MEASUREMENT: Over level of stifle joint

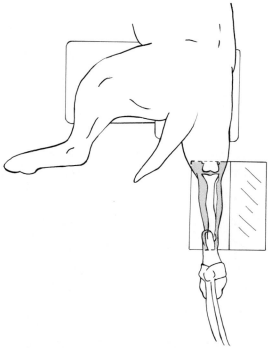

■ **FIG. 14.23** Correct positioning for the caudocranial view of the tibia and fibula.

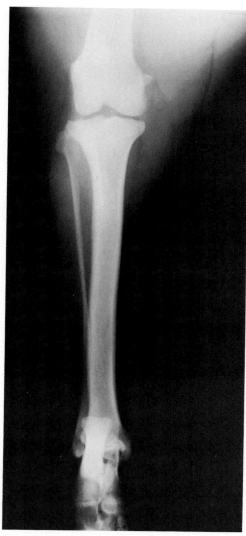

■ **FIG. 14.24** Radiograph of the caudocranial view of the tibia and fibula.

TARSUS

Lateral View

The patient is placed in lateral recumbency with the affected limb closest to the cassette. The tarsus is placed in a natural, slightly flexed position and centered to the cassette. The tarsus must remain in a true lateral position; a sponge wedge or tape can be used to eliminate any rotation of the limb. The opposite limb should be pulled cranially out of line of the x-ray beam.

BEAM CENTER: Middle of tarsus
MEASUREMENT: Over thickest area of tarsal joint

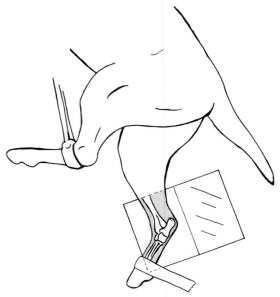

■ **FIG. 14.25** Correct positioning for the lateral view of the tarsus.

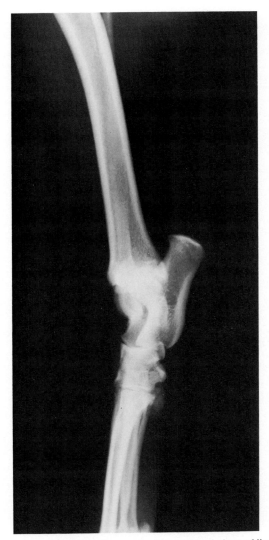

■ **FIG. 14.26** Radiograph of the lateral view of the tarsus.

Plantarodorsal and Dorsoplantar Views

The patient is placed in sternal recumbency with the affected limb extended as for the caudocranial view of the tibia and fibula. The tarsus is centered to the cassette. Foam blocks are placed under the caudal abdomen and pelvic region for patient comfort and to control rotation of the tarsus. A foam wedge should be placed under the stifle joint to achieve maximum extension of the tarsus. Keep in mind that if the stifle joint is in a true caudocranial position, the tarsus will naturally follow in a true plantarodorsal position.

The dorsoplantar view of the tarsus may be easier to facilitate in some cases in which an animal resists caudal extension of the hind limb. The patient is placed in sternal recumbency with the affected limb extended cranially alongside the body. The limb should be slightly abducted from the body wall to prevent any superimposition over the tarsus. A true dorsoplantar position is ensured by rotating the stifle medially in order to center the patella between the femoral condyles.

BEAM CENTER: Middle of tarsal joint
MEASUREMENT: Thickest area of tarsal joint

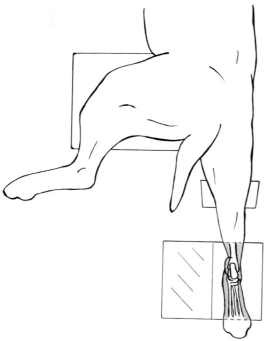

■ **FIG. 14.27** Correct positioning for the plantaro-dorsal view of the tarsus.

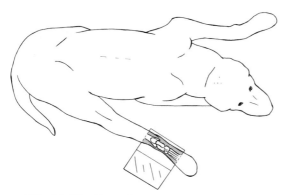

■ **FIG. 14.28** Correct positioning for the dorso-plantar view of the tarsus.

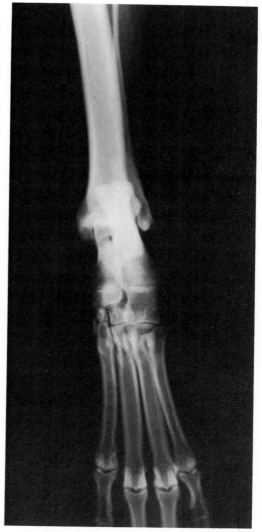

■ **FIG. 14.29** Radiograph of the plantarodorsal view of the tarsus.

METATARSUS-PHALANGES

Lateral View

The patient is placed in lateral recumbency with the affected metatarsus centered to the cassette. The opposite limb can be pulled caudally or cranially out of view of the x-ray beam. The joint is positioned in a natural flexed position. A sponge pad can be placed under the stifle joint to maintain a true lateral position of the metatarsus. The field of view should include the tarsal joint, metatarsus, and phalanges.

BEAM CENTER: Midmetatarsal region
MEASUREMENT: Distal tarsal joint

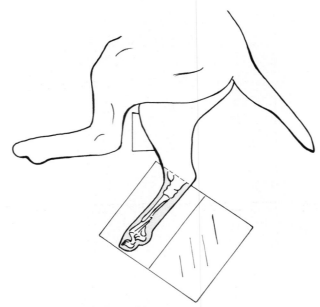

■ **FIG. 14.30** Correct positioning for the lateral view of the metatarsus and phalanges.

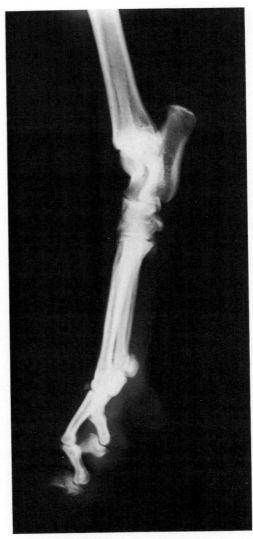

■ **FIG. 14.31** Radiograph of the lateral view of the metatarsus and phalanges.

Dorsoplantar and Plantarodorsal Views

For the dorsoplantar view, the patient is placed in sternal recumbency and the limb of interest is pulled cranially and slightly abducted from the body wall. The metatarsus is centered to the cassette. To achieve a true dorsoplantar view, the stifle joint of the affected limb is rotated laterally and secured with tape. The field of view should include the tarsus, metatarsus, and phalanges.

The plantarodorsal view is positioned the same as the plantarodorsal view of the tarsus.

BEAM CENTER: Midmetatarsal region
MEASUREMENT: Distal tarsal joint

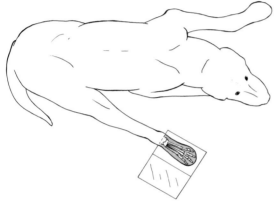

■ **FIG. 14.32** Correct positioning for the dorso-plantar view of the metatarsus and phalanges.

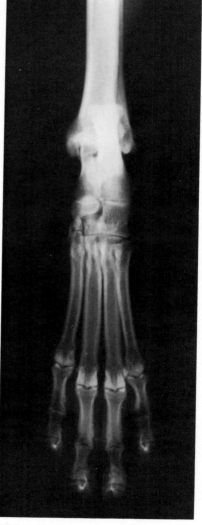

■ **FIG. 14.33** Radiograph of the dorsoplantar view of the metatarsus and phalanges.

BIBLIOGRAPHY

Douglas SW, Herrtage ME, Williamson HD: *Principles of Veterinary Radiography*, 4th ed. Bailliere Tindall, Philadelphia, 1987.

Habel RE: *Applied Veterinary Anatomy*, 2nd ed. RE Habel, Ithaca, NY, 1978.

Kleine LJ, Warren RG: *Small Animal Radiography*. CV Mosby, St. Louis, 1982.

Morgan JP, Silverman S: *Techniques of Veterinary Radiography*, 4th ed. Iowa State University Press, Ames, 1987.

Ryan GD: *Radiographic Positioning of Small Animals*. Lea & Febiger, Philadelphia, 1981.

Schebitz H, Wilkins H: *Atlas of Radiographic Anatomy of the Dog and Cat*. WB Saunders, Philadelphia, 1986.

Smallwood JE, Shively MJ: Nomenclature for radiographic views of limbs. Equine Pract 1:41–45, 1979.

Ticer JW: *Radiographic Technique in Small Animal Practice*, 2nd ed. WB Saunders, Philadelphia, 1984.

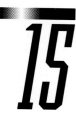

SMALL ANIMAL SKULL

SKULL

Introduction

In order to obtain a correctly positioned radiograph of the skull, a controlled patient is vital. Anesthesia is usually needed. If the animal is under general anesthesia, it may be necessary to remove the endotracheal tube in some views to avoid superimposing shadows over the area of interest. The key to a diagnostic radiograph of the skull is precision and symmetry. Any rotation, even slight, may inhibit an accurate diagnosis.

The anatomy of the skull is complicated, and radiography of the skull can be just as complex. Familiarity with the anatomy of the small animal skull will facilitate correct positioning of the various views (Figs. 15.1 and 15.2). Furthermore, because veterinary radiography deals with many breeds and species, the number of physical variations in skull anatomy adds to the complexity of positioning. Compare the skull of a collie with that of a Boston terrier—the difference is enormous. However, the principles presented here can be applied to any small animal breed and species.

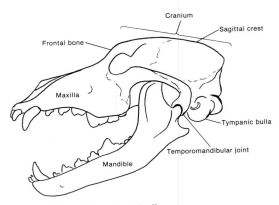

■ **FIG. 15.1** Lateral canine skull.

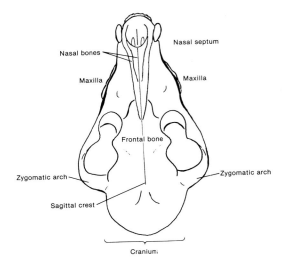

■ **FIG. 15.2** Ventrodorsal canine skull.

Lateral View

The patient should be placed in lateral recumbency with the affected side of the skull toward the cassette. To eliminate rotation of the skull, a foam pad of suitable thickness is placed under the ramus of the mandible. The nasal septum should be parallel to the surface of the cassette. From the view of the x-ray tube (bird's-eye view), the mandibular rami should be superimposed. Placing a pad under the cranioventral cervical region and pulling the front limbs caudally may assist in maintaining the skull in a true lateral position. The field of view should include the tip of the nose to the base of the skull.

BEAM CENTER: Lateral canthus of eye
MEASUREMENT: Over high point of zygomatic arch (for demonstration of nares, measurement should be taken at nasal notch)

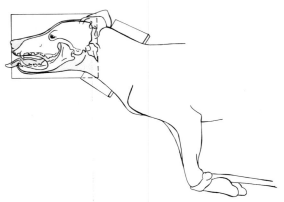

■ **FIG. 15.3** Correct positioning for the lateral view of the skull.

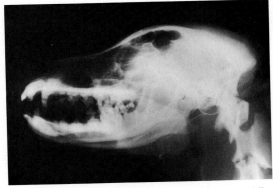

■ **FIG. 15.4** Radiograph of the lateral view of the skull.

Dorsoventral View

The patient is placed in sternal recumbency with the head resting on the cassette. Gentle pressure can be placed over the cervical region with a sandbag to keep the skull next to the cassette in a dorsoventral position. The front limbs can remain in a natural position alongside the head but out of view of the x-ray beam. Check the final positioning by looking in a rostrocaudal direction. The sagittal plane of the head should be perpendicular to the cassette. If the head consistently rotates to one side or the other, a strip of adhesive tape can be placed over the cranium in the desired position. The field of view should include the tip of the nose to the base of the skull.

BEAM CENTER: Lateral canthus of eye
MEASUREMENT: Over high point of cranium

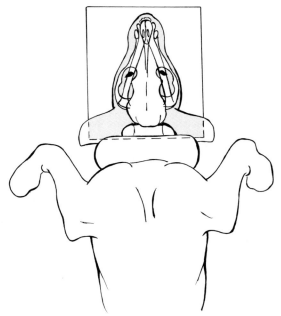

■ **FIG. 15.5** Correct positioning for the dorsoventral view of the skull.

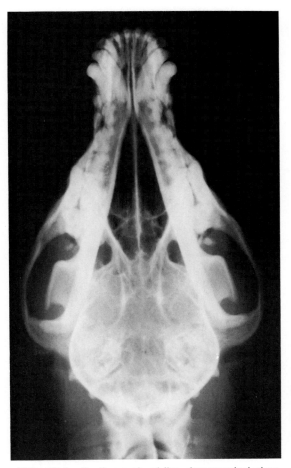

■ **FIG. 15.6** Radiograph of the dorsoventral view of the skull.

Ventrodorsal View

The patient is placed in dorsal recumbency. A V trough or sandbags can be used to keep the animal in position. The front limbs are extended caudally and secured. A foam pad should be placed under the mid-cervical region to gain proper positioning of the skull on the cassette. The nose must remain parallel to the cassette, and the skull must be balanced in a true ventrodorsal position. Rotation of the skull is a problem with animals that have a prominent external occipital protuberance. A thin sponge pad placed under the cranium will help prevent this type of rotation. The field of view should include the tip of the nose to the base of the skull.

BEAM CENTER: Lateral canthus of eye
MEASUREMENT: Lateral canthus of eye

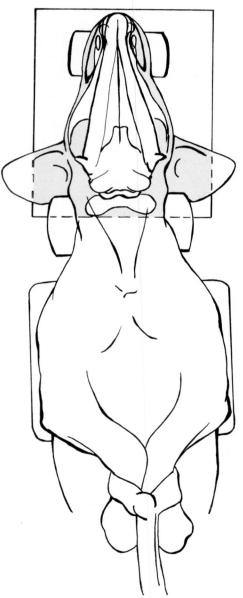

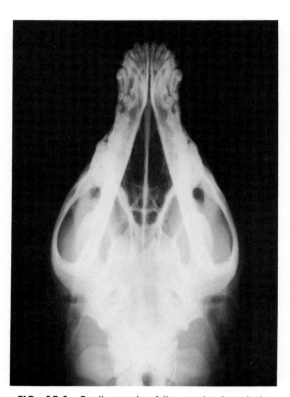

■ **FIG. 15.8** Radiograph of the ventrodorsal view of the skull.

■ **FIG. 15.7** Correct positioning for the ventrodorsal view of the skull.

FRONTAL SINUSES

Rostrocaudal View

The patient is placed in dorsal recumbency with the nose pointing upward. The front legs should be pulled caudally alongside the body. The nose is positioned perpendicular to the cassette. A length of roll gauze or tape can be tied around the nose to stabilize the patient in this position. The frontal sinuses should be centered to the cassette, and the field of view should include the entire forehead of the patient. The collimator light should be aimed in conjunction with the angle of the nose off vertical to be centered tangent to the sinuses.

BEAM CENTER: Through center of frontal sinuses, between eyes
MEASUREMENT: Over site of nasal sinuses ("nose stop")

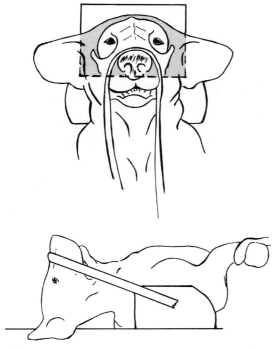

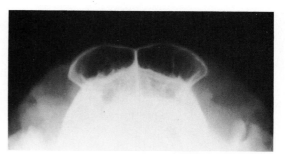

■ **FIG. 15.10** Radiograph of the rostrocaudal view of the front sinuses.

■ **FIG. 15.9** Correct positioning for the rostrocaudal view of the frontal sinuses.

CRANIUM

Rostrocaudal View

The patient is placed in dorsal recumbency with the nose pointing upward and the front limbs pulled caudally alongside the body. This view is very similar to the frontal sinus projection except the angle of the nose is directed slightly in a caudal direction. With a length of roll gauze or tape, the nose is pulled caudally approximately 10 to 15 degrees. If an endotracheal tube is in place, care must be taken not to crimp the tube while flexing the animal's neck. The cranium should be centered to the cassette, and the field of view should include the entire cranium.

BEAM CENTER: Midpoint between eyes
MEASUREMENT: Site of frontal sinuses

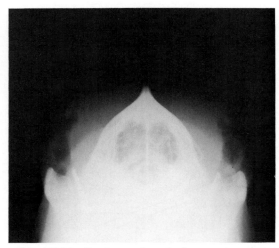

■ **FIG. 15.12** Radiograph of the rostrocaudal view of the cranium.

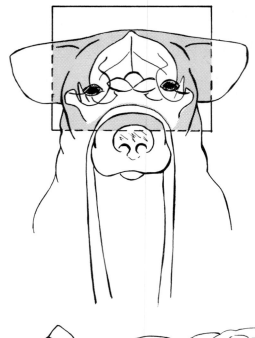

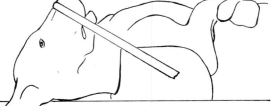

■ **FIG. 15.11** Correct positioning for the rostrocaudal view of the cranium.

NASAL CAVITY

Ventrodorsal Open-Mouth View

The patient is placed in dorsal recumbency with the front legs extended caudally alongside the body. The maxilla should remain parallel to the cassette and secured with a strip of tape placed inside the mouth, with the ends of the tape adhered to the table on either side of the patient's head. A length of roll gauze or tape is tied around the mandible and pulled in a caudal direction so that the mouth is wide open. The mouth may also be propped open with a tongue depressor placed between the canine teeth of the upper and lower arcades. Keep in mind that the tongue depressor may cast a slightly superimposing shadow over the nasal cavity. If an endotracheal tube is in place, it should be tied to the mandible or removed before exposure to prevent superimposition of this structure over the area of interest.

The x-ray tube should be angled 10 to 15 degrees so that the x-ray beam is directed inside the mouth. The nasal cavity should be centered to the cassette, and the field of view should include the entire maxilla from the tip of the nose to the pharyngeal region.

BEAM CENTER: Through level of third upper premolar
MEASUREMENT: Over level of third upper premolar

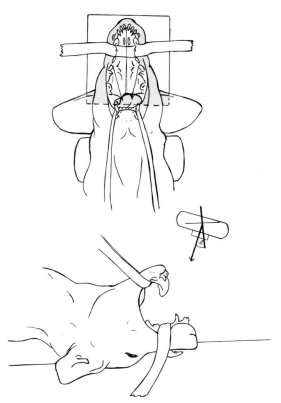

■ **FIG. 15.13** Correct positioning for the ventrodorsal open-mouth view of the nasal cavity.

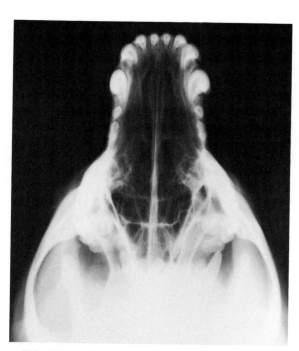

■ **FIG. 15.14** Radiograph of the ventrodorsal open-mouth view of the nasal cavity.

TYMPANIC BULLAE

Rostrocaudal Open-Mouth View

The patient is placed in dorsal recumbency with the nose pointing upward and the front legs pulled in a caudal direction alongside the body. The mouth is held open with gauze or other suitable mouth speculum. The nose should be pulled approximately 5 to 10 degrees in a cranial direction, and the mandible pulled caudally. The amount of cranial pull on the maxilla will vary with the shape of the skull of the breed. The bullae should be projected free from the mandible and the hard palate of the maxilla. The field of view should include the entire nasopharyngeal region of the skull.

BEAM CENTER: At level of commissure of lips
MEASUREMENT: At level of commissure of lips

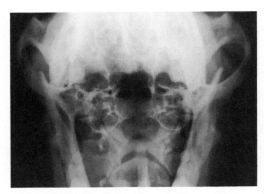

FIG. 15.16 Radiograph of the rostrocaudal open-mouth view of the tympanic bullae.

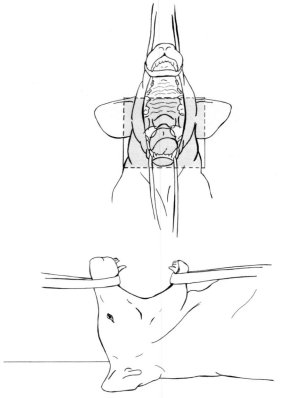

FIG. 15.15 Correct positioning of the rostrocaudal open-mouth view of the tympanic bullae.

Lateral Oblique View

The patient is placed in lateral recumbency with the unaffected tympanic bullae toward the cassette. The front legs should be extended caudally slightly to facilitate the skull to lie in a natural oblique position. In most instances, the skull will have a natural lie of 8 to 12 degrees rotation from true lateral. This degree of rotation allows the tympanic bullae to offset one another and provides adequate isolation of the structures. This view of the bullae can also be used to examine an oblique projection of the temporomandibular joints.

BEAM CENTER: Over center of tympanic bullae
MEASUREMENT: At level of tympanic bullae

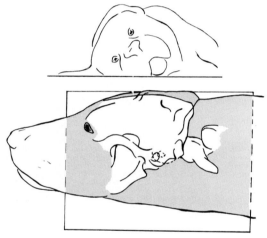

■ **FIG. 15.17** Correct positioning for the lateral oblique view of the tympanic bullae.

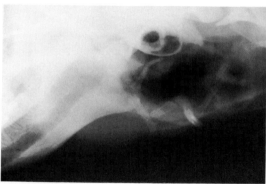

■ **FIG. 15.18** Radiograph of the lateral oblique view of the tympanic bullae.

TEMPOROMANDIBULAR JOINT

Ventrodorsal Oblique View

The patient is placed in lateral recumbency with the affected side toward the cassette. The skull is initially placed in a true lateral position. The cranium is then rotated approximately 20 degrees toward the cassette. A sponge wedge under the mandible will secure the skull in this position. This rotation prevents superimposition by the opposite temporomandibular joint and other surrounding structures. The ventrodorsal oblique projection can be taken with the mouth open or closed.

BEAM CENTER: Over center of temporomandibular joint
MEASUREMENT: Over lateral canthus of eye

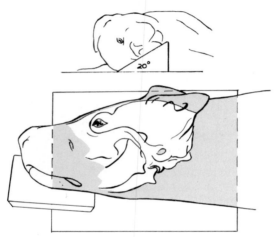

■ **FIG. 15.19** Correct positioning for the lateral oblique view of the temporomandibular joint.

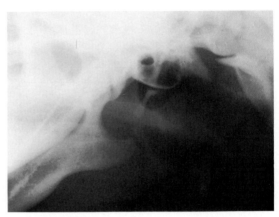

■ **FIG. 15.20** Radiograph of the lateral oblique view of the temporomandibular joint.

MAXILLA

Dorsoventral Intraoral View

The patient is placed in sternal recumbency with the head in straight alignment with the spine. A nonscreen packaged film is placed in the mouth to the level of the commissure of the lips. A cassette can be placed in the mouth but is difficult to insert because of its size. The corner edge of the film is introduced into the mouth first to allow more of the maxilla to be radiographed. Because the source-image distance (SID) is reduced as a result of the film being elevated off the table, the x-ray tube should be raised accordingly to compensate.

BEAM CENTER: Over site of interest
MEASUREMENT: At level of commissure of lips

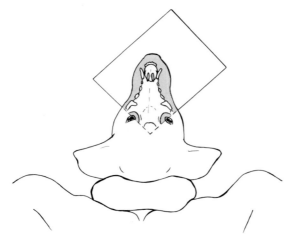

■ **FIG. 15.21** Correct positioning for the dorsoventral intraoral maxilla.

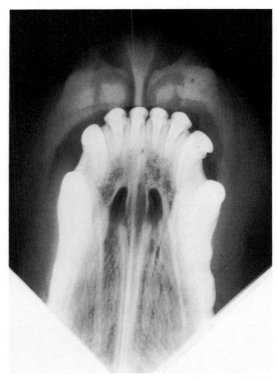

■ **FIG. 15.22** Radiograph of the dorsoventral intraoral maxilla.

Upper Dental Arcade

Open-Mouth Ventrodorsal Oblique View

The patient is placed halfway on its back with the maxillary arcade of interest closest to the cassette. The head is rotated approximately 45 degrees to the cassette and stabilized with a sponge wedge pad or cotton. The rotation of the head eliminates superimposition of the contralateral arcade. The mouth should be maintained in an open position with a tongue depressor or other suitable radiolucent mouth gag.

BEAM CENTER: Over third premolar
MEASUREMENT: At proximal hard palate

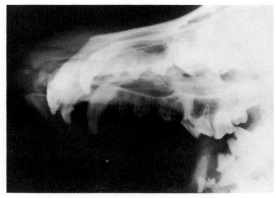

■ **FIG. 15.24** Radiograph of the ventrodorsal open-mouth oblique view of the maxilla (upper dental arcade).

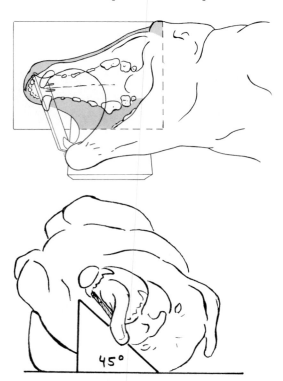

■ **FIG. 15.23** Correct positioning for the ventrodorsal open-mouth oblique view of the maxilla (upper dental arcade).

MANDIBLE

Ventrodorsal Intraoral View

The patient is placed in dorsal recumbency with the head extended in a cranial direction. A nonscreen packaged film is placed in the mouth with the corner edge of the film introduced first. The film is inserted until the edges of the film reach the commissure of the lips. The tongue should be pulled cranially to eliminate unequal density over the mandibular area. Because the SID is reduced as a result of the film being elevated off the table, the x-ray tube should be raised accordingly to compensate.

BEAM CENTER: Over site of interest
MEASUREMENT: At commissure of lips

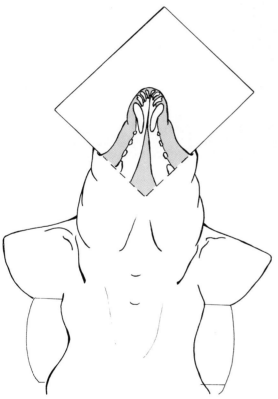

FIG. 15.25 Correct positioning of the ventrodorsal intraoral view of the mandible.

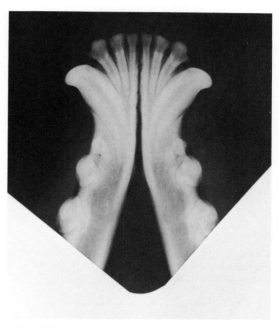

FIG. 15.26 Radiograph of the ventrodorsal intraoral view of the mandible.

Lower Dental Arcade

Open-Mouth Lateral Oblique View

The patient is placed in lateral recumbency with the affected mandible closest to the cassette. A radiolucent mouth gag is placed to separate the upper and lower arcades. The cranium should be rotated approximately 20 degrees away from the tabletop and maintained in this position with a sponge wedge pad or cotton.

BEAM CENTER: Over site of interest
MEASUREMENT: At level of first molar

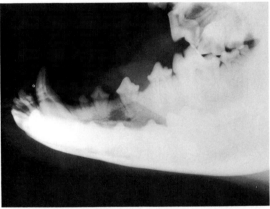

■ **FIG. 15.28** Radiograph of the dorsoventral oblique open-mouth view of the mandible (lower dental arcade).

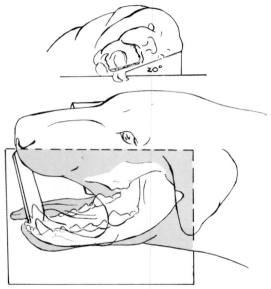

■ **FIG. 15.27** Correct positioning for the dorsoventral oblique open-mouth view of the mandible (lower dental arcade).

TEETH

Lateral Intraoral View

The most accurate method of visualizing a tooth and tooth root is with intraoral nonscreen dental film.

The patient is placed in lateral recumbency with the nonaffected side on the table and the area of interest uppermost. The film is inserted into the mouth and placed against the medial border of the maxilla or mandible behind the affected tooth. Difficulty may be encountered when trying to insert the film against the medial border of the maxilla and mandible because of the normal anatomy of the canine and feline mouth. That is, the hard palate of the dog and cat is relatively flat, which makes positioning the film difficult. The film is maintained in position with a pair of forceps. If necessary, the angle of the x-ray tube or skull of the patient should be altered to keep the film perpendicular to the x-ray beam.

BEAM CENTER: Over site of interest

MEASUREMENT: At site of interest (exposure factors are usually approximated and are dependent on patient's size—consult film manufacturer)

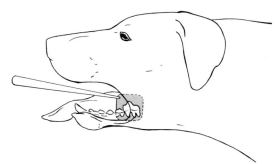

■ **FIG. 15.29** Correct positioning for a lateral intraoral view of the teeth using nonscreen dental film.

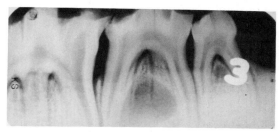

■ **FIG. 15.30** Radiograph of a lateral intraoral view of the teeth using nonscreen dental film.

BIBLIOGRAPHY

Douglas SW, Herrtage ME, Williamson HD: *Principles of Veterinary Radiography*, 4th ed. Bailliere Tindall, Philadelphia, 1987.

Habel RE: *Applied Veterinary Anatomy*, 2nd ed. RE Habel, Ithaca, NY, 1978.

Kleine LJ, Warren RG: *Small Animal Radiography*. CV Mosby, St. Louis, 1982.

Ryan GD: *Radiographic Positioning of Small Animals.* Lea & Febiger, Philadelphia, 1981.

Schebitz H, Wilkins H: *Atlas of Radiographic Anatomy of the Dog and Cat.* WB Saunders, Philadelphia, 1986.

Smallwood JE, Shively MJ: Nomeclature for radiographic views of limbs. Equine Pract 1:41–45, 1979.

Ticer JW: *Radiographic Technique in Small Animal Practice*, 2nd ed. WB Saunders, Philadelphia, 1984.

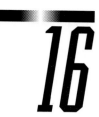

SMALL ANIMAL SPINE

INTRODUCTION

In order to obtain a diagnostic radiograph of the vertebral column, two factors need to be considered. First, the vertebral column must always be as parallel to the tabletop as possible. Second, the disk spaces of the spine must be near perpendicular to the tabletop and in parallel alignment with the central axis of the primary x-ray beam. These criteria can be met by a number of means.

On rare occasions, no manual assistance may be needed to achieve correct positioning of animal patients placed in recumbency. However, because it is usually necessary to alter the lateral recumbent position of the animal, positioning devices such as foam sponges, sandbags, or cotton may be helpful. Usually, efforts to improve the patient's positioning center around elevating the sternum and hind legs and providing support for the skull and midcervical and midlumbar regions (Figs. 16.1 and 16.2). Remember, any positioning device that is superimposed on an area of interest must be radiolucent.

Another method that can be used to achieve correct positioning is manual traction. By pulling the front and rear legs in opposite directions for views of the thoracolumbar spine, the vertebral column naturally extends to a near parallel position and the intervertebral disk spaces are opened. This positioning method is contraindicated for patients that have spinal column injuries such as fractures or luxations.

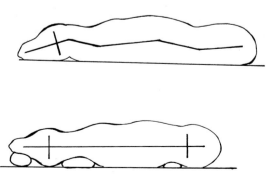

■ **FIG. 16.1** Positioning alterations necessary for a lateral spine. Sponges are used to support the midcervical, midlumbar, and skull regions to keep the spine parallel to the table.

■ **FIG. 16.2** Positioning alterations necessary for a lateral spine. Sponges are used to support the sternum and between the hind legs to prevent rotation of the spine.

CERVICAL SPINE

Ventrodorsal View

The patient is placed in dorsal recumbency with the head extended cranially and the front limbs pulled caudally alongside the body. The patient must be restrained in a true ventrodorsal posture, and the cervical spine must be parallel to the cassette. A sponge pad or cotton can be placed under the midcervical region to eliminate any distortion in this area. The field of view should include the base of the skull, the entire cervical spine, and the first few thoracic vertebrae.

For large patients that weigh over 50 pounds, it may be necessary to radiograph the cervical spine in two separate areas. Two radiographs are required because of the extreme difference in thickness between the caudal and the cranial cervical spine. For example, the first area should include the base of the skull and C-1 to C-4, centering the x-ray beam at C2-3. The second area should include C-4 to T-1, centering the x-ray beam at C5-6.

BEAM CENTER: Over C4-5 intervertebral space
MEASUREMENT: C5-6 intervertebral space

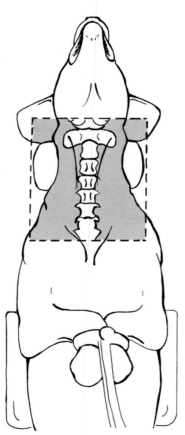

■ **FIG. 16.3** Correct positioning for the ventrodorsal view of the cervical spine.

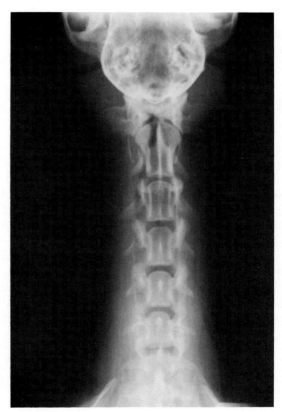

■ **FIG. 16.4** Radiograph of the ventrodorsal view of the cervical spine.

Extended Lateral View

The patient is placed in lateral recumbency with the head and neck extended and the front limbs pulled in a caudal direction. Gentle traction should be placed on the cervical region by pulling the head of the patient in a cranial direction. This traction can be accomplished manually by stretching the cervical spine, or a length of roll gauze can be tied around the nose behind the canine teeth and pulled cranially. A foam wedge pad is placed under the mandible to eliminate skull obliquity. To position the cervical spine so that it is parallel to the cassette, it may be necessary to place a sponge wedge pad or cotton under the midcervical region. The field of view should include the base of the skull, the entire cervical spine, and a few thoracic vertebrae.

For large patients that weigh over 50 pounds, it may be necessary to radiograph the cervical spine in two sections, making sure to overlap the two views. For example, the first section of the spine should include the base of the skull to C-4, centering the x-ray beam at the C2-3 interspace. The second section will then include C-4 to T-1, centering the x-ray beam at the C5-6 interspace.

BEAM CENTER: Intervertebral space of C-4 and C-5
MEASUREMENT: Over level of C-7 (thoracic inlet)

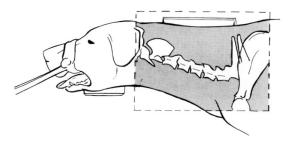

■ **FIG. 16.5** Correct positioning for the lateral view of the cervical spine.

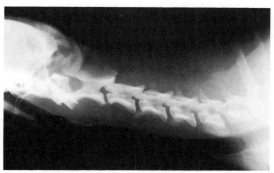

■ **FIG. 16.6** Radiograph of the lateral view of the cervical spine.

Flexed Lateral View

The patient is placed in lateral recumbency with the front limbs pulled in a caudal direction. A length of roll gauze or rope is tied around the mandible behind the canine teeth, and the free end of the line is placed between the forelimbs. Gentle traction is placed on the free end of the gauze, and the head is pulled caudally toward the humeri. Care must be taken not to hyperflex the neck, which may cause tracheal trauma or collapse of an endotracheal tube. It may be necessary to elevate the vertebrae with a sponge wedge pad or cotton to the level of the thoracic spine. An appropriate size cassette should be used so that the field of view includes the base of the skull to the first few thoracic vertebrae.

BEAM CENTER: C3-4 intervertebral space
MEASUREMENT: Over level of C-7 (thoracic inlet)

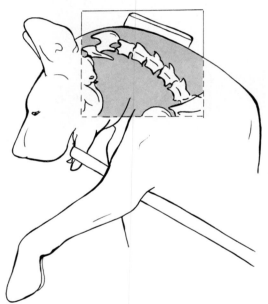

■ **FIG. 16.7** Correct positioning for the flexed lateral view of the cervical spine.

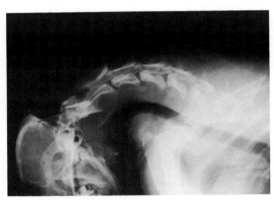

■ **FIG. 16.8** Radiograph of the flexed lateral view of the cervical spine.

Hyperextended Lateral View

The patient is placed in lateral recumbency with the front limbs extended caudally. The head and neck region is extended in a dorsal direction until resistance is met. A foam wedge pad or cotton is placed under the mandible to alleviate skull obliquity and under the midcervical region to align the vertebrae. The field of view should include the base of the skull to the first few thoracic vertebrae.

BEAM CENTER: C3-4 intervertebral space
MEASUREMENT: Over level of T-1 (thoracic inlet)

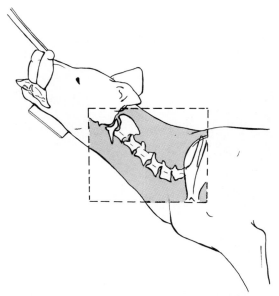

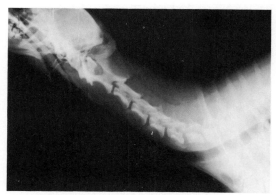

■ **FIG. 16.10** Radiograph of the extended lateral view of the cervical spine.

■ **FIG. 16.9** Correct positioning of the extended lateral view of the cervical spine.

THORACIC SPINE

Ventrodorsal View

The patient is placed in dorsal recumbency with the front limbs extended cranially. The rear limbs can assume a normal position. The animal must be maintained in a true ventrodorsal position so that the sternum is superimposed on the thoracic spine. A V trough placed under the lumbar region can assist in maintaining this position. The field of view should include all of the thoracic vertebrae from C-7 to L-1.

BEAM CENTER: Over level of caudal border of scapula (T-6)
MEASUREMENT: At highest point of sternum

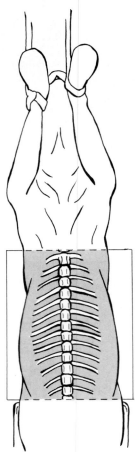

■ **FIG. 16.11** Correct positioning for the ventrodorsal view of the thoracic spine.

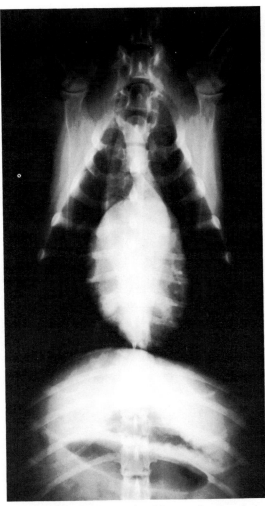

■ **FIG. 16.12** Radiograph of the ventrodorsal view of the thoracic spine.

Lateral View

The patient is placed in lateral recumbency with the front and rear limbs moderately extended in opposite directions away from the body. The sternum is elevated with a sponge wedge pad to eliminate any rotation of the thoracic vertebrae. To ensure proper positioning, the sternum should be the same distance to the tabletop as the thoracic spine. The thoracic spine is centered to the cassette, and the field of view should include the area from the 7th cervical vertebral body to the 1st lumbar vertebral body.

BEAM CENTER: Over 7th thoracic vertebral body
MEASUREMENT: At level of 7th rib

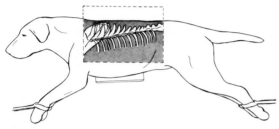

■ **FIG. 16.13** Correct positioning for the .lateral view of the thoracic spine.

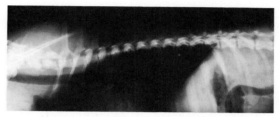

■ **FIG. 16.14** Radiograph of the lateral view of the thoracic spine.

THORACOLUMBAR SPINE

Ventrodorsal View

The patient is placed in dorsal recumbency with the front limbs extended cranially. The hind limbs can assume a normal position. The patient must be maintained in a true ventrodorsal position with the sternum superimposed over the thoracic spinal column. A V trough may be helpful in stabilizing the animal. The spine is centered to the cassette, and the field of view should include all of the thoracic and lumbar vertebrae.

BEAM CENTER: Over thoracolumbar junction
MEASUREMENT: At thoracolumbar junction

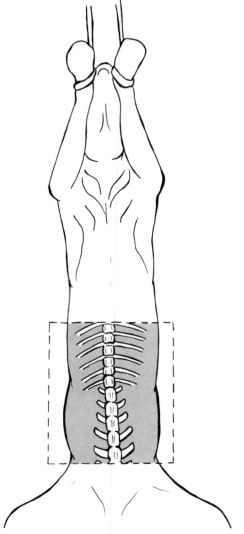

■ **FIG. 16.15** Correct positioning for the ventrodorsal view of the thoracolumbar spine.

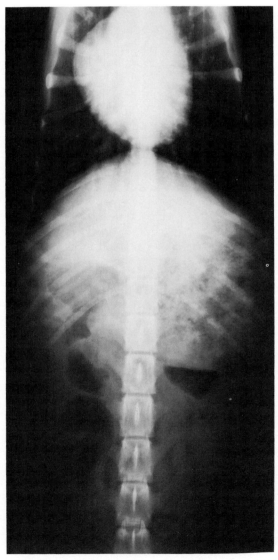

■ **FIG. 16.16** Radiograph of the ventrodorsal view of the thoracolumbar spine.

Lateral View

The patient is placed in lateral recumbency with the front and rear limbs pulled in opposite directions away from the body. A sponge wedge pad is placed under the sternum so that it is elevated to the same horizontal plane as the thoracic vertebrae. The spine should be centered to the cassette, and the field of view should include the entire thoracolumbar spine.

BEAM CENTER: Over thoracolumbar junction
MEASUREMENT: At thoracolumbar junction

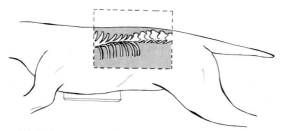

■ **FIG. 16.17** Correct positioning for the lateral view of the thoracolumbar spine.

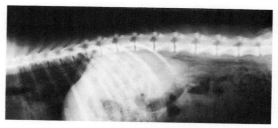

■ **FIG. 16.18** Radiograph of the lateral view of the thoracolumbar spine.

LUMBAR SPINE

Ventrodorsal View

The patient is placed in dorsal recumbency with the front limbs extended cranially and the rear limbs in a normal position. To maintain a true ventrodorsal position, a V trough can be placed under the thoracic region. The spine should be centered to the cassette, and the field of view should include the entire lumbar spine from the 13th thoracic vertebral body to the 1st sacral vertebral body.

BEAM CENTER: Over 4th lumbar vertebral body
MEASUREMENT: At level of 1st lumbar vertebral body

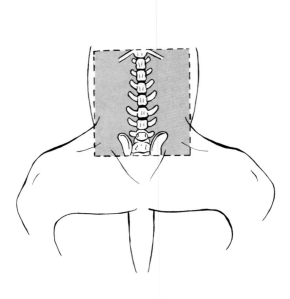

■ **FIG. 16.19** Correct positioning for the ventrodorsal view of the lumbar spine.

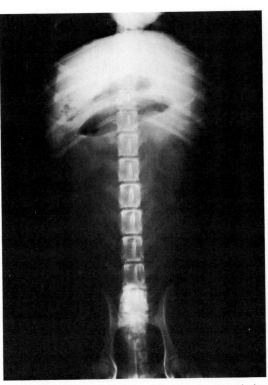

■ **FIG. 16.20** Radiograph of the ventrodorsal view of the lumbar spine.

Lateral View

The patient is placed in lateral recumbency with the front and rear limbs in moderate extension. A sponge wedge pad should be placed under the sternum to eliminate any rotation of the lumbar spine. It may be necessary to place a sponge pad or cotton under the midlumbar region to achieve proper alignment. The lumbar spine is centered to the cassette, and the field of view should include the entire lumbar vertebrae from the 13th thoracic vertebral body to the 1st sacral vertebral body.

BEAM CENTER: Over level of 4th lumbar vertebral body
MEASUREMENT: At level of 1st lumbar vertebral body

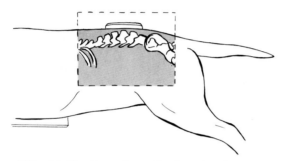

■ **FIG. 16.21** Correct positioning for the lateral view of the lumbar spine.

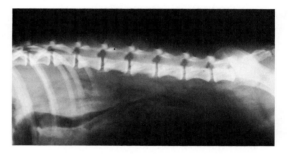

■ **FIG. 16.22** Radiograph of the lateral view of the lumbar spine.

SACRUM

Ventrodorsal View

The patient is placed in dorsal recumbency with the rear limbs in a normal position. A V trough can be placed under the thoracic region to maintain a true ventrodorsal position. The sacrum is centered to the cassette. The x-ray tube is directed at a 30-degree angle toward the head and centered over the sacrum. The field of view should include the area from the 6th lumbar vertebral body to the iliac crests.

Positioning for the lateral sacrum is the same as for the lateral pelvis.

BEAM CENTER: Over level of sacrum
MEASUREMENT: At level of sacrum

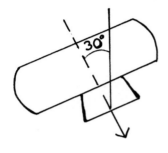

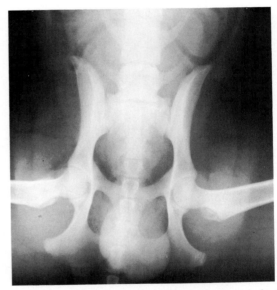

■ **FIG. 16.24** Radiograph of the ventrodorsal view of the sacrum.

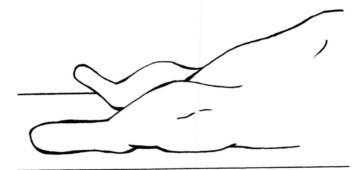

■ **FIG. 16.23** Correct positioning for the ventrodorsal view of the sacrum.

CAUDAL SPINE

Ventrodorsal View

The patient is placed in dorsal recumbency with the rear limbs in a normal position. The body can be maintained in a true ventrodorsal position with the aid of a V trough placed under the thoracic region. The tail is extended in a caudal direction and centered in the middle of the cassette. For animals that have a natural curl to the tail, it may be necessary to tape the tail to the cassette.

BEAM CENTER: Over area of interest
MEASUREMENT: At proximal tail

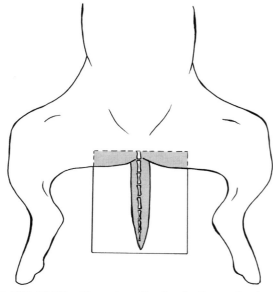

■ **FIG. 16.25**   Correct positioning for the ventrodorsal view of the caudal spine.

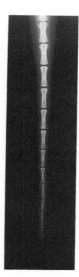

■ **FIG. 16.26**   Radiograph of the ventrodorsal view of the caudal spine.

Lateral View

The patient is placed in lateral recumbency with the tail extended in a caudal direction. It may be necessary to raise the cassette and maintain it on a foam block of appropriate thickness. Elevating the cassette allows the tail to remain parallel to the tabletop and in alignment with the rest of the spine. The tail is centered to the cassette.

BEAM CENTER: Over area of interest
MEASUREMENT: At proximal tail

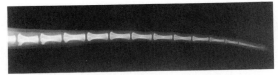

■ **FIG. 16.28** Radiograph of the lateral view of the caudal spine.

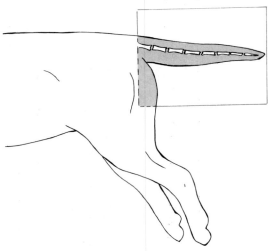

■ **FIG. 16.27** Correct positioning for the lateral view of the caudal spine.

BIBLIOGRAPHY

Douglas SW, Herrtage ME, Williamson HD: *Principles of Veterinary Radiography,* 4th ed. Bailliere Tindall, Philadelphia, 1987.

Habel RE: *Applied Veterinary Anatomy,* 2nd ed. RE Habel, Ithaca, NY, 1978.

Kleine LJ, Warren RG: *Small Animal Radiography.* CV Mosby, St. Louis, 1982.

Ryan GD: *Radiographic Positioning of Small Animals.* Lea & Febiger, Philadelphia, 1981.

Schebitz H, Wilkins H: *Atlas of Radiographic Anatomy of the Dog and Cat.* WB Saunders, Philadelphia, 1986.

Smallwood JE, Shively MJ: Nomenclature for radiographic views of limbs. Equine Pract 1:41–45, 1979.

Ticer JW: *Radiographic Technique in Small Animal Practice,* 2nd ed. WB Saunders, Philadelphia, 1984.

SMALL ANIMAL
SOFT TISSUE

CHAPTER OUTLINE

- PHARYNX
- THORAX
- ABDOMEN

INTRODUCTION

The term soft tissue is used for the areas of the body that surround the skeletal structures. Unlike radiography of bone tissue, visualization of soft tissue can be difficult because it involves only slight differences in radiographic density. Production of a soft tissue radiograph that has high contrast between the various adjacent soft structures is nearly impossible without the use of contrast media. In order to achieve the correct contrast, density, and visualization, a number of factors must be considered:

1. To attain a long scale of contrast with good visualization of the internal soft tissue structures, a relatively high kilovoltage and low milliamperage-seconds is used.

2. A grid is necessary for areas of dense tissue to maintain image clarity and radiographic detail.

3. An exposure time of 1/30 second or less is necessary for radiography of the thorax to minimize motion due to cardiac and respiratory movement.

4. Proper preparation is necessary for abdominal radiography. The patient should be fasted for 12 to 24 hours and given a cleansing enema at least 1 hour prior to radiography.

5. Exposure of the thorax and abdomen must be taken on the correct phase of respiration: thorax = inspiration, abdomen = expiration.

211

PHARYNX

Lateral View

The patient is placed in lateral recumbency with the forelimbs pulled in a caudal direction. The head and neck are extended cranially and placed in a true lateral position. A sponge wedge pad placed under the mandible helps eliminate obliquity of the skull and frees the larynx from the mandible to allow better visualization of the laryngeal region. The air passages of the upper respiratory tract act as a negative contrast agent and permit the soft tissue structures of the pharyngeal region to be differentiated. The field of view should include the entire area of the neck between the lateral canthus of the eye and the 3rd cervical vertebral body.

BEAM CENTER: Over pharynx
MEASUREMENT: At level of base of skull

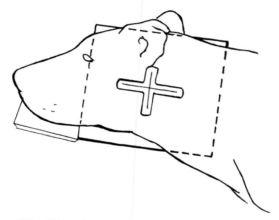

■ **FIG. 17.1** Correct positioning for the lateral view of the pharynx.

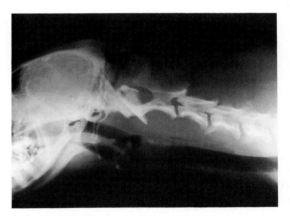

■ **FIG. 17.2** Radiograph of the lateral view of the pharynx.

THORAX

Dorsoventral View

The dorsoventral view of the thorax is preferred for the evaluation of the heart because the heart is closer to the sternum and is in near normal suspended position within the thorax. Unfortunately, larger dogs may be difficult to position for the dorsoventral projection because of their deep chests. The dorsoventral view requires great care to ensure that the sternum is superimposed over the vertebral column. If this position is impossible to execute, it may be necessary to attempt a ventrodorsal projection.

The patient is placed in sternal recumbency with the thoracic vertebrae superimposed over the sternum. The forelegs are pulled slightly forward to prevent the elbows from tucking under the thorax. The rear legs are allowed to flex in a natural crouching position. This crouched position may be difficult for the canine patient with hip dysplasia, and it may be necessary to consider the ventrodorsal view. The head is lower and placed between the two forelimbs. The field of view should include the entire thorax. The rule is "the thorax is inside the rib cage"; if you include all of the ribs, you will x-ray the whole thorax.

The exposure must be taken at the peak of inspiration to allow complete radiographic visualization of the lung tissue. The patient's breathing should be observed several times before making the exposure. This allows the radiographer ample time to make the exposure at the proper phase of respiration.

BEAM CENTER: Over caudal border of scapula
MEASUREMENT: At level of caudal border of scapula

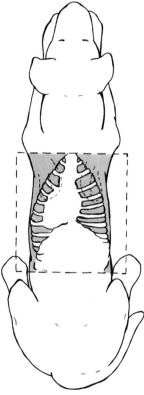

■ **FIG. 17.3** Correct positioning for the dorsoventral view of the thorax.

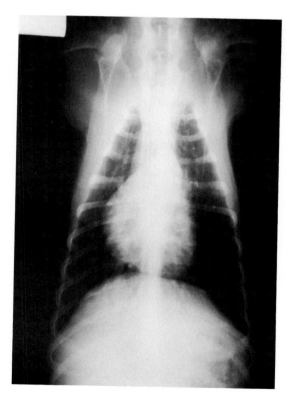

■ **FIG. 17.4** Radiograph of the dorsoventral view of the thorax.

Ventrodorsal View

The ventrodorsal view of the thorax is advocated when a full view of the lung fields is necessary. This projection provides a better view of the accessory lung lobes and caudal mediastinum. Although it is easier to control a patient in ventrodorsal position, this view is contraindicated for patients that have obvious respiratory distress. Placing such an animal on its back would be dangerous and could possibly cause further respiratory compromise.

The patient is placed in dorsal recumbency with the forelimbs extended cranially. The hind limbs can assume a normal position. Great care must be taken to ensure that the patient is in a true ventrodorsal posture. The sternum must be superimposed over the spine. If rotation is encountered, a V trough or sandbags placed under the pelvic region may be helpful. The field of view should include the entire thorax. The rule is "the thorax is inside the rib cage"; if you include all of the ribs, you will x-ray the whole thorax.

The exposure is taken at the peak of inspiration. The patient's breathing should be observed several times before making an exposure. This allows the radiographer ample time to make the exposure at the proper phase of respiration.

BEAM CENTER: Over caudal border of scapula
MEASUREMENT: At level of caudal border of scapula

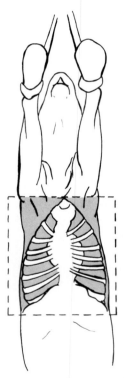

■ **FIG. 17.5** Correct positioning for the ventrodorsal view of the thorax.

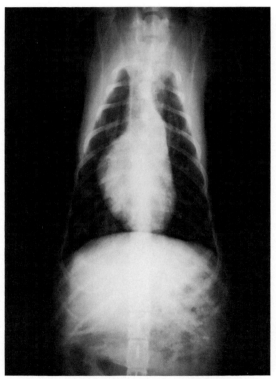

■ **FIG. 17.6** Radiograph of the ventrodorsal view of the thorax.

Lateral View

A right lateral study of the thorax has been recommended for a more accurate view of the cardiac silhouette. Not all veterinary radiologists agree with this recommendation, and some prefer a left lateral thorax. We will not argue either point here. In some instances it will be necessary to expose both right and left lateral projections when subtle lung metastasis is suspected.

The patient is placed in lateral recumbency, left or right side down, with the front limbs extended cranially. Extension of the forelimbs helps to eliminate superimposition of the triceps and humeri over the cranial aspect of the thorax. The hind limbs should be pulled slightly in a caudal direction to maintain a proper degree of symmetry of the thoracic cage. The head is extended slightly to avoid displacement of the trachea. The sternum is elevated with the use of a foam wedge pad to a level above the x-ray table equal to that of the thoracic vertebrae. Elevating the sternum will prevent rotation of the thorax. The field of view should include the entire thoracic cavity from the line of the manubrium sterni caudally to the 1st lumbar vertebral body. The rule is "the thorax is inside the rib cage"; if you include all of the ribs, you will x-ray the whole thorax.

The exposure should be taken at the peak of inspiration.

BEAM CENTER: Over caudal border of scapula
MEASUREMENT: At level of caudal border of scapula

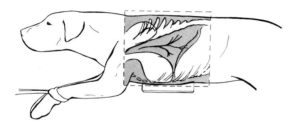

■ **FIG. 17.7** Correct positioning for the lateral view of the thorax.

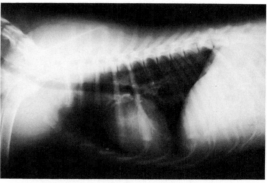

■ **FIG. 17.8** Radiograph of the lateral view of the thorax.

Lateral View with Horizontal Beam

The lateral view with a horizontal beam is used to confirm the presence of fluid or free air in the thoracic cavity and to facilitate quantifying the amount present. Two positions can be utilized: (1) the standing lateral and (2) the sternally recumbent lateral. The standing lateral is not as desirable because of superimposition of the humeral soft tissues over the cranial thorax in a natural standing posture.

For the sternally recumbent lateral, the patient is placed in sternal recumbency on top of a foam pad that is approximately 5 to 10 cm thick. The height of elevation is determined by the size of the animal and the cassette used. The forelimbs and head are gently extended in a cranial direction. The hind limbs are allowed to assume a natural crouched position. The cassette is placed in a vertical position against the lateral side of the patient. A commercially available cassette holder or positioning devices are helpful to support the cassette in place. The thorax should be centered to the cassette, and the field of view should include from the manubrium sterni caudally to the 1st lumbar vertebral body. The field of view should include the entire thorax. The rule is "the thorax is inside the rib cage"; if you include all of the ribs, you will x-ray the whole thorax. (Note: The same projection can be performed for the abdomen.)

BEAM CENTER: Over caudal border of scapula
MEASUREMENT: At level of caudal border of scapula

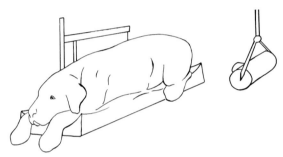

■ **FIG. 17.10** Correct positioning for the recumbent lateral view of the thorax using a horizontal x-ray beam.

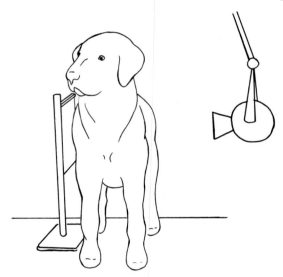

■ **FIG. 17.9** Correct positioning for the standing lateral view of the thorax using a horizontal x-ray beam.

Lateral Decubitus View (Ventrodorsal View with Horizontal Beam)

The lateral decubitus projection, along with the standing lateral, is used to confirm quantitative thoracic fluid or air. This study is made with the animal in lateral recumbency with a horizontal x-ray beam directed ventrodorsally. The position is further specified according to the side that is down (i.e., left decubitus).

The patient is placed in lateral recumbency on top of a 5- to 10-cm thick foam pad. The foam pad is necessary to elevate the patient off the tabletop and allow visualization of both sides of the thorax. The forelimbs and the head are extended cranially. The hind limbs are pulled slightly in a caudal direction to keep the spine of the patient close to the cassette. The thorax is centered to the cassette, which is placed behind the patient in a vertical posture. The field of view should include the entire thorax. (Note: The same projection can be performed for the abdomen.)

BEAM CENTER: Over caudal border of scapula
MEASUREMENT: At level of caudal border of scapula

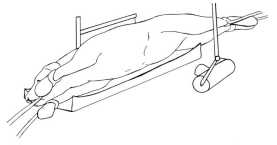

■ **FIG. 17.11** Correct positioning for the ventrodorsal decubitus view of the thorax using a horizontal x-ray beam.

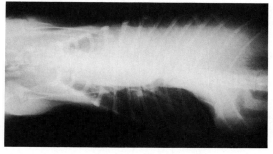

■ **FIG. 17.12** Radiograph of the ventrodorsal decubitus view of the thorax (exhibiting fluid) using a horizontal x-ray beam.

ABDOMEN

Ventrodorsal View

The patient is placed in dorsal recumbency with the hind limbs positioned in normal flexion. A V trough or sandbags placed under the thoracic region may be helpful in maintaining a true ventrodorsal posture. The field of view should include the entire abdomen from the diaphragm to the level of the femoral head. With larger patients, it may not be possible to include the entire abdomen on one cassette. In this case, two radiographs should be taken: one of the cranial abdomen and the other including the caudal abdomen.

The exposure for an abdominal radiograph is taken during the expiratory pause so that the diaphragm is in a cranial position and not placing any compression on the abdominal contents.

BEAM CENTER: Over caudal aspect of 13th rib (for feline patients, center two to three fingerbreadths caudal to the 13th rib)
MEASUREMENT: At level of caudal aspect of 13th rib

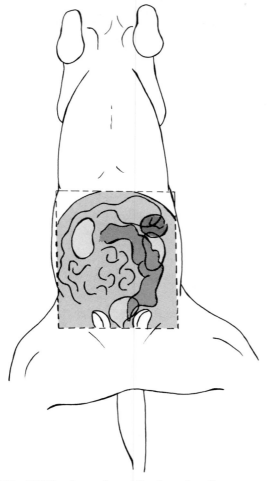

■ **FIG. 17.13** Correct positioning for the ventrodorsal view of the abdomen.

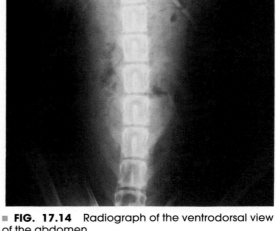

■ **FIG. 17.14** Radiograph of the ventrodorsal view of the abdomen.

Lateral View

The patient is placed in right lateral recumbency with the hind limbs extended in a caudal direction. The right lateral view is chosen to facilitate longitudinal separation of the kidneys. Pulling the hind limbs caudally helps eliminate superimposition of the femoral muscles over the caudal portion of the abdomen. A foam pad of suitable thickness is placed between the femurs to eliminate rotation of the pelvis and caudal abdomen. Another foam pad should be placed under the sternum to elevate it to the same level as the thoracic spine. The abdomen should be centered to the cassette, and the field of view should include the diaphragm caudally to the femoral head.

The exposure is made during the expiratory pause so that the diaphragm is displaced cranially.

BEAM CENTER: Over caudal aspect of 13th rib (for feline patients, center two to three fingerbreadths caudal to 13th rib)
MEASUREMENT: At level of caudal aspect of 13th rib

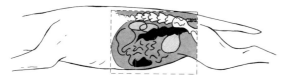

■ **FIG. 17.15** Correct positioning for the lateral view of the abdomen.

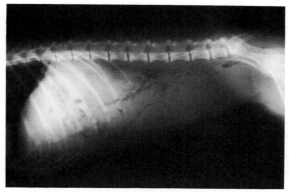

■ **FIG. 17.16** Radiograph of the lateral view of the abdomen.

BIBLIOGRAPHY

Douglas SW, Herrtage ME, Williamson HD: *Principles of Veterinary Radiography*, 4th ed. Bailliere Tindall, Philadelphia, 1987.

Habel RE: *Applied Veterinary Anatomy*, 2nd ed. RE Habel, Ithaca, NY, 1978.

Kirk RW: *Current Veterinary Therapy: Small Animal Practice—Thoracic Radiography*. WB Saunders, Philadelphia, 1986.

Kleine LJ, Warren RG: *Small Animal Radiography*. CV Mosby, St. Louis, 1982.

Ryan GD: *Radiographic Positioning of Small Animals*. Lea & Febiger, Philadelphia, 1981.

Schebitz H, Wilkins H: *Atlas of Radiographic Anatomy of the Dog and Cat*. WB Saunders, Philadelphia, 1986.

Smallwood JE, Shively MJ: Nomenclature for radiographic views of limbs. Equine Pract 1:41–45, 1979.

Ticer JW: *Radiographic Technique in Small Animal Practice*, 2nd ed. WB Saunders, Philadelphia, 1984.

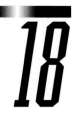

SPECIAL PROCEDURES

GLOSSARY

ANGIOCARDIOGRAPHY: An intravenous radiographic contrast study evaluating the vascular system and chambers of the heart.

ANGIOGRAPHY: An intravenous radiographic contrast study evaluating the vascular system.

ANTEGRADE URETHROGRAM: A method of urethrography in which the contrast medium is voided from the urinary bladder.

ARTHROGRAPHY: A radiographic contrast technique evaluating the articular cartilage, joint space, and joint capsule.

BARIUM SULFATE: A common positive contrast medium that is available in various forms and is often used as a suspension in gastrointestinal evaluations.

CHOLECYSTOGRAPHY: An oral or intravenous radiographic contrast study evaluating the bile ducts and gallbladder.

CONTRAST MEDIUM: A substance that is either radiolucent or radiopaque that can be administered to increase radiographic contrast within an organ or system.

CYSTOGRAPHY: Radiographic contrast studies evaluating the urinary bladder.

DOUBLE CONTRAST: A radiographic contrast technique which uses a combination of positive and negative contrast media simultaneously.

DOUBLE-CONTRAST CYSTOGRAM: A radiographic study of the urinary bladder involving distending the bladder with a gas and then adding a small amount of positive iodinated contrast medium.

ESOPHAGRAPHY: A radiographic contrast study performed to evaluate esophageal function and morphology.

EXCRETORY UROGRAPHY: An intravenous radiographic contrast study of the kidney and ureters.

FISTULA: An abnormal tube-like passage within body tissue.

FISTULOGRAPHY: A positive or negative radiographic contrast study used to determine the depth and origin of a fistulous tract.

GASTROGRAPHY: A radiographic contrast study performed to evaluate the size, shape, position, and morphology of the stomach.

INTRAVENOUS PYELOGRAM (IVP): A radiographic contrast study of the kidney structure and collection system.

INTRAVENOUS UROGRAM (IVU): A radiographic contrast study of the kidney structure and collection system.

LOWER GASTROINTESTINAL STUDY: Commonly referred to as a **barium enema**; a radiographic contrast study evaluating the rectum, colon, and cecum.

LYMPHOGRAPHY: A radiographic contrast study evaluating lymphatic vessels and lymph nodes.

continued

G L O S S A R Y   *Continued*

MYELOGRAPHY: A radiographic contrast study evaluating the subarachnoid space surrounding the spinal cord.

NEGATIVE CONTRAST AGENTS: Gases that are more radiolucent to x-rays than are soft tissue and have a black appearance on a radiograph.

NEPHROGRAM: A phase of an excretory urogram characterized by the diffuse opacification of the renal parenchyma.

PARASYMPATHOLYTIC AGENTS: Drugs that eliminate the influence of the parasympathetic nervous system.

PNEUMOCYSTOGRAM: A negative-contrast radiographic technique evaluating the urinary bladder.

PNEUMOPERITONEOGRAPHY: A negative-contrast radiographic study consisting of the introduction of a gas into the peritoneal cavity.

POSITIVE CONTRAST AGENTS: Substances containing elements of high atomic number that are more radiopaque to x-rays than are tissue and bone and have a white appearance on a radiograph.

POSITIVE CONTRAST CYSTOGRAM: A radiographic study of the bladder involving distention of the bladder with positive iodinated contrast medium.

PYELOGRAM: A phase of an excretory urogram characterized by the opacification of the renal collection system.

RETROGRADE URETHROGRAM: A method of urethrography by which the contrast medium is infused via a catheter placed at the distal end of the urethra.

SIALOGRAPHY: A radiographic contrast study evaluating the salivary glands and ducts.

TRI-IODINATED COMPOUNDS: A common component of iodinated positive contrast media that contains three atoms of iodine per molecule.

UPPER GASTROINTESTINAL STUDY (UGI): A radiographic contrast study evaluating the stomach and small intestines.

URETHROGRAPHY: A radiographic contrast study evaluating the urethra.

VAGINOGRAPHY: A radiographic contrast study evaluating the female reproductive organs.

INDICATIONS

Special radiographic procedures are used to supplement or confirm information garnered from routine survey radiographs. Under normal circumstances, soft tissue structures or organs are difficult or impossible to identify on plain films owing to lack of contrast. A **contrast medium** is a substance that is either radiolucent or radiopaque that can be administered to an animal to increase radiographic contrast within an organ or system. With the use of a contrast medium, soft tissue structures can be visualized and the structure under investigation can be evaluated for size, shape, and position. In addition, defects in the mucosal surface of an organ or luminal contents can be identified. In some instances it is possible to evaluate organ function or assess the physiologic condition. Although contrast studies can be extremely helpful for a complete diagnosis, at no time should a special procedure replace routine survey radiography.

CONTRAST MEDIA

There are two basic categories of contrast media: positive and negative. **Positive contrast agents**, such as barium or iodine compounds, contain elements of high atomic number. These agents absorb more x-rays than do soft tissue or bone. Positive contrast media are radiopaque to x-rays and appear white on a radiograph. These compounds can be used to fill or outline a hollow organ (e.g., urinary bladder and alimentary tract) or they can be injected into a blood vessel (sterile, water-based compounds only) for immediate visualization of the vascular supply or for subsequent excretion evaluation. **Negative contrast agents** consist of gases (e.g., oxygen and carbon dioxide) that have a low specific gravity. Substances with a low specific gravity are more radiolucent to x-rays than is soft tissue and have a black appearance on a radiograph.

Many different compounds are used as radiographic contrast media. In addition, various manufacturers market identical contrast agents under different names and concentrations. Although it is virtually impossible to become familiar with all of the contrast agents available, it is possible to place them into one of three general categories: (1) positive-contrast iodinated preparations, (2) positive-contrast barium sulfate preparations, and (3) negative-contrast gases. Each category has basic characteristics that are used to classify contrast agents. These characteristics allow a better understanding of each individual medium available.

The majority of agents currently available are intended for human use; however, some products are specifically approved by the U.S. Food and Drug Administration for animals. The choice of contrast agent should be made on the basis of the type of study to be performed, the condition of the patient, the possible side effects, and the judgment of the veterinarian that it is the best available product for use.

Iodine Preparations

The iodine compounds are divided into two subcategories: water-soluble agents and viscous/oily agents.

Water-Soluble Agents

Water-soluble iodine preparations make up the largest group of contrast agents. Most water-soluble iodine preparations are opaque to x-rays, pharmacologically inert, low in viscosity for rapid intravenous injection, low in toxicity, rapidly excreted by the kidneys, and chemically stable so no iodine is released in the body.

The choice of radiographic contrast agent is a matter of personal preference. The **tri-iodinated compounds** are widely accepted because they are well tolerated by the body and provide excellent contrast. Tri-iodinated compounds contain three atoms of iodine per molecule. They are supplied as sodium or meglumine salts of iothalamic diatrizoic or metrizoic acids, or as a mixture of these two salts.

In general, sodium salts are less viscous. The meglumine salts reduce toxicity, minimize high sodium concentrations, and lessen tissue irritability. These contrast agents are normally injected into a vascular system for immediate visualization of the system or subsequent demonstration of the excretory system. In addition, water-soluble agents can be infused into the bladder via a urinary catheter to visualize the urinary mucosa and bladder shape and size.

Possible toxicity is a concern of any pharmaceutical. The ionic (salt) preparations all have a local irritant effect and should be administered intravascularly or infused into an organ. Because of this property, iodine agents are contraindicated for myelography and arthrography. An intravenous injection of an iodinated contrast agent can cause side effects such as mild discomfort and nausea in an animal patient. Although extremely rare, more severe reactions such as cardiac arrest, hypovolemia, and anaphylaxis have been cited in a few clinical cases in the past. In general, sodium salts are more toxic than meglumine salts but are included in the compound to reduce viscosity for easier administration.

Low-osmolar contrast media, such as metrizamide, iopamidol, and iohexol, are nonionic and reduce adverse side effects due to hyperosmolarity. Although expensive, these contrast agents are suitable for intravascular studies as well as myelographic studies.

Water-soluble contrast agents are sometimes indicated for gastrointestinal use in patients that have a suspected perforation. If this type of contrast agent were to enter the alimentary tract through a perforation, it would be rapidly absorbed due to its solubility. These agents are not used routinely, however, because of their fast transit time and hypertonicity. The iodine agents lose their contrast because they rapidly absorb fluid in the alimentary tract and become progressively dilute. With these agents, mucosal detail is poor. In some cases, the contrast agent is absorbed into the vascular system and excreted through the urinary system, giving rise to a confusing radiologic pattern.

Oily/Viscous Agents

Oily/viscous agents have very little application in veterinary radiography. Their use is limited to lymphography.

Oily contrast media consist of iodized oils. The oil contains a suspension of propyliodone in either water or arachidic oils. Because of their viscous nature and insolubility in water, they are not resorbed in the body and produce fat embolism. The iodized oils cannot be administered intravascularly. In addition, the agent does not mix with cerebrospinal fluid during myelography. The oils tend to coagulate within the spinal canal and fail to outline lesions clearly. Current practice does not include oily media for myelography. If the agent is not removed, the absorption rate within the spinal canal is extremely slow. The absorption rate is estimated at approximately 1 ml/year.

Barium Preparations

Barium sulfate is a positive contrast suspension and is the medium of choice for radiographic studies of the gastrointestinal tract. Because it is completely insoluble, it is not diluted by alimentary secretions and is not absorbed through the intestines. Barium is available in various forms (e.g., liquid, paste, and powder for reconstitution with water).

The primary disadvantage of barium sulfate is that if it should pass through a perforation in the alimentary tract into the thorax or abdomen, it would not be absorbed or eliminated. The barium can remain indefinitely and could potentially produce a granulomatous reaction. In cases in which a perforation is suspected, it is advisable to use a water-soluble contrast medium. If, however, the water-soluble study is negative, a barium study should follow to avoid missing a perforation.

Morbidity and mortality are no worse than those with a leakage of gastrointestinal contents, if the barium is surgically flushed out of the abdominal cavity within 6 to 8 hours. Barium that is inadvertently aspirated into the trachea is usually cleared by cough. If the medium reaches the small bronchi and alveoli, it is unlikely to be removed.

Negative Contrast Agents — Gases

Gases used for negative-contrast radiographic studies include air, oxygen, nitrogen, nitrous oxide, and carbon dioxide. Of all the gases available, air, oxygen, and carbon dioxide are most frequently used. Carbon dioxide has an advantage over room air in that it is better absorbed into the body when administered into a hollow organ; room air can cause air emboli.

Gases are inexpensive, relatively safe, and easy to administer. Negative contrast media enhance the contrast between the various soft tissues but produce less mucosal detail than positive contrast media. Some special procedures call for the use of both negative and positive contrast media, or **double contrast**. A double-contrast study gives optimum mucosal detail and avoids the masking of small anomalies by large volumes of positive contrast media.

PATIENT PREPARATION

Proper patient preparation is vital to a diagnostic radiographic study. Prior to the study, the gastrointestinal tract should be emptied by withholding food for 12 to 24 hours and, if necessary, administering a cleansing enema. The presence of any gastrointestinal contents can detract from a quality study and may obstruct view of certain areas of interest as a result of superimposition. Keep in mind that cathartics and enemas often produce gastrointestinal gas. To reduce the amount of gas present in the gastrointestinal tract during a study, the cathartic should be administered 4 to 12 hours prior to the radiographic procedure, and a radiographic study should not be administered within an hour of enema administration.

Evacuation of the gastrointestinal tract should be as atraumatic as possible, especially when working with an acutely ill patient. When an enema is contraindicated because of the poor condition of the patient, it is usually sufficient to fast the animal. If the patient's health is such that fasting would compromise the health further, mild nongranular nourishment such as baby food or other commercially available foods (e.g., Hill's a/d, Clinicare) can be given.

Many special radiographic procedures require the use of sedation or anesthesia. Caution must be used so that the procedure is not compromised by the anesthetic. For example, general anesthesia is contraindicated for a gastrointestinal study owing to subsequent slowed motility. If sedation is necessary, it should be limited to the use of a phenothiazine tranquilizer such as acepromazine maleate. Phenothiazine tranquilizers have only minimal effects on gastrointestinal motility or transit time. The use of **parasympatholytic agents** such as atropine should also be avoided for certain studies because of the anticholinergic effect.

CONTRAST STUDIES OF THE GASTROINTESTINAL TRACT

A patient presenting with diarrhea or vomiting is not uncommon in veterinary medicine. If medical management has failed and survey radiographs are inconclusive, a contrast study may be indicated.

Radiographic studies of the gastrointestinal tract consist of the introduction of contrast media either by oral administration or via an orogastric tube. Radiographs are then taken at intervals to evaluate changes in morphology, the rate of gastric emptying, and small bowel transit time. The studies described here do not include the use of fluoroscopy because the majority of veterinary practices do not have this type of equipment.

Esophagraphy

Esophagography is performed to evaluate esophageal function and morphology. An esophagram is indicated for patients with a history of regurgitation of undigested food, acute gagging, or dysphagia. This study consists of administering a positive contrast medium orally and exposing a number of radiographs during and after the swallow of the contrast agent. Liquid barium sulfate is usually the contrast medium of choice. Barium sulfate is also available in a thick paste form that is more difficult to swallow but that provides good mucosal coating of the esophagus. Barium may be mixed with canned and/or hard food to evaluate the function of the esophagus or for a partial obstruction that might be missed during a plain liquid barium swallow.

Precautions

When introducing a contrast medium orally, proper care must be taken to minimize the possibility of the patient aspirating the agent into the lungs. If a perforation or rupture is suspected, an iodinated contrast medium should be used rather than a barium compound. Beware of iodinated contrast agents if aspiration is likely. The hypertonicity of these agents, if the ionic variety is used, can cause massive fluid shifts into the lung. The iodinated contrast medium is readily absorbed by the body if it enters the thoracic cavity, whereas barium would not be absorbed and could remain indefinitely. A foreign substance such as barium could stimulate granuloma formation within the thoracic cavity.

T E C H N I Q U E   O U T L I N E

CONTRAST MEDIA:
70 to 100% barium sulfate (liquid and paste) or iodinated oral contrast

EQUIPMENT/SUPPLIES:
Optional canned/hard pet food

PATIENT PREPARATION:
None necessary

PROCEDURE

I.   Expose survey radiographs.

II.   Place patient in lateral recumbency on x-ray table.

III.   Slowly infuse liquid contrast medium into patient's cheek.

IV.   Expose several radiographs of the thorax to monitor the passage of contrast medium. The field of view should include the entire esophagus from the pharyngeal region to the stomach.) (Note: The first radiograph should be exposed within seconds of swallowing.)

V.   Repeat steps III and IV with the patient in dorsal recumbency.

VI.   Place the patient in lateral recumbency once again.

VII.   Slowly administer barium paste, and expose the radiograph during the swallow.

VIII.   If abnormalities are still not detected, mix the liquid contrast medium with canned and/or hard pet food and administer per os.

IX.   Radiographs are repeated; right and left lateral views may be indicated. Ventrodorsal views are contraindicated for patients with a dilated esophagus full of contrast medium. Placing the patient on its back may result in aspiration.

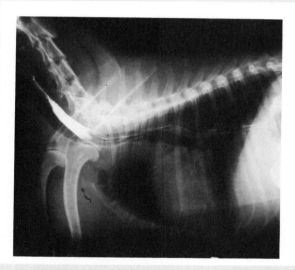

■ **FIG. 18.1** Radiograph of a lateral view of an esophagram immediately after administration of liquid barium.

Upper Gastrointestinal Study

An **upper gastrointestinal study (UGI)** is performed to evaluate the stomach and small intestines. A UGI series may be indicated for patients that have recurrent unresponsive vomiting, abnormal bowel movements, suspected foreign body or obstruction, chronic weight loss, or persistent abdominal pain.

The contrast medium is administered orally (per os or via stomach tube), and radiographs are taken during the passage of the agent. The UGI series is performed in a systematic manner so that the maximum amount of information can be obtained. Both positive and negative contrast media can be used if the stomach is the target. However, most studies are performed with the use of a positive contrast medium such as barium sulfate.

Precautions

If the patient is suspected of having a gastrointestinal perforation, barium sulfate is contraindicated. If barium were to enter the abdominal cavity, it would not be absorbed and may induce granuloma formation. In the instance of a perforation, an oral iodinated contrast medium should be used. Unfortunately, iodinated contrast media do not produce as much radiographic contrast. Iodine compounds tend to become diluted as they pass through the bowel because they draw extracellular fluid from the digestive tract. In addition, because of their osmotic activity, they are not recommended for use in dehydrated patients.

TECHNIQUE OUTLINE

CONTRAST MEDIA:
30 to 60% liquid barium sulfate or iodinated oral contrast

EQUIPMENT/SUPPLIES:
60-ml catheter-tip syringes
Orogastric tube

PATIENT PREPARATION:
Fast for 12 to 24 hours
Enema if necessary 2 to 4 hours prior to study
Sedate if necessary
(acepromazine maleate, 0.05 to 0.1 mg/kg IV)

PROCEDURE

I. Expose survey radiographs.

II. Administer barium to distend the stomach with contrast.
   A. Route: Per os by placing the positive contrast into the oral cavity and allowing the patient to swallow, or via orogastric tube. To ensure correct placement of the orogastric tube, infuse a small amount of water. If the tube is incorrectly placed and is located in the trachea, the patient should cough, signaling the technologist of incorrect placement.
   B. Dose: 4 to 8 ml/kg body weight.

III. Expose dorsoventral, ventrodorsal, right, and left lateral radiographs immediately after contrast administration.

IV. Expose right lateral ventrodorsal or dorsoventral radiographs at intervals until contrast reaches the large bowel (suggested times: 15, 30, 60 and 90 minutes).

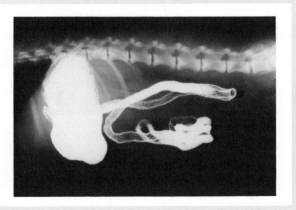

■ **FIG. 18.2** Lateral view of an upper gastrointestinal study exposed 5 minutes after the administration of barium.

T E C H N I Q U E   O U T L I N E   *Continued*

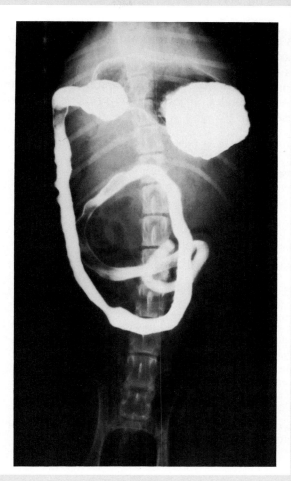

■ **FIG. 18.3** Ventrodorsal view of an upper gastrointestinal study exposed 5 minutes after the administration of liquid barium.

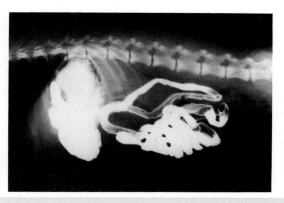

■ **FIG. 18.4** Lateral view of an upper gastrointestinal study exposed 30 minutes after the administration of liquid barium.

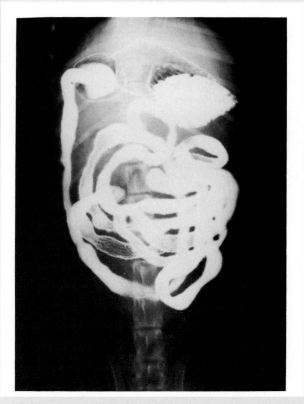

■ **FIG. 18.5** Ventrodorsal view of an upper gastrointestinal study exposed 30 minutes after the administration of liquid barium.

Gastrography

Gastrography is a relatively quick, simple technique to evaluate the size, shape, position, and morphology of the stomach. A gastrogram is indicated if the patient is experiencing acute or chronic vomiting, blood in the vomitus, or cranial abdominal pain.

The contrast medium is administered orally, and subsequent radiographs are exposed with the animal in various positions. Three different contrast studies can be performed: (1) positive, (2) negative, and (3) double. The positive- and negative-contrast gastrograms are primarily performed to evaluate gastric shape and size. The double-contrast gastrogram is the most diagnostic for examination of the gastric mucosal lining.

Precautions

A double-contrast gastrogram is not recommended for animals with a history of gastric distention and volvulus. Barium sulfate is contraindicated for a patient suspected of having a gastroenteric perforation. In such instances, an oral iodine preparation should be used.

TECHNIQUE OUTLINE

CONTRAST MEDIA:
Barium sulfate (liquid)
Air or carbon dioxide

EQUIPMENT/SUPPLIES:
Orogastric tube
60-ml catheter-tip syringes

PATIENT PREPARATION:
Fast for 12 to 24 hours or evacuate stomach of all contents
Sedate patient if necessary
(Suggested sedatives: acepromazine maleate and glucagon (glucagon is a gastrointestinal hypotonic agent that induces gastric hypomotility))

PROCEDURE

I. Expose survey radiographs.

II. Administer contrast medium orally or via orogastric tube.
  A. Positive-contrast gastrogram.
    1. 4 to 8 ml barium/kg.
  B. Negative-contrast gastrogram.
    1. 5 to 8 ml air or carbon dioxide/kg.
  C. Double-contrast gastrogram.
    1. 2 ml barium/kg.
    2. Air to follow barium: 10 to 20 ml air or carbon dioxide/kg.
    3. If patient regurgitates air, add additional air.
    4. Roll patient on its long axis.

III. Expose dorsoventral, ventrodorsal, left, and right lateral radiographs.

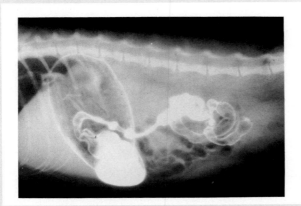

■ **FIG. 18.6** Lateral view of a double-contrast gastrogram.

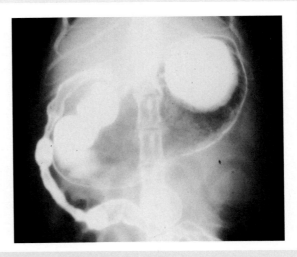

■ **FIG. 18.7** Ventrodorsal view of a double-contrast gastrogram.

Lower Gastrointestinal Study

A **lower gastrointestinal study (barium enema)** consists of the introduction of contrast medium via a catheter into the rectum, colon, and cecum. This study is indicated when full distention of the large intestine is necessary. Positive-, negative-, and double-contrast studies can be performed to evaluate the large intestine. A positive-contrast barium enema is indicated for a patient having abnormal bowel movements characterized by excessive mucus, bright-red blood in feces, pain during defecation, or diarrhea in high frequency. A barium enema can be used to detect intussusception, rectal mass, abdominal mass, stricture, or colonic obstruction.

Oral administration of a positive contrast medium does not fully distend the large bowel completely; thus, rectal administration is necessary. Unfortunately, many animals will not tolerate rectal infusion of contrast media without the use of chemical restraint. In most circumstances, anesthesia is required.

Precautions

Barium sulfate is contraindicated if the patient has a suspected perforation. In this case, an iodinated contrast medium should be used. Iodine compounds have the advantage of mixing well with the fluid of the colon, coating the mucosa without excessive distention, and allowing finer detail of the intestinal mucosal lining.

It is vital that the patient be properly prepared before the procedure. Any feces or ingesta left in the colon could create a confusing artifact. In addition to fasting the patient and administering a cleansing enema, it may be necessary to administer an oral cathartic such as a stool softener or mineral oil.

All colon examinations such as proctoscopy and rectal palpation should be performed at least 12 hours in advance, and enemas should be given at least 4 hours in advance. Rectal/colon examinations induce colonic spasms and gas accumulation. The collection of gas in the gastrointestinal tract can cause radiographic artifacts during a barium enema. Enema solution should consist of warm water or saline to cleanse the colon. Soapy water should not be used because of the irritating effects on the large bowel mucosa.

TECHNIQUE OUTLINE

CONTRAST MEDIA:
30 to 60% barium sulfate or
Iodinated compound

EQUIPMENT/SUPPLIES:
Bardex or Foley balloon-tip
catheter
60-ml catheter-tip syringes
Contrast agent reservoir (enema
bag or can or commercially
available set)
Examination gloves
Lubricant
Hemostat

PATIENT PREPARATION:
Low-residue diet 48 hours prior
to study
Fast for 24 hours prior to study
Enema until clear, 12 hours in
advance
Mild oral cathartic if necessary
Anesthesia if necessary

PROCEDURE

I. Expose survey radiographs; ensure that the large bowel is clear of all fecal matter.

II. With the patient in lateral recumbency, gently insert the lubricated catheter tip into the rectum and inflate the balloon so that it is located just inside the internal anal sphincter.

III. Attach the catheter end to the infusion device (bucket or bag) or syringe.

IV. Slowly inflate the contrast medium.
   A. Positive contrast media should be warmed to body temperature.
   B. Dose is approximately 10 to 15 ml/kg.

V. Clamp catheter with a clamp or hemostat.

VI. With catheter in place, expose lateral radiograph to evaluate distention of the large bowel.

VII. Add more contrast media if necessary.

VIII. When desired distention of the large bowel is attained, expose ventrodorsal, right, and left lateral radiographs (oblique views if necessary).

IX. After study is completed, evacuate the contrast agent from the large bowel as completely as possible. This is accomplished by lowering the contrast reservoir below the patient level and allowing gravity to empty the contrast from the bowel.

continued

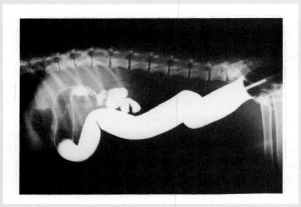

■ **FIG. 18.8** Lateral view of a barium enema.

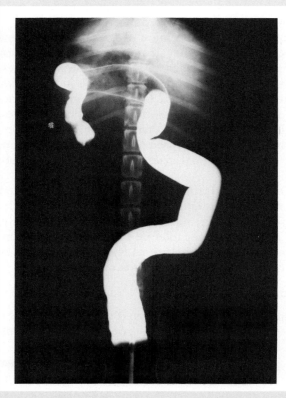

■ **FIG. 18.9** Ventrodorsal view of a barium enema.

CONTRAST STUDIES OF THE URINARY SYSTEM

Contrast studies of the upper and lower urinary system are excellent for the evaluation of the kidneys, ureters, bladder, and urethra. Urography and cystography are relatively inexpensive and highly diagnostic techniques that can be performed in any veterinary practice that has the proper equipment.

A radiographic study of the urinary system may be indicated for a patient with hematuria, proteinuria, crystalluria, polyuria, isosthenuria, or dysuria. The clinical signs of the patient will dictate the contrast study needed. Unfortunately, each study has its limitations; a number of different studies may be necessary to evaluate the entire urinary system.

Excretory Urography

Excretory urography consists of an intravenous injection of sterile water-soluble iodinated contrast medium and exposure of radiographs at subsequent intervals. The iodinated contrast medium circulates through the venous blood, is filtered out of the blood, and collects in the kidneys. An excretory urogram, also referred to as an **intravenous urogram (IVU)** or an **intravenous**

pyelogram **(IVP)**, is a very useful radiographic study for the evaluation of kidney structure and collection system. However, an IVP is not used to evaluate renal function quantitatively.

The excretory urogram is divided into two phases: (1) **nephrogram** and (2) **pyelogram**. Radiographs taken immediately after the injection of contrast medium exhibit the agent uniformly perfused throughout the renal vasculature. The diffuse opacification of the renal parenchyma is characteristic of the nephrogram phase. This phase demonstrates the vascular supply and perfusion of the kidney and documents the presence of functional renal tissue, particularly if it persists beyond the angiographic blush.

As the contrast agent is filtered into the renal collection system with the urine, the renal pelvis and recesses are opacified. This is known as the pyelogram phase. The pyelogram phase can be accentuated by placing abdominal compression (with a compression band or abdominal pressure wrap) on the caudal abdomen, which results in a cessation of urine flow to the bladder. This is neither necessary nor recommended because it can cause transient worsening of renal function under experimental circumstances.

Precautions

Any urine samples needed for laboratory data should be obtained prior to the injection of contrast media. Iodinated contrast agents will increase urine specific gravity to a variable degree and induce a false positive reaction for protein detected by sulfosalicylic acid.

Because the amount of iodinated contrast medium to be injected may be quite large, the placement of an indwelling catheter is suggested. An indwelling catheter facilitates injection and decreases the possibility of perivascular injection. Sedation is usually not necessary if the patient is cooperative.

Although rare, systemic reactions after an intravenous injection of iodinated contrast medium have been reported in animals. In clinical experience with dogs and cats at the Veterinary Teaching Hospital at the University of Minnesota, approximately 1 in 80 intravenous contrast injection procedures result in fatality. The incidence of mild reactions is unknown but is probably higher. Most severe acute reactions occur within the first 5 to 10 minutes and have an unpredictable outcome. They range in severity from mild (requiring no treatment) to fatal. The most frequently observed acute clinical signs in dogs and cats are vomiting, defecation, urination, and hypotension with or without collapse.

Several measures are suggested to prevent adverse reactions to contrast media. Because most reactions occur within minutes, preparation for emergency care should be made before the injection. The animal's disease state should be assessed, and dehydration corrected. An emergency resuscitation kit containing endotracheal tubes, Ambu bag, emergency drugs, and intravenous fluids should be available prior to injection. The patient's vital signs should be monitored during and after the injection to observe for any adverse reactions.

TECHNIQUE OUTLINE

CONTRAST MEDIA:
Water-soluble iodinated compound

PATIENT PREPARATION:
Fast 12 to 24 hours
Cleansing enema (administer 4 hours prior to study to minimize gas artifact)

PROCEDURE

I. Expose survey radiographs.

II. Place intravenous indwelling catheter in cephalic or saphenous vein.

III. Place the patient in dorsal recumbency.

IV. Infuse contrast medium.
   A. Concentration: 300 to 400 mg iodine/ml suggested.
   B. Dose: 3 ml/kg (90 ml maximum).
   C. Injection rate: rapid bolus (1 to 3 minutes for entire injection).

V. Expose ventrodorsal projection immediately after rejection for nephrogram phase.

VI. Subsequent lateral and ventrodorsal films are taken at 5, 10, and 20 minutes to show the pyelogram and drainage phases. (If a compression band is used, it is necessary to remove it before exposing the 20-minute drainage phase radiograph.)

VII. Cystography can be performed at this time.

continued

T E C H N I Q U E   O U T L I N E   *Continued*

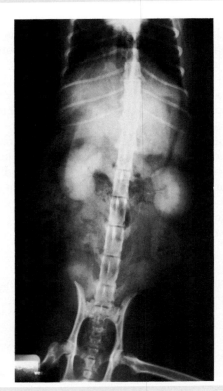

■ **FIG. 18.10** Ventrodorsal view of the nephrogram phase of an intravenous pyelogram.

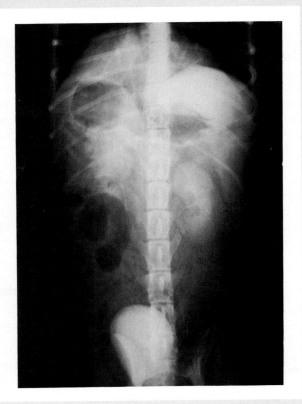

■ **FIG. 18.12** Ventrodorsal view of the pyelogram and drainage phase of an intravenous pyelogram.

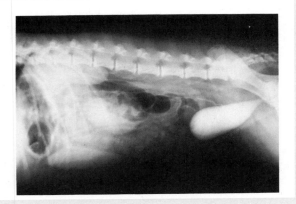

■ **FIG. 18.11** Lateral view of the pyelogram and drainage phase of an intravenous pyelogram.

Cystography

Cystography consists of the introduction of contrast media into the bladder via a urinary catheter. Positive, negative, and double contrast can be utilized for cystography. In addition, a cystogram can be performed in conjunction with an upper urinary tract study. A contrast study of the bladder is beneficial for the investigation of cystic calculi, mural lesions, bladder rupture, and other bladder wall abnormalities.

A cystogram is indicated for an animal exhibiting unresponsive clinical signs such as hematuria, crystalluria, bacturia, dysuria, anuria, and incontinence. At no time should cystography replace a clinical evaluation of the patient history, physical examination, and laboratory data. Radiographic findings from cystography can be used to confirm, refute, or correct diagnoses formulated by clinical evaluation.

Sedation is recommended for cystography because distention of the urinary bladder can be uncomfortable, especially for a patient with cystitis.

Precautions

Any urine samples needed for laboratory data should be obtained prior to the injection of contrast media. Iodinated contrast agents will increase urine specific gravity to a variable degree and induce a false positive reaction for protein detected by sulfosalicylic acid. Procedures using contrast agents can influence laboratory data obtained from the upper and lower urinary tracts for as long as 24 hours.

Every effort should be made to protect the patient from iatrogenic trauma that can be associated with urinary catheterization. Any induced trauma can predispose an animal to a bacterial infection. A gentle, meticulous technique helps prevent infection or damage to the delicate tissues of the genital tract, the urethra, and the urinary bladder. The smallest-diameter urinary catheter feasible for an objective study should be used. Catheters with flared distal ends are recommended to reduce the risk of migration of the catheter to a point of no return. The flared tip will also accommodate the tip of the syringe. Keeping a three-way valve (stopcock) on the distal end of the catheter will lessen concern about migration. Care should also be taken to ensure that the catheter is not overinserted into the bladder. A sharp-pointed catheter can penetrate the bladder wall if excessive force is used. Pliable catheters can become entangled in the bladder, making removal difficult.

The use of barium sulfate and sodium iodide is contraindicated for cystography. Although rare, complications with barium sulfate include barium casts and interstitial fibrosis secondary to vesicoureteral reflux. Barium also serves as a nidus for the formation of uroliths. In addition, granulomatous disease might occur secondary to a rupture of the bladder or urethra. Sodium iodide solution is not recommended for cystography because of its irritating effect on the mucosa of the bladder and urethra. Sodium iodide solution has been known to produce acute hemorrhagic cystitis, epithelial ulcerations, and submucosal hemorrhage. Tri-iodinated ionic compounds are the contrast agents of choice; they are versatile and can be used for excretory urograms as well as cystourethrograms.

Leakage of urine and contrast media around or through the catheter may occur during the procedure. It is important that any spill be cleaned off the equipment and patient immediately; contrast contaminants can cause confusing artifacts on a radiograph.

There are some indications that the injection of room air into a lower urinary tract might cause a fatal air embolism. This has been noted in patients suffering from active bladder hemorrhage. The air can enter the low-pressure venous system via bleeding capillaries. Although the occurrence of air embolism is rare, carbon dioxide or nitrous oxide should be used for patients with macroscopic hematuria. Carbon dioxide and nitrous oxide are 20 times more soluble in serum than air or oxygen and can be absorbed better in the body.

The dose of contrast medium necessary to distend the bladder of an animal for a cystogram will vary according to the size and condition of the bladder. With either agent, an iodinated compound or air, quantities of 10 to 300 ml are normally required to fill the bladder adequately. It is important to distend the bladder moderately in order to avoid artifactual thickening of the bladder wall or folding of the mucosa due to underdistention. In the same respect, the bladder should not be overdistended with contrast medium. Overdistention of the bladder could result in a retrograde reflux of the contrast agent into the ureters and renal pelvis or even cause a bladder rupture (Fig. 18.13).

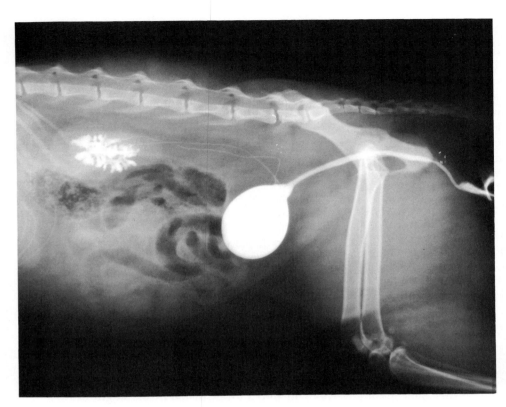

■ **FIG. 18.13** Lateral view of a cystogram showing overdistention of the bladder, resulting in ureteral reflux of contrast media.

T E C H N I Q U E   O U T L I N E

C O N T R A S T   M E D I A :
Any of the tri-iodinated contrast agents

E Q U I P M E N T / S U P P L I E S :
$3^1/_2$ to 5 French sterile polypropylene or red rubber urinary catheter (metal catheters are not recommended for female dogs because their rigid structure frequently causes trauma to the urethra or bladder)
Three way valve (stopcock)
Syringes ranging from 3 to 60 ml in volume
Sterile aqueous lubricant or sterile lidocaine gel to reduce discomfort and risk of iatrogenic trauma caused by urethral spasms
Germicidal soap and water
Gauze pads
Sterile gloves
Otoscope speculum (to aid in visualizing the urethral opening in female patients)

P R O C E D U R E

I.   Expose survey radiographs.

II.   Cleanse adjacent structures external to the urethral orifice with germicidal soap and water.

III.   Gently insert the lubricated catheter so that the tip is positioned in the trigone of the bladder.

IV.   Gently aspirate all urine out of the bladder.
   A.   Note the amount of urine withdrawn to give an estimate of the amount of contrast medium needed.

V.   If blood clots are present in the bladder, they should be flushed out with saline.

VI.   Infuse 5 to 10 ml of 2% lidocaine into the bladder, if necessary, to decrease spasticity. Unless spasticity is reduced, it may be difficult or impossible to distend the bladder.

VII.   Negative-contrast cystogram (**pneumocystogram**).
   A.   Slowly infuse negative contrast agent into the bladder via the urinary catheter.
      1.   Dose: Approximately 10 ml air/kg.
         a.   The dose will vary with the size of the animal; smaller dogs usually require a larger amount per kilogram than larger dogs to fill the bladder. Always palpate the bladder during infusion and stop when it is moderately turgid.

T E C H N I Q U E O U T L I N E *Continued*

PATIENT
PREPARATION:
Fast 12 to 24 hours
Cleansing enema (administer 4
hours prior to study to minimize
gas artifact)

    B. Expose lateral and ventrodorsal radiographs of the
caudal abdomen.
      1. An oblique view may be necessary, especially
of male dogs because of the superimposing os
penis over the bladder on the ventrodorsal
projection.

VIII. **Double-contrast cystogram.**
    A. This study can follow a negative-contrast cys-
togram, or the bladder should be distended with a
negative contrast agent.
      1. Dose: Approximately 10 ml air/kg.
        a. The dose will vary with the size of the animal;
smaller dogs usually require a larger amount
per kilogram than larger dogs to fill the
bladder.
    B. Infuse a small amount of positive contrast (tri-
iodinated) medium via the catheter into the
bladder.
      1. Cat: 1 to 2 ml positive contrast into the bladder.
      2. Dog: 1 to 3 ml positive contrast into the bladder.
        a. Amount depends on the size of the animal
and residual volume of the catheter.
    C. Expose lateral and ventrodorsal radiographs of the
caudal abdomen.
      1. An oblique view may be necessary, especially
of male dogs because of the superimposing os
penis over the bladder on the ventrodorsal
projection.

IX. **Positive-contrast cystogram.**
    A. Slowly infuse 10 to 15% positive (tri-iodinated)
contrast medium diluted with saline into the bladder
until distended.
      1. Dose: Approximately 10 ml/kg.
        a. The dose will vary with the size of the animal;
smaller dogs usually require a larger amount
per kilogram than larger dogs to fill the
bladder. Always palpate the bladder during
infusion, and stop when it is moderately
distended.
    B. Expose lateral and ventrodorsal radiographs of the
caudal abdomen.
      1. An oblique view may be necessary, especially
of male dogs because of the superimposing os
penis over the bladder on the ventrodorsal
projection.

continued

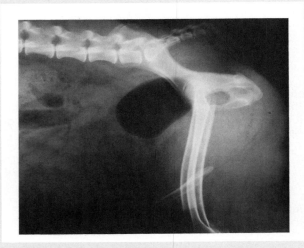

■ **FIG. 18.14** Lateral view of a negative-contrast cystogram.

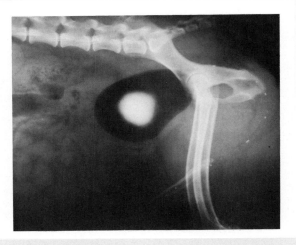

■ **FIG. 18.15** Lateral view of a double-contrast cystogram.

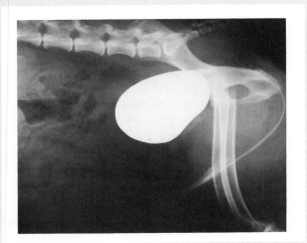

■ **FIG. 18.16** Lateral view of a positive-contrast cystogram.

Urethrography

Urethrography consists of filling the urethra with contrast medium to detect urethral trauma, stricture, obstruction, and other pathologic disturbances such as tumor invasion. Filling the urethra can be accomplished by either retrograde or antegrade infusion of contrast medium. A **retrograde urethrogram** can be performed with either positive or negative contrast media. An **antegrade urethrogram** study is best done with positive contrast media.

Precautions

Sedation is recommended for urethrography because there is slight patient discomfort. The retrograde study of the urethra requires the use of a balloon-tip catheter such as a Swan-Ganz. It is important that the balloon tip be placed just inside the urethral orifice to ensure that the majority of the urethra can be examined. A sufficient amount of contrast agent must be injected to fully distend the urethra. A urethra that is not fully distended may mimic a stricture lesion or other mucosal impingement. It is best to make the exposure during the infusion of the contrast medium toward the end of the injection. For male dogs, the bladder should be filled prior to the actual urethral injection.

Antegrade urethrography can conveniently be performed following a positive-contrast cystogram. It is important that the bladder be distended to create pressure to induce micturition. However, excessive pressure should never be placed on the urinary bladder, which could induce a bladder rupture. If a voiding urethrogram cannot be obtained, retrograde urethrography should be performed.

TECHNIQUE OUTLINE

CONTRAST MEDIA:
Water-soluble iodinated contrast agent or air, carbon dioxide, or nitrous oxide

EQUIPMENT/SUPPLIES:
12- to 20-ml syringes
Balloon-tip urinary catheter
Sterile lubricant

PATIENT PREPARATION:
Fast 12 to 24 hours
Cleansing enema (administer 4 hours prior to study to minimize gas artifact)

PROCEDURE

I. Expose survey radiographs.

II. Place the patient in lateral recumbency.

III. Retrograde urethrogram.
  A. Fill the lumen of the catheter with contrast medium before placement into the urethra.
  B. Insert the lubricated tip of the catheter 1 to 3 cm into the urethral orifice and inflate the balloon.
  C. Inject 3 to 20 ml of contrast medium into the urethra (amount of agent needed will vary with size of patient).
  D. Make the exposure during infusion toward the end of the injection.
  E. Repeat the injection for ventrodorsal and oblique projections, if necessary.

IV. Antegrade (voiding) urethrogram.
  A. With the bladder distended with a positive contrast agent, gentle pressure is placed on the bladder with a paddle or wooden spoon.
  B. Exposure is taken when urine is noted at the urethral orifice.

T E C H N I Q U E   O U T L I N E   *Continued*

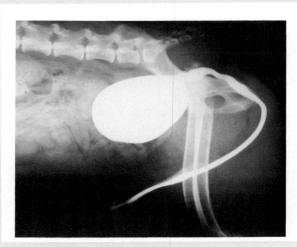

■ **FIG. 18.17** Lateral view of a retrograde cystourethrogram.

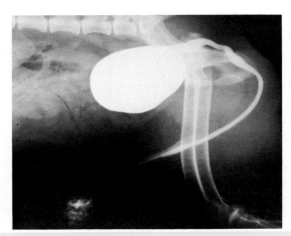

■ **FIG. 18.18** Lateral view of an antegrade cystourethrogram.

ADDITIONAL TECHNIQUES — A BRIEF OVERVIEW
Arthrography

Arthrography is a technique in which a contrast agent is injected through a needle into a true joint space and subsequent radiographs are exposed. A contrast medium placed within a joint cavity will demonstrate the articular surfaces and outline the joint capsule. This type of study may be indicated for a patient that is lame or has pain associated with a joint, where survey radiographs provided insufficient information. An arthrogram can be used to evaluate a ruptured joint capsule, the presence of a cartilaginous flap, meniscal injuries, and the necessity for surgery.

The positive or negative arthrogram can be performed with a water-soluble iodine compound or air (carbon dioxide or nitrous oxide). The iodinated contrast agent should be diluted with sterile saline to a 20 to 40% solution. If more-concentrated contrast solutions are used, they can completely obliterate the intracapsular ligaments or the damaged cartilage.

An arthrogram is contraindicated if there is an infection of the soft tissues surrounding the joint. In this circumstance, inserting the needle into a joint capsule could result in an injected joint. This could lead to severe infection of the joint. The use of air for a negative-contrast arthrogram may result in an air embolism. It may be appropriate to use carbon dioxide or nitrous oxide rather than air for a pneumoarthogram.

Angiography and Angiocardiography

Angiography consists of a bolus injection of iodinated positive contrast medium into a vascular system (e.g.,

cardiac or extremity) immediately followed by radiographic exposures. An angiogram may be used to demonstrate occlusion of a particular blood vessel, demonstrate pathologic lesions of the vascular system, or provide evidence of a tumor that was undefinable on survey radiographs.

A water-soluble iodine compound is the contrast medium of choice for angiography. For most procedures (e.g., angiography and **angiocardiography**), the contrast medium can be injected into a blood vessel proximal to the region of interest. Because the contrast agent will be rapidly transported away from the area under examination by the circulating blood, it is necessary to expose the radiographs during or immediately after the injection is made.

Ideally, the progress of a bolus injection of contrast medium should be followed in a series of radiographs exposed in rapid succession. This can be accomplished with a commercially available rapid film changer or, in a small veterinary practice, can be conveniently done with a sheet of sturdy clear plastic and a number of loaded cassettes (Fig. 18.19). The sheet of clear plastic is positioned on top of small wood blocks, and the patient is centered on top of the glass sheet. The cassettes are numbered, placed under the plastic sheet, and positioned in a single-file line, with each cassette abutting the next. As the contrast medium is injected, the exposures are taken. The cassettes are advanced as each exposure is made.

Cholecystography

Cholecystography consists of oral or intravenous administration of positive contrast medium that is ex-

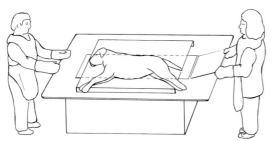

■ **FIG. 18.19** Simple cassette tunnel system for a nonselective cardioangiogram. A sheet of plastic is propped a couple of inches off of the table with wood or foam blocks. The cassettes are placed on the table and advanced after each exposure.

creted through the biliary system. The gallbladder and bile ducts and the degree of opacification can be useful in the evaluation of gallbladder function and health. Nonvisualization of the gallbladder after injection of the contrast medium indicates possible gallbladder disease, biliary obstruction, gallstones, hepatocellular dysfunction, or failure to absorb the contrast agent if orally administered. Although opinions vary, the intravenous route of administration is most predictable and most rapid.

The injectable contrast choleographic agents are recommended for the dog because the oral preparations have variable absorption and do not always provide a satisfactory study.

After the injection of the choleographic agent, radiographs should be taken at intervals of 15, 30, 60, and 120 minutes. The time required for complete opacification of the gallbladder will vary with each patient. Once the gallbladder is identified radiographically, a small, preferably fatty meal may be given to the patient and second radiographs are obtained. Feeding the patient a small meal will allow evaluation of the emptying of the gallbladder.

Fistulography

Fistulography consists of the injection of a positive or negative contrast medium into a fistula to determine the depth and origin of the tract. A **fistula** is any abnormal, tube-like passage within the body tissue. The occurrence of a fistula is usually the result of an injury or congenital deformity. The presence of a draining wound of undetermined origin may indicate the presence of a fistulous tract and the need for a fistulogram. Often, the site of the wound may be far removed from the site of the drainage.

The contrast medium of choice for a fistulogram is any water-soluble iodinated agent. The contrast agent is infused into the fistulous tract with a syringe and flexible catheter, preferably with a balloon tip. After the contrast medium is infused, radiographs of the area should be taken to document the flow of the agent.

Lymphography

Lymphography is the demonstration of the lymphatic system with the use of an injectable positive contrast medium. This type of study may be indicated to evaluate the cause of edema in the forelimb or hind limb of an animal.

Lymphography is usually limited to areas of the extremities, head, and cervical region owing to the inaccessibility of the lymphatic vessels in other areas of the body. The procedure involves identification and surgical exposure of a lymphatic duct and direct introduction of contrast medium into that duct. Immediately after the injection of the contrast agent, radiographs of the area are obtained.

The contrast medium used for lymphography is either a water-soluble or an oily iodinated agent. The advantage of the oily agent is that it remains within the lymph nodes for up to a month, which allows for repeated radiographic studies. Unfortunately, the oily iodinated compounds can cause local irritation and may be contraindicated for a patient suffering from lymphedema. Oily compounds could aggravate an already impaired lymphatic system.

Myelography

Myelography consists of introducing a positive contrast medium into the subarachnoid space of the spine and taking radiographs of the opacified region of the spine. A myelogram is indicated to highlight a lesion that is undetectable on survey radiographs. Positive contrast in the subarachnoid space can be used to identify compression of the spinal cord due to a mass, protruding disk, vertebral abnormality, or spinal cord swelling.

General anesthesia is required for myelography because of the sensitive nature of a subarachnoid injection. The site of injection should be surgically prepared, and a spinal needle introduced into the cisternal or lumbar space. The contrast medium is then slowly injected into the subarachnoid space. A proper dose of contrast agent is determined by the patient size and area under examination. After the injection, radiographs are taken of the areas of interest. Individuals should be familiar with injection sites, techniques of injection, and caveats (which are beyond the scope of this text) before administering myelography.

A number of contrast agents have been used for myelography in the past. Unfortunately, many have posed considerable problems. Because of the extreme sensitivity of the spinal tissues and the irritating effects of conventional ionic contrast agents, some patients suffered convulsions and death as a result of a subarachnoid injection of these media. Oily iodinated contrast agents have also been used but do not mix well with the spinal fluid and tend to coagulate and have an extremely slow absorption time. Currently, a low-osmolar, nonionic, water-soluble contrast medium is the standard choice for myelography.

Pneumoperitoneography

Pneumoperitoneography consists of the introduction of negative contrast (gas) into the peritoneal cavity in an attempt to obtain better contrast within the abdomen. This type of study is beneficial for the evaluation of the liver, spleen, stomach, distal colon, kidneys, urinary bladder, uterus, and abdominal wall.

Carbon dioxide and nitrous oxide are the preferred gases for pneumoperitoneography because of their rapid absorption in the body. Room air does not absorb as readily and has an increased incidence of resulting in air embolism.

This study usually requires a sedated patient. Any gas in the peritoneal cavity can be uncomfortable and may cause the patient to struggle. An injection site on the midline halfway between the umbilicus and the pubis should be surgically prepared. A plastic or metal catheter with a stylet is inserted into the peritoneal cavity, and the stylet is withdrawn. With a syringe, a test aspiration is made to ensure that the catheter placement is within the peritoneal cavity. Once the placement of the catheter is confirmed, negative contrast is injected until the abdominal wall is moderately distended. Abdominal distention can be evaluated by thumping the abdominal wall. A dull thud or the sound of a flat bongo drum indicates proper distention. Once distended, standard projections of the abdomen are obtained.

Sialography

Sialography involves injection of a positive contrast medium into the salivary ducts and glands. This type of study is beneficial for the evaluation of salivary duct patency and gland morphology. The parotid, zygomatic, mandibular, and sublingual salivary ducts can be examined by means of this technique. The most frequent use of sialography in veterinary radiography is for the confirmation of a salivary mucocele.

The procedure requires that the patient is sedated. A blunt-ended needle is inserted into the salivary duct, and a small amount of water-soluble contrast medium is infused. Lateral and dorsoventral radiographs of the skull are obtained to visualize the salivary system.

Vaginography

Vaginography consists of the introduction of a positive contrast medium into the vagina and cervix. Uterus and fallopian tubes may opacify if the cervix is open, as in estrus. This study can be used to evaluate the morphology of the vaginal vault and possibly the reproductive tract. A vaginogram may be indicated for a female patient to investigate infertility or a possible mass lesion.

A vaginogram is performed on an anesthetized patient. A balloon-tip syringe is inserted into the vulva, and the cuff is inflated just inside the vaginal vault. Once the catheter is in the correct position, a water-soluble iodinated contrast medium is infused into the vagina until back pressure is felt on the syringe. The amount necessary to distend the vagina will vary according to patient size. Lateral and ventrodorsal abdominal radiographs are taken to record the infusion of the contrast medium.

BIBLIOGRAPHY

Allan GS, Dixon RT: Cholecystography in the dog: The choice of contrast media and optimal dose rates. JAVRS 16:98–103, 1975.

Feeney DA, Walter PA, Johnston GR: The effect of radiographic contrast media on the urinalysis. *In* Kirk RW (ed): *Current Therapy IX: Small Animal Practice.* WB Saunders, Philadelphia, 1986.

Harvey CE: Sialography in the dog. JAVRS 10:18–27, 1969.

Lavin-Cunliffe LM: Feline cystography and urethrography: Technical use in practice. Vet Tech 10:364–373, 1989.

Morgan JP, Silverman S: *Techniques in Veterinary Radiography,* 4th ed. Iowa State University Press, Ames, 1987.

Osborne CA, Jessen CR: Double-contrast cystography in the dog. J Am Vet Med Assoc 154:1100, 1971.

Park RD: Contrast studies of the lower urinary tract. Vet Clin North Am 4:863, 1974.

Prior JE, Schaffer B, Skelly JF: Direct lymphangiography in the dog. J Am Vet Med Assoc, 140:943–946, 1962.

Suter PF, Carb AV: Shoulder arthrography in dogs—radiographic anatomy and clinical application. J Small Anim D 10:407–413, 1969.

Ticer JW: *Radiographic Techniques in Small Animal Practice,* 2nd ed. WB Saunders, Philadelphia, 1984.

Webbon PM, Clark KW: Bronchography in normal dogs. J Small Anim D 18:327–332, 1972.

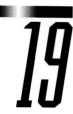

LARGE ANIMAL RADIOGRAPHY

INTRODUCTION

Working with the large animal patient requires much patience and time. Any procedure performed must be well thought out before the start. The radiographer must expect the unexpected. Successful large animal radiography is the result of having a plan prior to the examination, teamwork during the examination, and patience throughout.

Whereas the differences between large and small animals are great, the principles of radiography are essentially the same. All directional terms and positions that apply to a dog and cat apply to a horse and cow. The two major differences are size and posture. In large animal radiography, unless the animal is young and/or small enough to be placed on an x-ray table, the patient is in a standing position. The size and posture of the patient necessitate special consideration in the areas of patient restraint, equipment, patient preparation, radiation safety, and positioning devices.

SPECIAL CONSIDERATIONS

Patient Restraint

A large animal is often startled by unfamiliar objects, especially those brought close to its body. A good pre-lude to a radiographic examination of a large animal is an official introduction of the patient to the x-ray machine. Allowing the horse or cow to gently sniff the machine and cassette may eliminate fear of the unknown. Always avoid sudden movement or loud noises, which may startle the animal. Continually reassure the patient in a calm voice.

In a standing position, the large animal patient is relatively unrestrained. Because of this, there is a greater risk of injury to personnel and to the x-ray machine. The x-ray tube is particularly vulnerable because it has to be positioned close to the animal's leg and is liable to be kicked.

Several methods can be used to restrain a large animal for a radiographic examination, including a twitch, stocks, or sedation. Sedation is a common method of restraint. The patient is given a small amount of chemical sedative to allow the radiographer freedom to move the x-ray machine without startling the animal, resulting in movement. If sedation is not possible or if the patient is restless, movement can be restricted if an attendant holds up one of the animal's legs. When attempting to radiograph a limb, the opposite limb is raised. Although rare, it may be necessary to place the patient under general anesthesia. Many attendants are required for this endeavor to manipulate the patient and to position the equipment when the large animal is anesthetized. The veterinarian will need to assess the situation and determine the type of restraint necessary.

Equipment

The radiographic machinery required for large animals must have adequate power and easy maneuverability. It is necessary for the x-ray tube to be able to be moved horizontally around the standing patient and vertically to expose an area as low as the level of the floor. The x-ray machines used for radiography of large animals fall into three categories: (1) small portable unit, (2) mobile unit, and (3) mounted unit.

The portable unit is commonly used by equine and bovine veterinary practitioners who make "house calls." The portable unit is small and light enough that it can be easily moved from one location to another (see Fig. 2.4). The average power capacity of a portable unit is limited to a maximum milliamperage (mA) setting of 20 and a maximum kilovoltage (kVp) of 90. Owing to the low mA capability, exposure times of 0.1 second or greater are usually necessary. Long exposure times increase the likelihood of motion during exposure. Because line voltage varies from barn to barn, exposures are not always consistent with portable units. The collimation on a portable unit also will vary, and the collimator may not always have a light to visualize the field of exposure. Thus, it is often easy to expose an area larger than necessary. This can pose a special problem with radiation safety—that is, the exposure of personnel to excessive radiation.

Mobile units have the advantage of having more power. The capacity of an average mobile unit ranges from 100 to 300 mA and up to 120 kVp. The higher mA capacity allows for shorter exposure times. The main disadvantage of this unit is its weight and thus lack of maneuverability. The mobile unit has large wheels to allow ambulation but tends to be cumbersome and difficult to move on uneven floor surfaces (see Fig. 4.2).

Large, permanently mounted x-ray units are commonly utilized by veterinary specialty and referral practices. The power capacity may exceed 1000 mA. For large animal radiography, these units are commonly mounted on the ceiling with a series of overhead rails. The overhead rails allow the x-ray tube to be moved vertically and horizontally around the patient (see Fig. 2.18B). Unfortunately, ceiling units that have overhead rails may be noisy and distracting to a fearful patient. In addition, the size of the x-ray tube housing may limit its use for studies of the feet. This is because even if the tube is on the floor, the focal spot may be 6 to 8 inches off the floor, resulting in obliquity of the views.

Patient Preparation

Careful preparation of the patient is necessary for an artifact-free radiograph. For all examinations, the haircoat should be brushed or washed to remove obvious dirt, bedding, or other surface artifacts. The areas of interest should also be wiped dry with a towel to remove any water or other remaining liquid contaminants. For radiography of the equine foot, a number of steps are necessary to prevent extraneous radiographic shadows over the areas under examination. The first step is to remove the shoe of the patient and trim back any overgrown portions of the hoof. Next, the sole and clefts should be picked and scrubbed clean. The final step is to pack the sole of the foot with a radiolucent material such as methylcellulose, softened soap, or PlayDoh. Packing the sole prevents the appearance of an air artifact superimposed over the areas of interest.

Radiation Safety

All rules of radiation safety discussed in Part I of this text also apply to large animal radiography. A few extra rules of safety must be considered, however, because of the size and posture of the patient and the considerably high exposure factors needed.

The attendants holding the patient and holding the cassette next to the anatomy must be wearing appropriate lead attire. Because the attendants' attention is focused on the patient rather than the x-ray beam, it is the responsibility of the radiographer to ensure that they are a safe distance from the primary beam. Cassette holding devices are helpful to reduce exposure to the attendants. The device usually consists of a clamp that is attached to the cassette and is then held at length by a handle (Fig. 19.1).

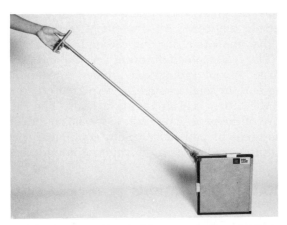

■ **FIG. 19.1** A cassette holder used for equine radiography.

Positioning Devices

At times, it may be necessary to raise the animal's foot because the x-ray tube cannot be dropped to the level of the floor. A positioning block can be used to raise the foot into position and serve as a cassette holder as well (Fig. 19.2). The block is usually constructed of wood built to suit the particular x-ray unit. A slot can be cut into the wood to serve as a cassette holder. The foot of the patient can be placed directly onto the block to raise it into position next to the cassette, or the cassette can be placed beside the block.

Another device that is often needed is a cassette tunnel. A tunnel can be constructed of a radiolucent wood or hard plastic but must be durable enough to withstand the weight of the patient. For a dorsoventral oblique view of the coffin or navicular bone, it is necessary for the patient to be standing on top of the cassette. A cassette cannot withstand such weight without sustaining damage. A tunnel device can make the examination possible without damaging the equipment (Fig. 19.3).

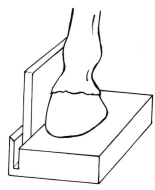

■ **FIG. 19.2** For equine pedal radiography, it may be necessary to raise the patient's foot off of the ground in order to radiograph that area. A wood block is commonly used for this purpose. The wood block pictured here has a slot designed to hold a cassette next to the limb of interest.

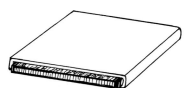

■ **FIG. 19.3** A cassette tunnel.

DISTAL PHALANX (PEDAL BONE)

Lateral View

The patient's foot is placed on a wood block to elevate it to a level where the central x-ray beam can be directed horizontally toward the pedal bone. The placement of the foot must be as close to the edge of the block as possible so that the cassette is as close to the medial aspect of the foot as possible. The object-film distance must be minimal. To prevent motion, it may be helpful to have an attendant hold the patient's leg of interest over the carpus or elevate the opposite limb so that the limb being examined is completely weight bearing. The cassette is placed on the medial side of the foot either directly on the floor or in the cassette groove in the wood block. The field of view should include the entire hoof. (Note: This same position is used to examine the lateral navicular bone. The beam center is directed at the palmar aspect of the coronary band.)

BEAM CENTER: Over hoof wall just below coronary band

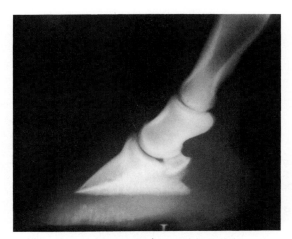

■ **FIG. 19.5** Radiograph of the lateral view of the distal phalanx.

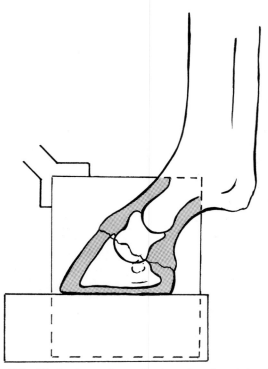

■ **FIG. 19.4** Correct positioning for the lateral view of the distal phalanx.

Dorsopalmar/Dorsoplantar View

The patient's foot is placed on a wood block so that it is elevated to the level of the horizontal central x-ray beam. The heel of the foot should be placed on the edge of the block or cassette groove. The cassette is placed directly behind the foot on the floor or in the cassette groove and held perpendicular to the floor. It may be helpful to raise the opposite limb so that full weight is placed on the limb of interest. This will decrease the possibility of motion. The field of view should include the entire hoof.

BEAM CENTER: Over middle of pedal bone just below coronary band

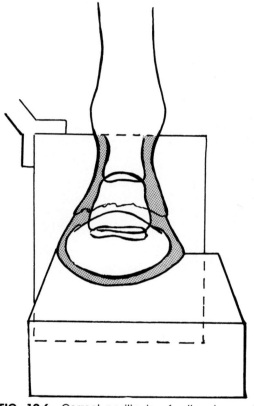

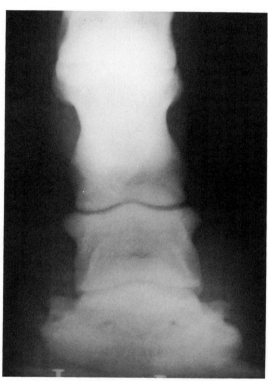

■ **FIG. 19.7** Radiograph of the dorsopalmar view of the distal phalanx.

■ **FIG. 19.6** Correct positioning for the dorsopalmar/dorsoplantar view of the distal phalanx.

Dorsopalmar/Dorsoplantar Oblique View

The cassette is placed in a tunnel cassette holder, and the foot of the patient is positioned on top of the tunnel. The foot should be in the center of the cassette so that the entire hoof and pedal bone are included in the field of view. It may be necessary to raise the opposite limb to ensure that the limb of interest is weight bearing. The x-ray tube is angled 45 degrees to the ground and directed at the hoof wall. (Note: This same view can be used to visualize the navicular bone. Because of the superimposition of the navicular bone over the 2nd phalanx, higher exposure factors are necessary to visualize this area, and an angle of 65 degrees off horizontal should be used.)

BEAM CENTER: Over middle point of hoof wall just below coronary band

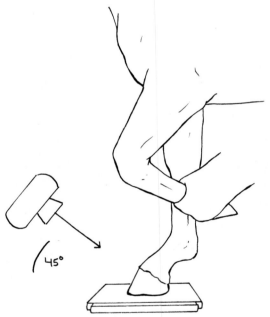

FIG. 19.8 Correct positioning for the dorsopal-mar/dorsoplantar oblique view of the distal pha-lanx.

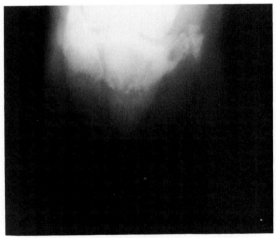

FIG. 19.9 Radiograph of the dorsopalmar oblique view of the distal phalanx.

NAVICULAR BONE

Dorsopalmar/Dorsoplantar Oblique View

The foot of the patient can be placed (1) on a cassette within a cassette tunnel as shown for the dorsopalmar/dorsoplantar oblique view of the distal phalanx or (2) on a block with specially designed grooves that hold the hoof in an angled position. With the patient standing on the cassette, the x-ray beam is angled 65 degrees toward the middle of the 2nd phalanx. When the block is used, the toe of the hoof is placed in a vertical groove so that the dorsal wall of the hoof is positioned vertically. The cassette is placed behind the heels in a cassette groove. The opposite leg must bear the majority of the weight of the patient. The x-ray beam is directed parallel to the ground, and the field of view should include the 2nd and 3rd phalanges. With the foot on the block in this vertical position, a 45- to 65-degree-angle view of the navicular bone is projected onto the x-ray film.

BEAM CENTER: Over center of 2nd phalanx just above coronary band

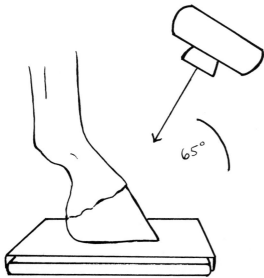

■ **FIG. 19.10** Correct positioning for the dorsopalmar oblique view of the navicular bone with the patient standing on a cassette tunnel.

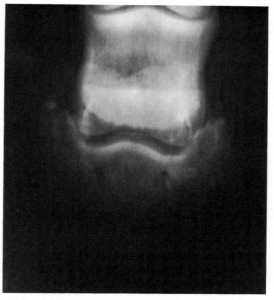

■ **FIG. 19.12** Radiograph of the dorsopalmar oblique view of the navicular bone.

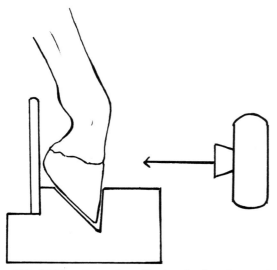

■ **FIG. 19.11** Correct positioning for the dorsopalmar oblique view of the navicular bone with the dorsal wall of the hoof held in a vertical position with the use of a wood block.

Flexor View

The foot of the patient is placed on top of a cassette within a cassette tunnel. If possible, the patient should be stepping back slightly so that the fetlock is in an extended position. The 1st phalanx is close to perpendicular to the ground in this position, allowing better visualization of the navicular bone. The x-ray tube is positioned directly behind the foot and angled approximately 65 degrees to the floor. Great care must be taken with the x-ray tube in this position immediately behind the limb. It may be necessary to reduce the source-image distance (SID) when placing the x-ray tube under the belly of a horse for views of the front navicular bone.

BEAM CENTER: Over middle of heel bulbs

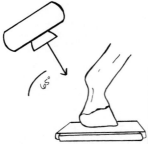
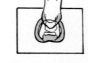

■ **FIG. 19.13** Correct positioning for the flexor view of the navicular bone.

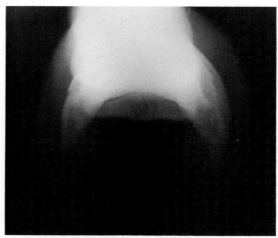

■ **FIG. 19.14** Radiograph of the flexor view of the navicular bone.

PROXIMAL PHALANGES

Lateral View (Short and Long Pastern)

The foot of the patient is placed on a wood block so that it is elevated slightly off the floor. The cassette is placed next to the medial aspect of the foot and should be on and perpendicular to the floor. The limb of interest should be weight bearing. It may be necessary to raise the opposite limb to eliminate motion. The x-ray beam is directed horizontally toward the phalanx. The field of view should include the 1st and 2nd phalanges for a general projection of the area.

BEAM CENTER: Over area of interest

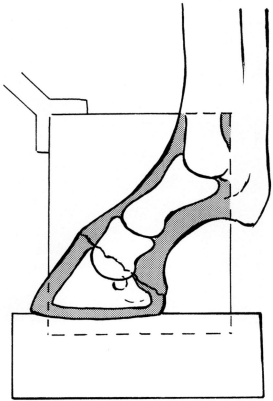

■ **FIG. 19.15** Correct positioning for the lateral view of the proximal phalanges.

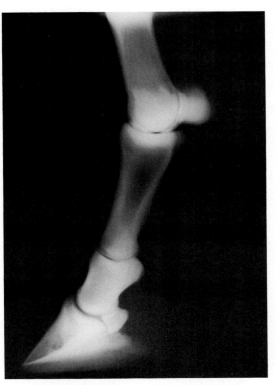

■ **FIG. 19.16** Radiograph of the lateral view of the proximal phalanges.

Dorsopalmar/Dorsoplantar View

The patient is positioned so that the limb under examination is weight bearing. The cassette is placed behind the limb parallel to the phalanges. It may be necessary to elevate the opposite limb to minimize motion. Depending on the angle of the foot and the placement of the cassette, it may be necessary to direct the x-ray tube at a 30- to 45-degree angle to the floor. The x-ray beam must be perpendicular to the cassette. The field of view should include the 1st and 2nd phalanges.

BEAM CENTER: Over area of interest

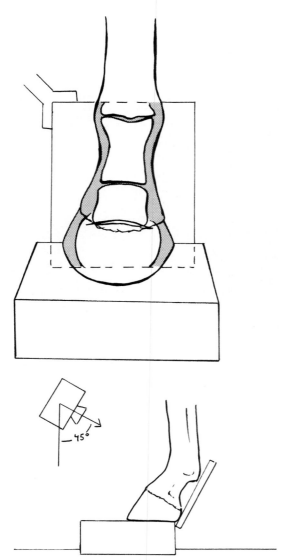

FIG. 19.17 Correct positioning for the dorsopalmar view of the proximal phalanges.

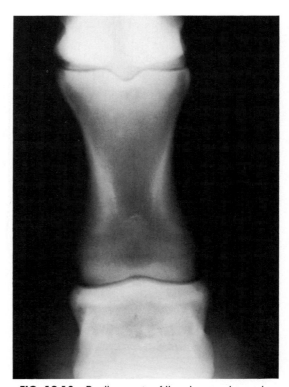

FIG. 19.18 Radiograph of the dorsopalmar view of the proximal phalanges.

FETLOCK JOINT

Dorsopalmar/Dorsoplantar View

The foot of the patient is placed with full weight on the floor directly under the body. The cassette is positioned on the floor directly behind the foot, touching the palmar or plantar aspect of the digit. The cassette should be held perpendicular to the floor. The opposite limb may be elevated if necessary to control the patient. The field of view should include the entire fetlock joint and a small portion of the bones proximal and distal to the joint. (Note: Aiming the x-ray beam at a slight tilt downward will minimize the sesamoid superimposition on the joint surfaces.)

BEAM CENTER: Through joint at right angle to cassette

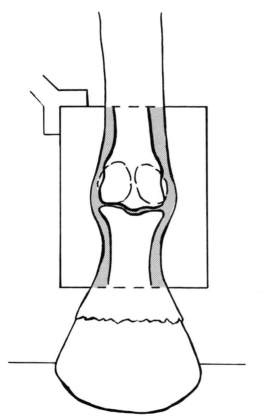

FIG. 19.19   Correct positioning for the dorsopalmar view of the fetlock joint.

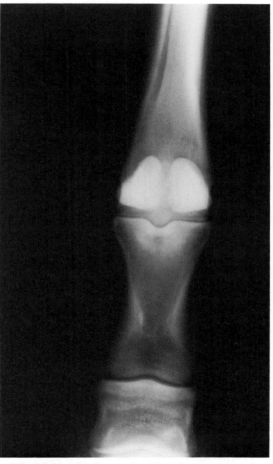

FIG. 19.20   Radiograph of the dorsopalmar view of the fetlock joint.

Lateral View

The foot of the patient is placed in a weight-bearing position directly under the body. The cassette is placed on the floor on the medial side of the foot of interest. The cassette should remain perpendicular to the floor. It may be necessary to raise the opposite limb to control the patient. The field of view should include the fetlock joint and a small portion of the bones proximal and distal to the joint.

BEAM CENTER: Through joint at right angle to cassette

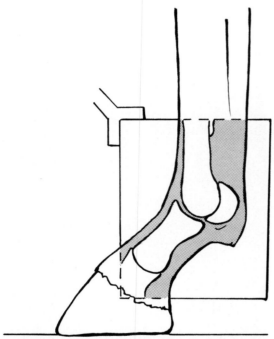

■ **FIG. 19.21** Correct positioning for the lateral view of the fetlock joint.

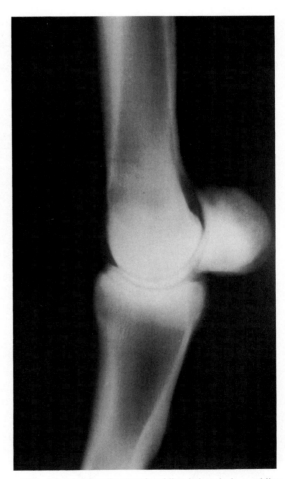

■ **FIG. 19.22** Radiograph of the lateral view of the fetlock joint.

Flexed Lateral View

The limb of interest is elevated, and the fetlock joint is flexed. The attendant holding the limb must be properly protected with lead gloves and apron. The cassette is positioned against the medial aspect of the joint. It is important that the cassette remain perpendicular to the floor. The limb should remain under the patient's body and not be abducted laterally. The x-ray beam is directed horizontally and parallel to the floor toward the cassette. The field of view should include the fetlock joint and a portion of the bones proximal and distal. The primary x-ray beam should be collimated so that the attendants' hands holding the limb are not exposed.

BEAM CENTER: Through joint at right angles to cassette

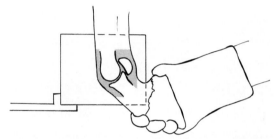

■ **FIG. 19.23** Correct positioning for the flexed lateral view of the fetlock joint.

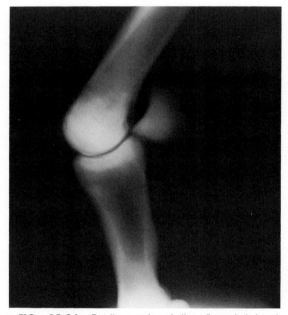

■ **FIG. 19.24** Radiograph of the flexed lateral view of the fetlock joint.

Oblique Views (Lateral and Medial)

The foot of the patient is placed in a normal weight-bearing position under the body. Depending on the oblique view desired, the x-ray tube is angled 30 to 45 degrees to either side of the dorsal midline of the foot. The precise angle of the tube will vary between patients and the area under investigation. The cassette is placed on the floor against the palmar or plantar aspect of the foot. The cassette is positioned so that the front of the x-ray beam is directed at a right angle to the cassette front. This view of the fetlock allows visualization of the medial and lateral sesamoid bones on the palmar/plantar aspect of the limb.

BEAM CENTER: Through middle of joint at 30- to 45-degree angle from dorsal midline of joint

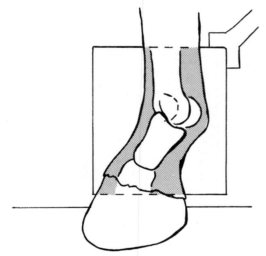

■ **FIG. 19.25** Correct positioning for the dorsomedial-palmarolateral oblique view of the fetlock.

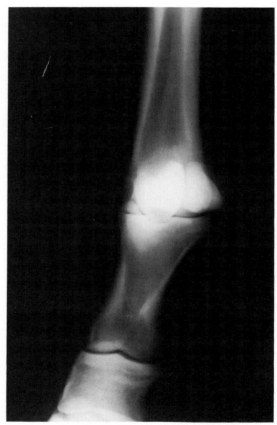

■ **FIG. 19.26** Radiograph of the dorsomedial-palmarolateral oblique view of the fetlock.

METACARPUS/METATARSUS

Dorsopalmar/Dorsoplantar View

The patient is allowed to stand in a normal position, bearing weight on the limb under investigation. The cassette is placed against the palmar or plantar aspect of the limb and is held perpendicular to the floor. The x-ray beam is directed parallel to the ground and at a right angle to the cassette. A large enough cassette should be used that the field of view includes the joints proximal and distal to the metacarpus or metatarsus (a 7 × 17 inch cassette is recommended).

BEAM CENTER: Over midpoint of metacarpus or metatarsus

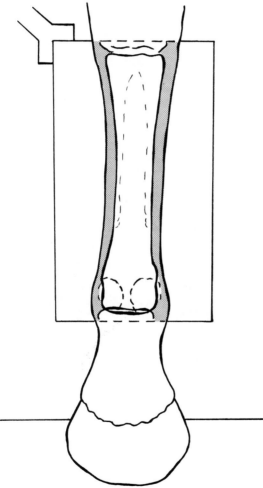

■ **FIG. 19.27** Correct positioning for the dorsopalmar view of the metacarpus.

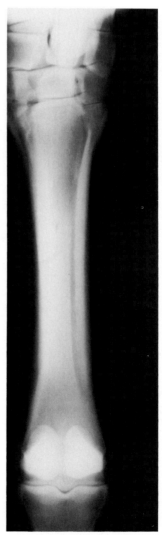

■ **FIG. 19.28** Radiograph of the dorsopalmar view of the metacarpus.

Lateral View

With the patient standing in a natural weight-bearing position, the cassette is placed medially against the limb. The cassette should remain perpendicular to the floor. The x-ray tube is positioned laterally, and the x-ray beam is directed at a right angle to the cassette. The cassette should be large enough that the field of view includes the joints proximal and distal to the metacarpus or metatarsus.

BEAM CENTER: Over midpoint of metacarpus or metatarsus

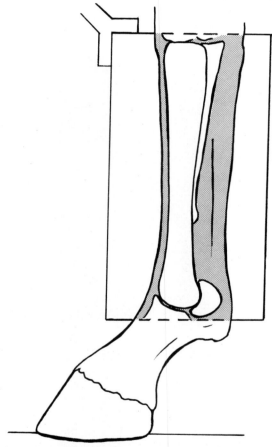

■ **FIG. 19.29** Correct positioning for the lateral view of the metacarpus.

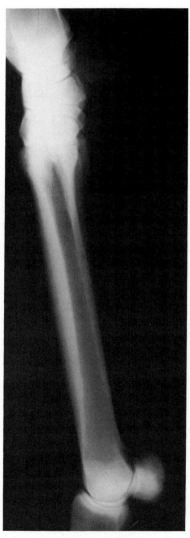

■ **FIG. 19.30** Radiograph of the lateral view of the metacarpus.

Oblique Views (Lateral and Medial)

For an unobstructed examination of the splint bones (2nd and 4th metacarpals/metatarsals) of the horse, oblique views are necessary. The patient is allowed to stand normally, bearing weight on the limb of interest. The cassette is placed either medial or lateral to the palmar or plantar aspect of the limb. For visualization of the lateral splint bone, the cassette is positioned at an approximate 45-degree angle medially. For the medial splint bone, the cassette is positioned laterally approximately 45 degrees. The field of view should include the metacarpus or metatarsus and the joints proximal and distal.

BEAM CENTER: At middle of metacarpus/metatarsus, approximately 45 degrees lateral or medial to a true dorsopalmar/dorsoplantar projection

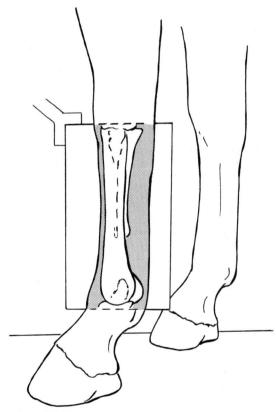

■ **FIG. 19.31** Correct positioning for the oblique view of the metacarpus for visualization of the splints.

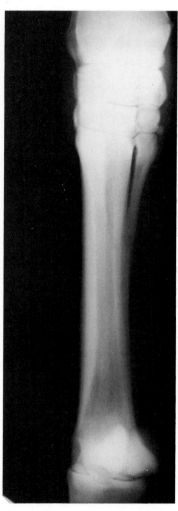

■ **FIG. 19.32** Radiograph of the oblique view of the metacarpus (splints).

CARPUS JOINT

Dorsopalmar View

The patient should be standing in a normal position with full weight placed on the limb of interest. The cassette is placed against the palmar aspect of the carpus and held perpendicular to the floor. It may be necessary to elevate the opposite limb to eliminate patient motion. The x-ray beam is directed perpendicular to the cassette. The field of view should include the entire carpus joint and a portion of the bones proximal and distal.

BEAM CENTER: Over middle of carpus joint at true dorsopalmar plane. A helpful guideline for determining a true dorsopalmar direction is to draw an imaginary line from the middle of the hoof wall to the radius. Center the beam on that imaginary line.

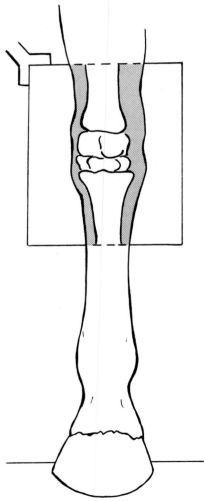

■ **FIG. 19.33** Correct positioning for the dorsopalmar view of the carpus.

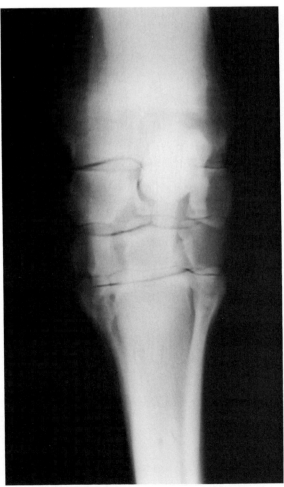

■ **FIG. 19.34** Radiograph of the dorsopalmar view of the carpus.

Lateral View

The patient is placed in a normal position with full weight placed on the limb to be examined. The cassette is placed against the medial aspect of the carpus and held perpendicular to the floor. The x-ray beam is directed perpendicular to the cassette. The field of view should include the carpus joint and a small portion of the bone proximal and distal.

BEAM CENTER: Over lateral aspect of limb in middle of carpus joint

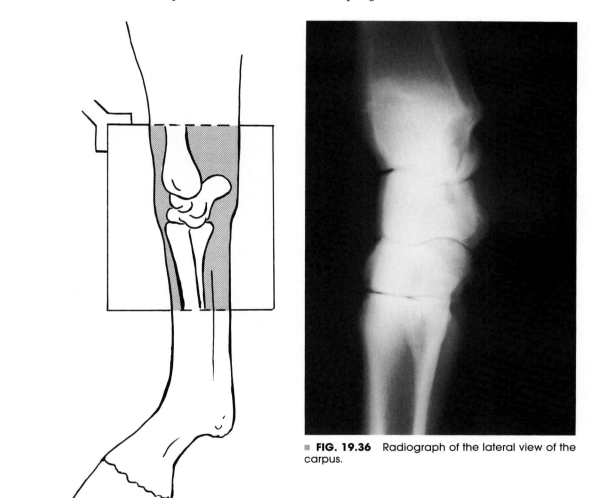

■ **FIG. 19.35** Correct positioning for the lateral view of the carpus.

■ **FIG. 19.36** Radiograph of the lateral view of the carpus.

Flexed Lateral View

The limb of interest is elevated, and the carpus is flexed. The attendant holding the limb should be properly attired in lead and out of line of the primary beam. The cassette is placed against the medial aspect of the carpus and held perpendicular to the floor. It is important to prevent abduction of the limb and to keep the carpus directly under the body. The x-ray beam is directed perpendicular to the cassette. The field of view should include the entire carpus joint.

BEAM CENTER: Over lateral aspect of limb in middle of carpus joint

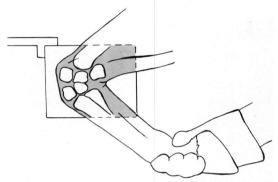

■ **FIG. 19.37** Correct positioning for the flexed lateral view of the carpus.

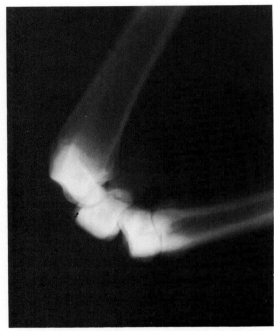

■ **FIG. 19.38** Radiograph of the flexed lateral view of the carpus.

Oblique Views (Lateral and Medial)

The patient is placed in a normal weight-bearing posture. The cassette is positioned against the palmar aspect of the carpus toward the medial or lateral side. The cassette must be held perpendicular to the surface of the floor, with the carpus centered to the cassette. The x-ray beam is directed perpendicular to the cassette. The field of view should include the entire carpus and a portion of the adjacent bones distal and caudal.

BEAM CENTER: Through middle of carpus angled approximately 45 degrees from dorsal midline of joint

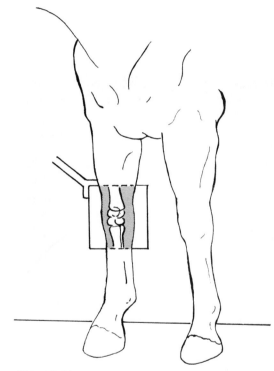

■ **FIG. 19.39** Correct positioning for the dorsomedial-palmarolateral oblique view of the carpus.

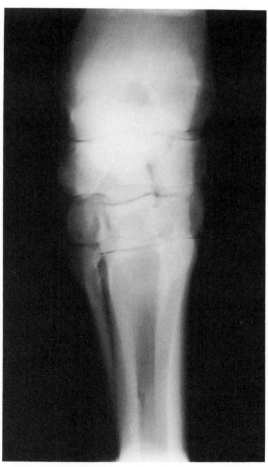

■ **FIG. 19.40** Radiograph of the dorsomedial-palmarolateral oblique view of the carpus.

Skyline View

The limb of the patient is elevated, and the carpus joint is flexed so that the metacarpus is parallel to the floor. The cassette is placed firmly against the dorsal surface of the proximal metacarpal region. The cassette should be as close to parallel to the floor as possible. The x-ray beam is directed toward the dorsal surface of the carpus. The angle of the x-ray beam will vary according to the row of carpal bones under examination. The x-ray beam is directed at a near perpendicular angle to the cassette to highlight the proximal row of carpal bones. To highlight the distal row, the beam is angled approximately 30 degrees to the cassette. The field of view should include the dome of the carpus.

BEAM CENTER: Through row of carpal bones of interest

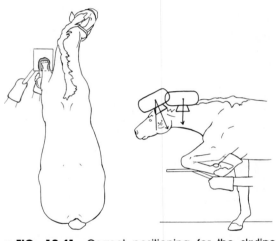

■ **FIG. 19.41** Correct positioning for the skyline view of the carpus.

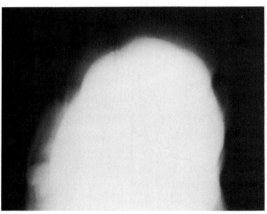

■ **FIG. 19.42** Radiograph of the skyline view of the carpus.

TARSUS JOINT

Dorsoplantar View

The patient is placed in a normal standing posture, bearing weight on the limb of interest. The limb should be rotated slightly lateral ("toe out") so that the x-ray tube does not need to be positioned directly under the body. The cassette is placed firmly against the plantar aspect of the tarsus and held perpendicular to the floor. Great care must be taken when working around the rear legs of large animals. Never stand directly behind the patient but, rather, stand off to the side when holding the cassette in place. To prevent patient motion, the front limb of the opposite side can be elevated. The x-ray beam is directed perpendicular to the cassette, and the field of view should include the entire tarsus and a portion of the adjacent bones distal and proximal.

BEAM CENTER: Through middle of joint at a true dorsoplantar plane. A guideline for determining a true dorsoplantar direction is to draw an imaginary line from the middle of the hoof wall to the tibia. Center the beam on this imaginary line.

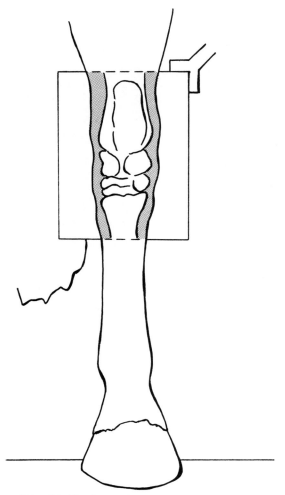

FIG. 19.43 Correct positioning for the dorsoplantar view of the tarsus.

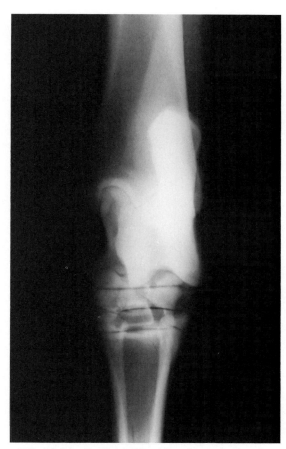

FIG. 19.44 Radiograph of the dorsoplantar view of the tarsus.

Lateral View

The patient should be standing in a normal weight-bearing position. The cassette is placed against the medial aspect of the tarsal joint and held perpendicular to the floor. The tarsal joint should be centered to the cassette, and the x-ray beam directed perpendicular to the cassette. The field of view should include the entire tarsal joint and a small portion of the adjacent bones distal and proximal.

For an alternate lateral projection of the tarsus, the joint can be elevated and flexed. The x-ray beam is directed in the manner just described. This view allows better visualization of the tibiotarsal joint.

BEAM CENTER: Over middle of tarsal joint approximately 4 inches distal from calcaneal tuberosity

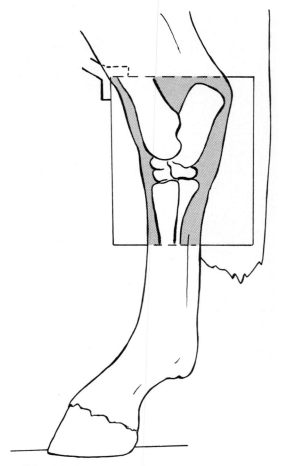

■ **FIG. 19.45** Correct positioning for the lateral view of the tarsus.

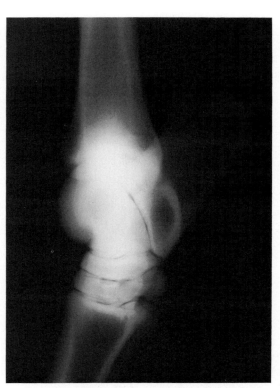

■ **FIG. 19.46** Radiograph of the lateral view of the tarsus.

Oblique Views (Lateral and Medial)

The patient is placed in a normal weight-bearing stance. The cassette is held firmly against the medial or lateral aspect of the plantar surface of the tarsus. The x-ray tube is positioned in front of the limb of interest, and the x-ray beam is angled approximately 45 degrees lateral or medial from the dorsal midline. The field of view should include the entire tarsal joint and a small portion of the bones distal and proximal.

BEAM CENTER: Over middle of tarsal joint approximately 4 inches from calcaneal tuberosity

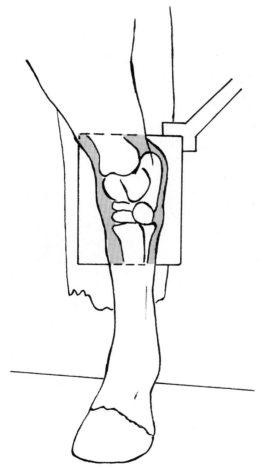

FIG. 19.47 Correct positioning for the dorsolateral-plantaromedial oblique view of the tarsus.

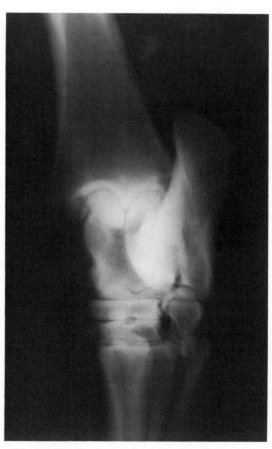

FIG. 19.48 Radiograph of the dorsolateral-plantaromedial oblique view of the tarsus.

ELBOW JOINT

Craniocaudal View

The elbow joint is difficult to radiograph while the animal is in a standing position because of its proximity to the ventral body wall. Although it is not always feasible, general anesthesia is preferred. With the patient anesthetized and placed in lateral recumbency, the limb can be abducted and extended away from the body wall for radiography.

With the patient in a standing position, the affected limb should be extended as far cranial as possi-

ble. The long edge of the cassette is pressed firmly against the thorax at the caudal aspect of the elbow. By pressing the cassette into the rib cage, the medial portion of the elbow should be in the field of view. The x-ray beam is directed through the cranial aspect of the joint, perpendicular to the cassette.

BEAM CENTER: Over middle of joint over cranial midline

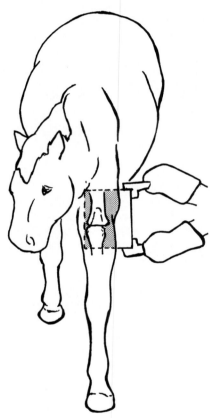

FIG. 19.49 Correct positioning for the craniocaudal view of the elbow.

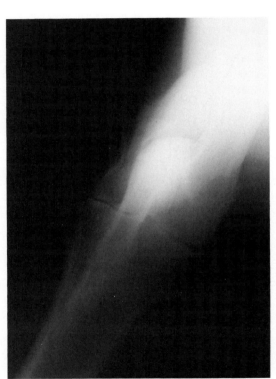

FIG. 19.50 Radiograph of the craniocaudal view of the elbow.

Lateral View

With the patient in a standing position, the limb of interest should be extended as far cranial as possible. To achieve full extension, the limb should be elevated and manually pulled forward. The success of this view is dependent on the extension of the limb. The cassette is placed firmly against the lateral aspect of the limb, with the elbow joint centered to the cassette. The cassette should remain perpendicular to the floor, and the x-ray beam is directed horizontally toward the medial side of the joint. The field of view should include the entire elbow joint.

BEAM CENTER: Over middle of elbow joint

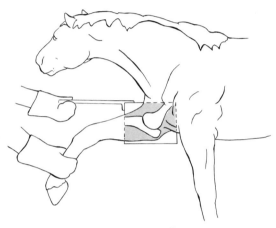

■ **FIG. 19.51** Correct positioning for the lateral view of the elbow.

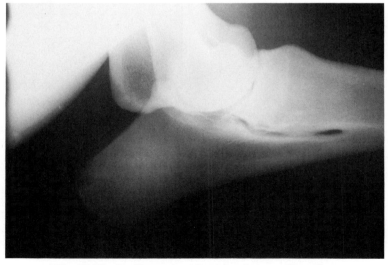

■ **FIG. 19.52** Radiograph of the lateral view of the elbow.

SHOULDER JOINT

Lateral View

To attain a quality projection of the shoulder joint, general anesthesia and placement of the patient in lateral recumbency are recommended. Because general anesthesia is not always practical, a standing lateral view is possible if the patient will allow the necessary manipulation of the limb.

With the patient standing, the affected limb is elevated and pulled cranially. Extending the limb will pull the shoulder joint away from the ventral body wall. The cassette is placed firmly against the lateral aspect of the shoulder joint. The x-ray beam is directed horizontally toward the medial side of the joint and perpendicular to the cassette.

BEAM CENTER: Over shoulder joint

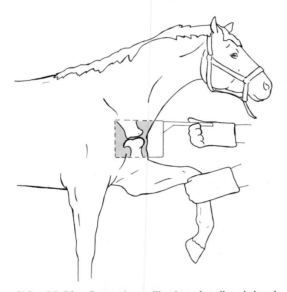

■ **FIG. 19.53** Correct positioning for the lateral view of the shoulder.

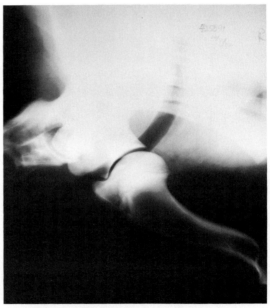

■ **FIG. 19.54** Radiograph of the lateral view of the shoulder.

STIFLE JOINT

Caudocranial View

Radiography of the stifle joint is difficult because of the thickness of the surrounding tissue. Because of the depth of the muscle in the femoral region, the caudocranial projection demonstrates little above the joint space.

The patient should be in a natural standing posture, and the x-ray tube positioned caudal to the stifle joint. If possible, the limb of interest should be stepped back in a caudally extended, weight-bearing position. Extending the limb facilitates placement of the cassette. The cassette is placed cranial to the stifle and tilted so that the long edge is snug against the body wall. The x-ray beam is directed perpendicular to the cassette.

Great care must be taken because of the sensitivity of the patient in this region of the body. The attendant holding the cassette and the radiographer positioning the x-ray tube should be prepared to move if the patient becomes agitated. It may be helpful to elevate the opposite limb to minimize motion and the risk of being kicked. Sedation is highly recommended.

BEAM CENTER: Over stifle joint, approximately 4 inches distal to patella

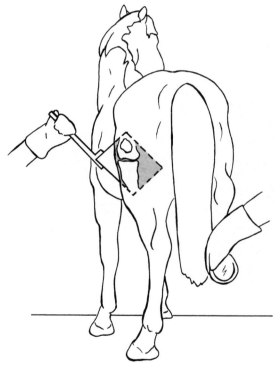

■ **FIG. 19.55** Correct positioning for the caudocranial view of the stifle joint.

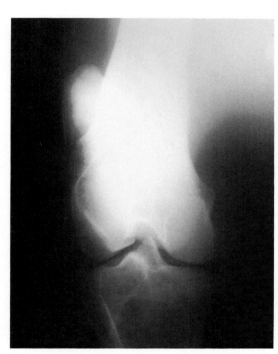

■ **FIG. 19.56** Radiograph of the caudocranial view of the stifle joint.

Lateral View

With the patient is a natural standing posture, the cassette is angled and cautiously placed against the medial side of the stifle joint. Gentle force should be used to push the flat edge of the cassette as far into the flank as possible. Most patients object to this placement of the cassette, and it may be necessary to elevate the opposite limb to prevent motion. The x-ray tube is positioned lateral to the stifle, and the x-ray beam is directed perpendicular to the cassette.

BEAM CENTER: Over stifle joint space, approximately 4 inches distal to patella

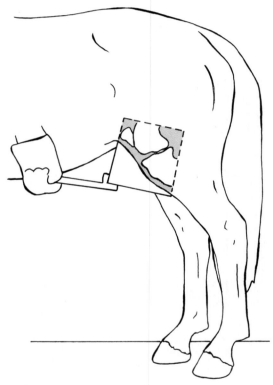

■ FIG. 19.57 Correct positioning for the lateral view of the stifle joint.

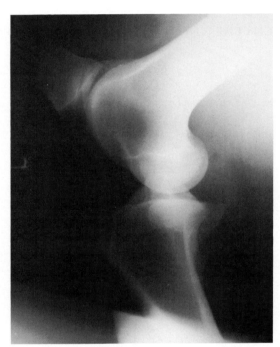

■ FIG. 19.58 Radiograph of the lateral view of the stifle joint.

PELVIS

Ventrodorsal View

General anesthesia is required for this radiographic study of a large animal patient. Due to the thickness of this area, the use of a grid is suggested. The mA and kVp necessary for this region require the use of a high-powered x-ray machine such as a mobile or ceiling-mounted unit.

The patient is placed in dorsal recumbency with the hind limbs flexed in a "frog-leg" position. The cassette is positioned under the patient, with the pelvis centered to the cassette. It may be necessary to expose the pelvis in two or three sections. The use of a cassette tunnel would ease the changing of the cassettes. The x-ray tube is positioned over the ventral region of the pelvis and is centered to the cassette. A 5:1 crisscross grid is also helpful provided that the x-ray machine output is adequate.

Beam Center: Over area of interest. If more than one projection is needed, each centering point should be marked with a felt pen or tape. Marking the centering points allows adjustments to be made from the previously exposed site.

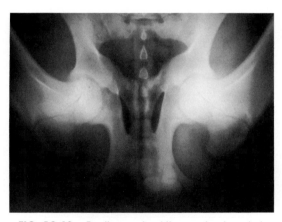

FIG. 19.60   Radiograph of the ventrodorsal view of the pelvis.

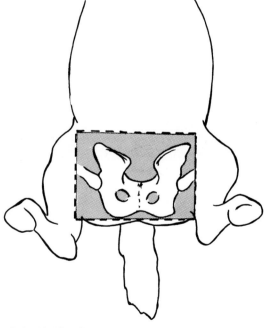

FIG. 19.59   Correct positioning for the ventrodorsal view of the pelvis.

SKULL

Lateral View

Before beginning the examination, the halter of the patient should be checked. If it has any metal on it, it should be removed and replaced with a rope halter. A rope halter usually does not have metal clips and buckles, which could impose radiographically on an area of interest.

The patient is positioned in a natural standing posture, and the head held without rotation. The cassette is placed against the lateral side of the skull on which the lesion excises. The x-ray tube is positioned on the opposite lateral side. The x-ray beam is directed perpendicular to the cassette.

BEAM CENTER: Over area of interest

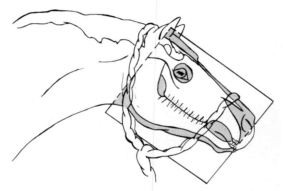

■ **FIG. 19.61** Correct positioning for the lateral view of the skull.

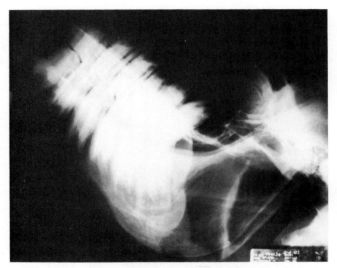

■ **FIG. 19.62** Radiograph of the lateral view of the skull.

Guttural Pouch/Larynx/Pharynx

Lateral View

The positioning of the caudal skull and laryngeal region is essentially the same as for the routine skull views. The fundamental difference is the placement of the cassette and the x-ray beam center point. The cassette is placed on the lateral side of the skull, with the caudal skull centered to the cassette. The x-ray tube is positioned on the opposite lateral side of the skull.

BEAM CENTER: Caudal to vertical ramus of mandible (over guttural pouch region)

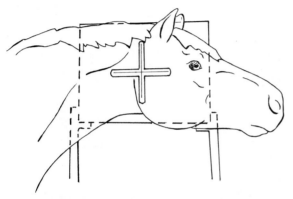

■ **FIG. 19.63** Correct positioning for the lateral view of the guttural pouch, larynx, and pharynx.

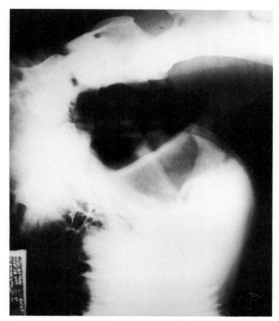

■ **FIG. 19.64** Radiograph of the lateral view of the guttural pouch, larynx, and pharynx.

Dorsoventral View

Sedation is highly recommended for this view of the skull. With the patient in a normal standing posture, the head is lowered as far as possible. The cassette is placed against the ventral side of the skull under the mandible. The x-ray tube is positioned over the head with the x-ray beam directed perpendicular to the cassette.

BEAM CENTER: At midline of skull over area of interest

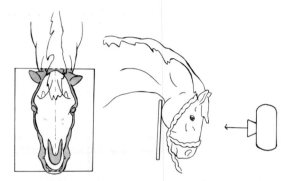

■ **FIG. 19.65**   Correct positioning for the dorsoventral view of the skull.

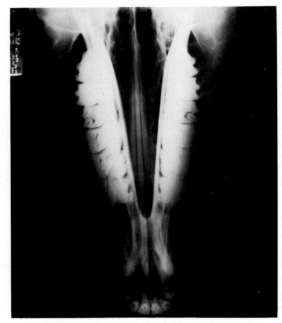

■ **FIG. 19.66**   Radiograph of the dorsoventral view of the skull.

Teeth (Mandibular and Maxillary)

Oblique Views

Cheek teeth are difficult to visualize on the routine lateral and ventrodorsal views because of superimposition of the opposite arcades. An oblique view is necessary to isolate the arcade of interest.

The patient is positioned as for the lateral view with the cassette placed against the lateral side of interest. The cassette remains perpendicular to the floor, and the x-ray beam is angled. For visualization of the maxillary teeth, the x-ray tube is angled down approximately 30 degrees from the parallel plane of the floor and centered over the teeth of interest. For the mandibular teeth, the x-ray tube is angled up approximately 45 degrees from the parallel plane and centered over the area of the lesion.

Views of the incisors can be radiographed by placing the cassette inside the mouth. The x-ray tube is positioned either above or below the head for the corresponding view, and the x-ray beam is centered over the area of interest. Sedation is required for intraoral radiography.

BEAM CENTER: Over area of interest

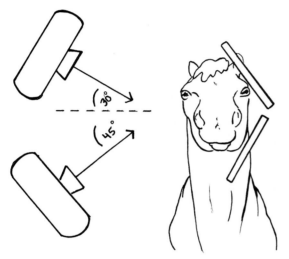

■ **FIG. 19.67** Correct positioning for the lateral oblique view of the cheek teeth.

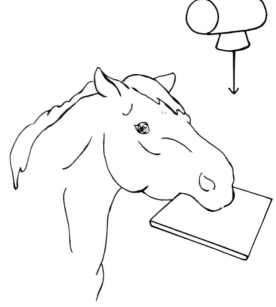

■ **FIG. 19.68** Correct positioning for the intraoral projection of the incisor teeth.

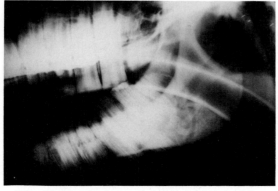

■ **FIG. 19.69** Radiograph of the lateral oblique view of the cheek teeth.

CERVICAL SPINE

Lateral View

In most circumstances, radiography of the cervical spine can be performed with the patient standing if the x-ray machine output is adequate. Because of the size of the patient, the cervical spine must be exposed in three views: (1) base of the skull, C-1, C-2, and C-3; (2) C-3, C-4, and C-5; and (3) C-5, C-6, and C-7.

The cassette is placed against the side of the cervical region. The x-ray tube is positioned on the opposite side of the patient with the x-ray beam directed perpendicular to the cassette. It is important to remember that the cervical spine runs along the ventral portion or the neck. Many times the spine is "missed" by centering the x-ray beam too far dorsally.

BEAM CENTER: Area 1: Over C-2
Area 2: Over C-4
Area 3: Over C-5

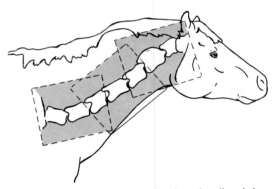

■ **FIG. 19.70** Correct positioning for the lateral view of the cervical spine.

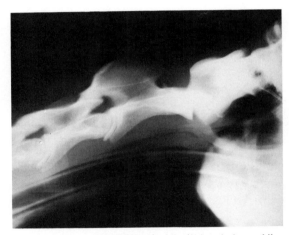

■ **FIG. 19.71** Radiograph of the lateral view of the cranial cervical spine.

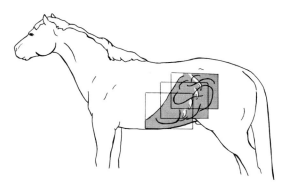

■ **FIG. 19.74** The three views of the lateral abdomen.

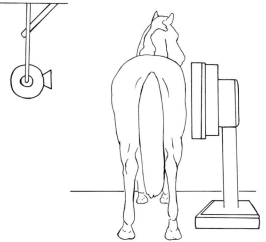

■ **FIG. 19.72** Drawing showing the placement of the cassette and x-ray tube for the lateral view of the thorax. A standing cassette holder with grid is used with the patient standing in front of the cassette.

ADDITIONAL AREAS—A BRIEF OVERVIEW

Areas of the body such as the thorax, abdomen, and thoracic spine can be radiographed only with special high-powered equipment. The ability to radiograph such areas is usually limited to highly specialized veterinary hospitals.

Thorax

Because of the size of the patient, four views of the thorax are usually required: (1) craniodorsal lateral, (2) caudodorsal lateral, (3) cranioventral lateral, and (4) caudodorsal lateral. The thorax can be radiographed with the patient standing. The cassette is placed in a standing mechanical cassette holder that has a built-in grid. A grid is necessary because of the high kVp used. It is important that the x-ray beam is centered to the grid before walking the patient into

position. The SID is normally increased to 80 inches. The patient is walked between the x-ray tube and the cassette. The lateral side of the patient should be as close to the cassette as possible. It is possible to radiograph the caudodorsal region with low-output equipment, short SID, and very fast intensifying screens, however (Figs. 19.72 and 19.73).

Abdomen

The same equipment and preparation are required for the abdomen as for the thorax. An abdomen can be radiographed with the patient in a standing position as well. A series of radiographs are recommended, starting cranioventral and extending caudodorsal (Fig. 19.74).

Thoracic Spine

A lower-powered unit can be used to visualize the dorsal spinous processes (withers) of the thoracic spine. If the ventral portion of the thoracic vertebrae has to be examined, higher exposure factors are needed to penetrate the thick tissues of this area. With a high-powered x-ray apparatus and a grid, it is possible to radiograph the thoracic spine. The patient positioning is similar to that for radiographs of the thorax except the x-ray beam is centered over the thoracic spine.

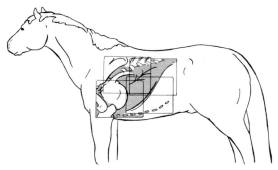

■ **FIG. 19.73** The four views of the lateral thorax.

BIBLIOGRAPHY

Dik KJ, Gunsser I: *Atlas of Diagnostic Radiology of the Horse: Parts I–III.* WB Saunders, Philadelphia, 1988.

Douglas SW, Herrtage ME, Williamson HD: *Principles of Veterinary Radiography,* 4th ed. Bailliere Tindall, Philadelphia, 1987.

Koblik PD, Toal R: Portable veterinary x-ray support systems for field use. J Am Vet Med Assoc 199:186–188, 1991.

Morgan JP, Silverman S: *Techniques in Veterinary Radiography,* 4th ed. Iowa State University Press, Ames, 1987.

Phillips DF: Radiology in your practice: Choosing the right equipment. Vet Med 587–598, 1987.

Smallwood JE, Shively MJ: Nomenclature for radiographic views of limbs. Equine Pract 1:41–45, 1979.

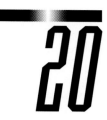

AVIAN AND EXOTIC RADIOGRAPHY

INTRODUCTION

Birds and exotic pets, including rodents, reptiles, and fish, have become very popular in recent years. Consequently, veterinary practitioners have experienced an increased demand for diagnostic and therapeutic care of these animals. Radiography is a valuable diagnostic technique because it is noninvasive and available for rapid interpretation. Fortunately, all principles pertaining to companion animal radiography can be applied to avian and exotic radiography. A few minor differences in equipment and technique are noted in this chapter.

SPECIAL CONSIDERATIONS

Equipment

The equipment necessary for avian and exotic radiography is essentially the same as for domestic animals. New high-detail film-screen systems enable most practitioners to radiograph exotic pets. Nonscreen film has been advocated in the past for radiographic studies of smaller exotic animals. Although nonscreen film produces high-detail radiographs, it is impractical at times because of the need for a long exposure time. A high-milliamperage x-ray machine, such as a 200- or 300-milliamperage (mA) unit, is recommended to allow the use of a short exposure time.

Exposure times of $\frac{1}{40}$ second or less are preferred in order to decrease the chance of a motion artifact on a radiograph. If the output of the machine is less than 200 mA, it may be necessary to decrease the source-image distance (SID) to compensate for the decreased output of the x-ray machine.

Maximum kilovoltage (kVp) is less important for avian and exotic radiography than for domestic animal radiography. Rather, the x-ray machine must have a low kVp setting and the ability to make small incremental changes in kVp. A grid is usually not needed. Scatter radiation must be minimized by using a beam-limiting device to collimate the x-ray beam to the smallest area possible. Because of the comparatively small patient size, negligible amounts of scatter radiation can greatly reduce the quality of a radiographic image.

Exposure Factors

Avian and exotic patients are usually not measured with a caliper to calculate the exposure. Normally, exposure factors are chosen according to the species and general size of the patient. Keep in mind that the exposure factors required for birds are less than those needed for reptiles of the same thickness. Soaring (flying) birds have very thin cortices and tubular bones. Compared with mammals, avian long bones have significantly less calcium and ossification, which makes them more radiolucent. Very slight exposure variations can produce marked alterations in radiographic images of birds.

The exposure factors listed in Table 20.1 are examples that can be used for an ultradetail rare-earth screen/medium (par)-speed film system. If a Plexiglass sheet is used for avian radiography, add 2 to 4 kVp to the exposure factors listed.

Patient Restraint

Three types of restraint are used for avian and exotic patients during radiography: (1) manual, (2) physical,

and (3) chemical. Regardless of the species and restraint device employed, the methods of restraint are similar. The head and torso are restrained first, then the wings (in the case of a bird), and the legs last. With larger rodent mammals, it is possible to use the same restraint methods as for a dog or cat.

Manual restraint involves an attendant (wearing lead attire) holding an animal in position while the exposure is taken. This method of restraint results in increased exposure to personnel and may be illegal in some states. Manual restraint should be avoided if at all possible.

T A B L E 20 . 1

Avian and Exotic Exposure Factors

PATIENT	kVp	mA	EXPOSURE TIME (SECONDS)	SID (INCHES)	mA-s
Psittacine					
Finch	42	300	1/60	40	5
Canary	44	300	1/60	40	5
Budgerigar	46–50	300	1/60	40	5
Cockatiel	50–55	300	1/40	40	7.5
Parrot	55–65	300	1/40	40	7.5
Raptor					
Small	50–55	300	1/40	40	7.5
Kestrel					
Saw-whet owl					
Screech owl					
Medium	55–60	300	1/30	40	10.0
Barred owl					
Red-tailed hawk					
Great horned owl					
Large	60–65	300	1/20	40	15.0
Eagle					
Extra Large	66	300	1/15	40	20.0
Trumpeter swan					
Rodents					
Small	42–46	300	1/40	40	7.5
Mouse					
Gerbil					
Hamster					
Medium	46–52	300	1/40	40	7.5
Rat					
Dwarf rabbit					
Ferret					
Large	54–60	300	1/40	40	7.5
Rabbit					
Guinea pig					
Reptiles					
Snake (small)	40–44	300	1/40	40	7.5
Snake (large)	45–55	300	1/40	40	7.5
Lizard	40–45	300	1/40	40	7.5
Turtle					
Small					
Lateral/DV	50–55	300	1/40	40	7.5
Craniocaudal	55–60	300	1/40	40	7.5
Large					
Lateral/DV	65–70	300	1/30	40	10.0
Craniocaudal	70–75	300	1/30	40	10.0

Physical restraint involves such devices as a plexiglass sheet, ropes, sandbags, and radiolucent adhesive tape. Birds can be restrained directly on a cassette; however, it is recommended that they be positioned on an intermediate surface, especially if several views of the same projection are scheduled. A thin radiolucent sheet of plexiglass slightly larger than the cassette often serves as an intermediate surface. The avian patient can be placed in position and secured with tape on the radiolucent sheet. The sheet can then be placed directly on the cassette (Fig. 20.1).

The type of tape used for physical restraint is important. Scotch tape and cloth medical tape should be avoided because they can damage or remove feathers, fur, or scales. Plexiglass tubes have been employed for the restraint of rodents and other laboratory animals. However, this method is not ideal for radiography because it is difficult to position a patient accurately in a tube. For example, it is not practical to expect a diagnostic radiograph of a rodent thorax if the front limbs are superimposed over the thoracic cavity.

Unfortunately, both manual and physical restraint methods have limitations. In many cases, physical restraint may result in excessive patient stress and possible injury from struggling. Injectable sedatives and inhalant anesthetics have greatly increased the feasibility and safety of radiographic procedures involving birds and exotic animals. In fact, chemical restraint has become the safest method in avian and exotic radiography. Chemical restraint is most often used in combination with other positioning techniques to obtain a properly positioned radiograph.

Patients must be evaluated individually to determine the appropriate restraint necessary. Manual or physical restraint should be used only with animals that are not prone to struggle and induce self-trauma. Supportive therapy, such as a heat lamp, may be helpful when anesthesia is used to keep the patient warm during and after the radiographic examination. Another technique to keep the avian patient warm during recovery is to gently roll the bird into a towel. This technique not only keeps the patient warm, it prevents thrashing and possible injury during anesthesia recovery. Careful judgment must be used with a critically ill patient. In some cases, it may be necessary to postpone radiography until the patient is stable.

AVIAN RADIOGRAPHY

Whole Body Ventrodorsal View

The avian patient is positioned on its back so that the sternum is superimposed over the spine. The wings are extended laterally and secured. If manual restraint is used, one hand grasps the head from the back, holding the mandibular articulation between the thumb and the forefinger. The other hand takes the feet and carefully extends them caudally. The wings should be abducted slightly from the body and held down by adhesive tape (Fig. 20.2).

Physical restraint for avian radiography is preferred. The patient is placed in dorsal recumbency as described, except the head is secured with adhesive tape. The neck is gently extended in a cranial direction and secured to the cassette with adhesive tape.

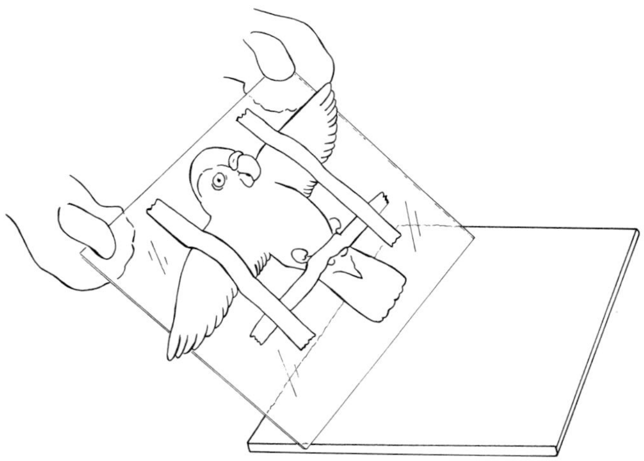

■ **FIG. 20.1** Example of restraint used for avian radiography. The bird is placed on a radiolucent sheet (clear plastic) and secured into position with adhesive tape. The radiolucent sheet is then placed onto the cassette.

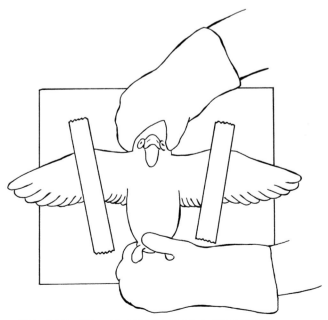

■ **FIG. 20.2** Manual restraint of an avian patient.

Care must be taken that the airway is not compromised by the tape across the neck region. The wings are abducted laterally and taped to the cassette in full extension. The legs are extended caudally, positioned symmetrically, and fastened to the cassette with masking tape. The tip of the tail can be secured to the cassette to provide additional restraint, if necessary.

BEAM CENTER: Over midline at caudal tip of sternum

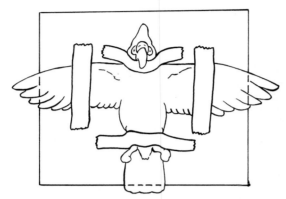

■ **FIG. 20.3** Correct physical restraint and positioning for the ventrodorsal view of the entire body of a bird.

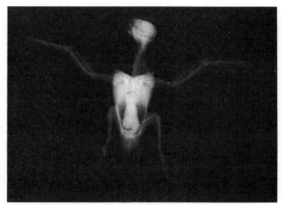

■ **FIG. 20.4** Radiograph of the whole body ventrodorsal view of a bird.

Whole Body Lateral View

The patient is placed in lateral recumbency, and the neck is secured to the cassette with masking tape. (Note: Right lateral views are taken to maintain consistency with comparable anatomic reference material.) The wings are extended dorsally directly above the body of the patient. The wing that is down on the cassette is positioned cranial to the other wing and secured with adhesive tape. The legs are extended ventrally away from the body wall and fastened with tape. The dependent leg is positioned cranial to the other leg. The limb closest to the cassette is always cranial to the contralateral limb so that each limb is identifiable on a lateral radiograph. The tail and body of the patient can be secured with tape if additional restraint is necessary.

BEAM CENTER: Over middle of body between spine and sternum at level of caudal tip of sternum

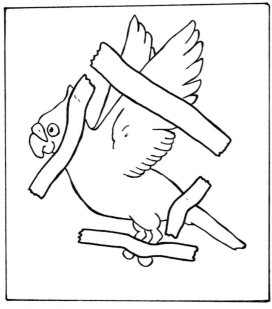

■ **FIG. 20.5** Correct positioning for the whole body lateral view of a bird.

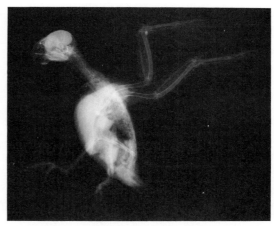

■ **FIG. 20.6** Radiograph of the whole body lateral view of a bird.

Wing — Caudocranial View

Manual positioning is necessary for the caudocranial view of the wing because of the awkward position required of the patient. Lead gloves are worn, and the bird is held upside-down so that the body is perpendicular to the cassette. The tip of the wing feathers is held gently, and the wing of interest is extended away from the body. The cranial edge of the wing is placed on the cassette. In order for the edge of the wing to be in contact with the cassette, it is helpful to allow the head of the patient to hang over the edge of the cassette. Exposure factors required for this view are approximately the same as those required for the entire body.

BEAM CENTER: Over area of interest

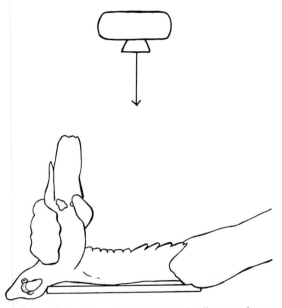

■ **FIG. 20.7** Correct positioning for the craniocaudal view of a bird's wing.

Gastrointestinal Contrast Study

A contrast study of the gastrointestinal tract can be valuable to the avian practitioner. Because visualization of many abnormalities on routine survey radiographs is difficult, the use of contrast media can be helpful in defining the location and size of a lesion. For example, because birds love to chew, they often suffer from gastrointestinal foreign bodies. In addition, stasis of the gastrointestinal tract is a common consequence when a bird is ill. Without the use of contrast media, diagnosis of such problems may be difficult or impossible.

TECHNIQUE OUTLINE

CONTRAST MEDIA:

20 to 30% barium sulfate (gastrografin is indicated if a perforation is susected but is not routinely used owing to its local mucosal irritant effect and rapid absorption through the intestinal walls)

PATIENT PREPARATION:

Fast approximately 4 hours (owing to the high metabolic rate of a bird, fasting longer than 4 hours could compromise the health of the patient)

PROCEDURE

I. Draw contrast medium into a syringe, warmed to approximately 80°F

II. Administer contrast to bird with a small feeding tube or urinary catheter.
   A. Force the patient's mouth open, and insert the feeding tube into the crop.
   B. For brids without a crop, pass the feeding tube into midesophageal region.
   C. Verify the position of the tube by palpation before injecting contrast because it is possible for it to be placed inadvertently into the trachea.
   D. To fill the gastrointestinal tract, administer 25 ml/kg of barium sulfate. For a small bird, such as a parakeet, 0.5 to 1.5 ml is adequate. Larger birds, such as parrots, may require up to 10 ml of contrast medium.

III. Expose lateral and ventrodorsal radiographs immediately after the administration of contrast. By 10 minutes after administration, the contrast should be past the crop and in the stomach. Radiographs are normally obtained in 30-minute intervals until the contrast medium has reached the cloaca. The amount of time it takes the barium to travel from the crop to the cloaca (transit time) will vary according to the size, species, and pathology of the patient. The average time ranges from 30 to 240 minutes. Small psittacines have the fastest transit time.

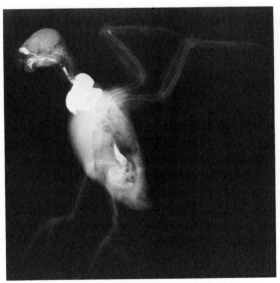

■ **FIG. 20.8** Lateral view of a barium series on a cockatiel. Note the small amount of barium aspiration in the trachea. All precautions should be taken to prevent the occurrence of barium aspiration.

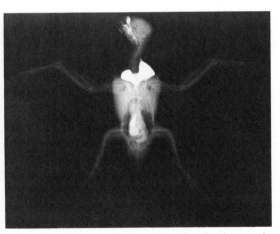

■ **FIG. 20.9** Ventrodorsal view of a barium series on a cockatiel. Note the small amount of barium aspirated in the trachea. All precautions should be taken to prevent the occurrence of barium aspiration.

RODENT RADIOGRAPHY

Rat

Whole Body Dorsoventral View

Positioning for a ventrodorsal projection can be performed in two ways: (1) by placing the small patient in a radiolucent tube or (2) by securing the patient to the cassette with adhesive tape. For whole body radiographs of larger rodents (guinea pigs and rabbits), the animal can be placed in the same positions as a small domestic animal (dog).

The radiolucent tube with the patient inside is placed on top of the cassette so that the animal is in sternal recumbency. The x-ray beam is directed vertically through the back of the rodent, and the field of view should include the entire body. A tube has disadvantages, however. A quality radiograph is compromised by superimposition of the legs under the body of the patient and by rotation. Superimposition and rotation decrease visualization of the thoracic and abdominal cavities.

Adhesive tape is the preferred method of restraint for a rodent because the extremities can be extended and rotation of the body can be eliminated. The patient is placed on top of the cassette in sternal recumbency. The head and legs are extended away from the body and secured with adhesive tape. It is important that the patient is in a true dorsoventral position, with the sternum superimposed over the spine. The x-ray beam is directed vertically through the back of the rodent, and the field of view should include the entire body.

BEAM CENTER: Over thoracolumbar spinal junction

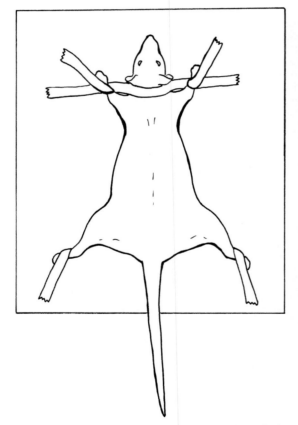

■ **FIG. 20.10** Correct positioning for the whole body dorsoventral view of a rodent.

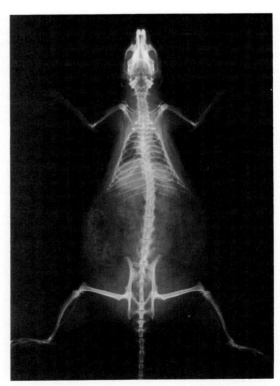

■ **FIG. 20.11** Radiograph of the whole body dorsoventral view of a rat.

Whole Body Lateral View

The advantage of using a radiolucent tube for small rodent radiography is that both the lateral and the ventrodorsal views can be obtained without manipulating the patient. With the patient positioned in the tube, the x-ray beam is directed horizontally toward the left side of the tube. The cassette is placed against the right side of the animal in the tube. It is necessary to elevate the radiolucent tube so that the entire body of the rodent can be visualized on the radiograph. Unfortunately, a tube may compromise a quality radiograph because of the superimposition of the legs over the thoracic and abdominal cavities (Fig. 20.12).

The best method of restraint is adhesive tape. The patient is placed in right lateral recumbency on top of the cassette. The front limbs and rear limbs are extended cranially and caudally, respectively, and se-

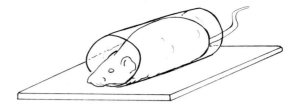

■ **FIG. 20.12** Correct usage of a radiolucent tube for rodent radiography.

cured. It may be necessary to place a length of adhesive tape over the neck if the patient is struggling. If manual restraint is employed, string or small forceps can be used to extend the limbs to decrease exposure to the attendants. The x-ray beam is directed vertically toward the rodent, and the field of view should include the entire body.

BEAM CENTER: Over thoracolumbar spinal junction

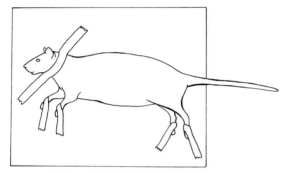

■ **FIG. 20.13** Correct positioning for the whole body lateral view of a rodent.

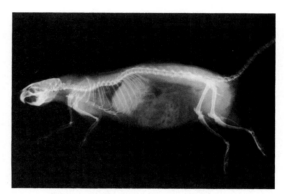

■ **FIG. 20.14** Radiograph of the whole body lateral view of a rat.

REPTILE RADIOGRAPHY

Turtle

Whole Body Dorsoventral View

Radiographic examinations of turtles can be difficult because of the presence of a shell. A number of views may be necessary to view the internal anatomy of the turtle adequately. The three routine views include (1) dorsoventral, (2) lateral, and (3) craniocaudal.

Under most circumstances, turtles are slow and docile. Normally, radiographic studies can be performed without sedation. Restraint devices such as adhesive tape or a radiolucent plastic box that the turtle is placed in can be used to restrict movement. In the case of a snapping turtle, sedation may be warranted if the patient becomes uncooperative.

To prepare a turtle for dorsoventral radiography, the patient is turned on its back. Just before the exposure is to be made, the patient is turned back on its ventral side. The turtle requires a few moments to become reoriented and will naturally extend its legs and head from the shell. At this moment, the exposure should be made. The field of view should include the entire body.

BEAM CENTER: Over center of shell

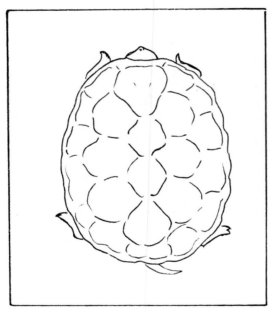

■ **FIG. 20.15** Correct positioning for the whole body dorsoventral view of a turtle.

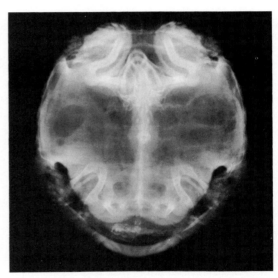

■ **FIG. 20.16** Radiograph of the whole body dorsoventral view of a turtle.

Whole Body Lateral View

The turtle is attached to a wood or plastic rack with adhesive tape. The ventral aspect of the body is in contact with the rack, and tape is wrapped around the circumference of the shell and rack. The rack is elevated into a vertical position so that the turtle is on its right side on top of the cassette. The x-ray beam is directed parallel to the rack through the patient from left to right.

With x-ray machines that have the capability of horizontal x-ray beam radiography, a lateral view can be taken with the patient in ventral recumbency. The turtle is placed on top of a sponge or wood block and secured with adhesive tape. The cassette is positioned vertically against the right side of the patient. The x-ray beam is directed parallel to the sponge or block through the patient from left to right.

BEAM CENTER: Over center of body

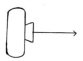
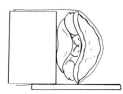

■ **FIG. 20.17** Correct positioning for a whole body lateral view of a turtle with the use of a rack.

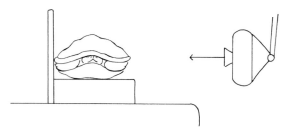

■ **FIG. 20.18** Correct positioning for the whole body lateral view of a turtle with the use of a horizontal x-ray beam.

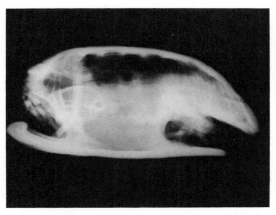

■ **FIG. 20.19** Radiograph of the whole body lateral view of a turtle.

Whole Body Craniocaudal View

The turtle is placed in ventral recumbency and fixed to a wood or plastic rack with adhesive tape. With the cassette on the table in horizontal position, the rack is elevated into a vertical posture. The caudal aspect of the turtle is placed against the cassette, and the head is pointed toward the x-ray tube. The x-ray beam is directed toward the head and should pass through the body from the head to the tail.

The craniocaudal view can also be performed with horizontal beam radiography. The patient is positioned in ventral recumbency on a sponge or wood block and secured with adhesive tape. The cassette is placed in vertical position against the caudal aspect of the patient. The x-ray beam is directed horizontal to the sponge through the body from the head to the tail.

BEAM CENTER: Through middle of head

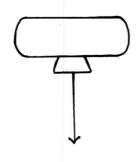

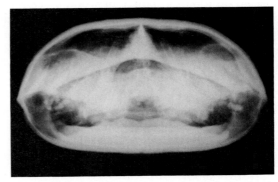

■ **FIG. 20.22** Radiograph of the whole body craniocaudal view of a turtle.

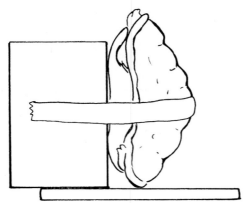

■ **FIG. 20.20** Correct positioning for the whole body craniocaudal view of a turtle using a rack.

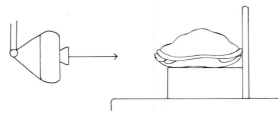

■ **FIG. 20.21** Correct positioning for the whole body craniocaudal view of a turtle using a horizontal x-ray beam.

Lizard

Whole Body Dorsoventral View

The size and disposition of a lizard determine the type of restraint necessary. Very calm and docile reptiles can be secured with adhesive tape, whereas restless or fractious reptiles require further restraint measures. Aggressive lizards and crocodiles should be radiographed with the snout tied to prevent injury to personnel. Smaller lizards usually require chemical and/or physical restraint. Larger lizards can usually be manually restrained. Sometimes it is sufficient to cover the animal with both hands and withdraw them just before the exposure is taken. For most species of lizards, it is necessary to restrain the tail as well.

The patient is placed in sternal recumbency on the cassette. The body is gently stretched, and the limbs are extended laterally and secured to the cassette. If necessary, the tail is secured with a length of adhesive tape. It is important that the patient be in a true dorsoventral position, with the sternum superimposed over the spine. The x-ray beam is directed vertically through the back of the patient, and the field of view should include the entire body.

BEAM CENTER: Over middle of body, to include thorax, abdomen, and entire skeletal system

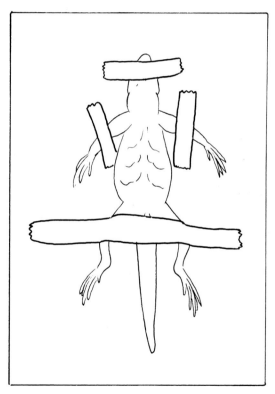

■ **FIG. 20.23** Correct positioning for the whole body dorsoventral view of a lizard.

Whole Body Lateral View

Restraint considerations are the same as for the whole body dorsoventral view of the lizard.

The patient is placed in right lateral recumbency against the cassette. The head and front limbs are extended cranially and secured either manually or with tape. The rear limbs are extended in a caudal direction and secured. If manual restraint is used, a firm grip may be necessary at first but can be relaxed after a few seconds. The x-ray beam is directed vertically through the left side of the patient, and the field of view should include the entire body.

BEAM CENTER: Over middle of body, to include thorax, abdomen, and vertebral column

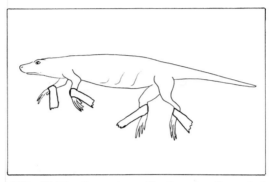

■ **FIG. 20.24** Correct positioning for the whole body lateral view of a lizard.

Snake

Whole Body Dorsoventral View

Radiography of snakes can be difficult because of their unique anatomy. In most cases, the entire body can be radiographed with the dorsoventral view. Small non-poisonous snakes can be placed directly on the cassette. If the patient is active, the snake can be placed in a double-open-ended cardboard or radiolucent plastic box. The box is then placed on top of the cassette, and the exposure is taken. A restless snake can also be secured in a long radiolucent tube. If directed, the snake will usually crawl in the tube on its own. The ends of the tube can be plugged with porous cork or other suitable material. In the case of a very restless or even fractious (poisonous) snake, sedation may be warranted.

Often the patient can be allowed to lay in a natural coiled position on the cassette without any restraint. With the patient in a coiled position, the entire body can be radiographed. If necessary, the patient can be placed in a plastic radiolucent tube and radiographed in segments. When radiographing a snake in segments, it is important to number or label each projection so that they can be viewed in proper sequence.

BEAM CENTER: Over area of interest

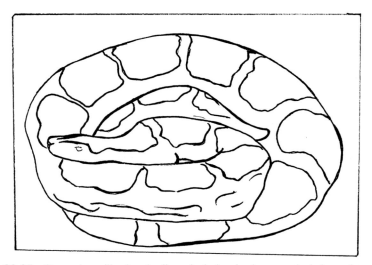

■ **FIG. 20.25** Correct positioning for the whole body dorsoventral view of a snake.

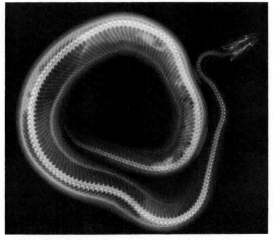

■ **FIG. 20.26** Radiograph of the whole body dorsoventral view of a snake.

Whole Body Lateral View

For longer snakes, it is necessary to radiograph the patient in segments or to concentrate on a certain segment of the body. When radiographing a snake in segments, it is important to number or label each projection so that they can be viewed in proper sequence. In either case, it is possible to fix the patient in position on the cassette with either manual or physical restraint. If a radiolucent tube is used, it is necessary to rotate the tube until the patient is in lateral recumbency.

BEAM CENTER: Over area of interest

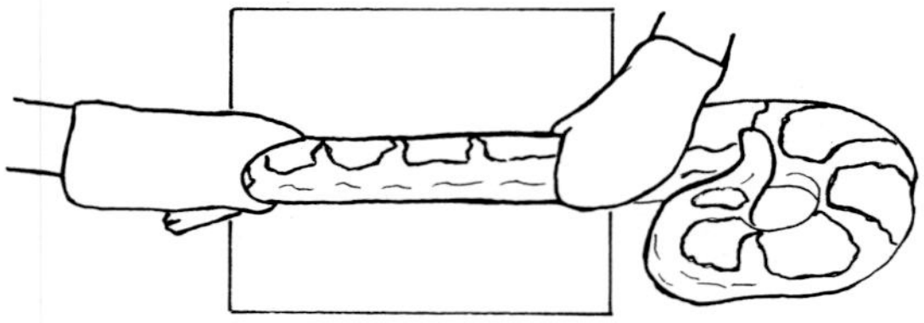

■ **FIG. 20.27** Correct positioning for a lateral view of a portion of a snake.

FISH RADIOGRAPHY

Lateral/Dorsoventral Whole Body View

Radiography of a fish can be challenging because the patient needs water to breathe. A dorsoventral view of a fish can be obtained by placing the patient in a Ziploc-type bag with enough water to allow respiration. The plastic bag is placed directly on top of the cassette, and the exposure is made when the fish is stationary.

A lateral view can be exposed in one of two ways. The first method requires the use of a horizontal x-ray beam. The plastic bag containing the fish and water is suspended beside the cassette, which is placed in a vertical position. The x-ray beam is directed horizon-

tally at the fish in the bag, and the field of view should include the entire body. To reduce and equalize the amount of water surrounding the fish, the bag can be compressed with a thin sheet of plexiglass.

An alternative method to obtaining a lateral view requires rapid preparation and exposure by the radiographer. The fish is wrapped in a wet paper towel and placed in lateral recumbency on the cassette. The exposure is taken quickly so that the patient can be returned to the water.

(Note: For amphibians, the same radiographic technique as for other exotics is suitable.)

BEAM CENTER: Over middle of body

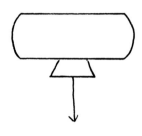

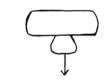

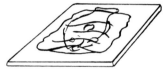

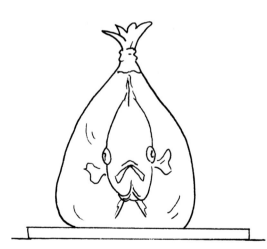

■ **FIG. 20.28** Correct positioning for a whole body dorsoventral view of a fish with the use of a bagful of water placed on a cassette.

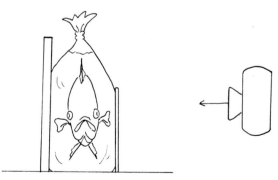

■ **FIG. 20.29** Correct positioning for a whole body lateral view of a fish with the use of a wet paper towel wrapped around the fish.

■ **FIG. 20.30** Correct positioning for a whole body lateral view of a fish with the use of a bagful of water placed next to a cassette in a vertical position. A horizontal x-ray beam is used.

BIBLIIOGRAPHY

Douglas SW, Herrtage ME, Williamson HD: *Principles of Veterinary Radiography*, 4th ed. Bailliere Tindall, Philadelphia, 1987.

Harrison GJ, Harrison LR: *Clinical Avian Medicine and Surgery*. WB Saunders, Philadelphia, 1986.

McMillan MC: Avian gastrointestinal radiography. Compend Cont Educ 5:273–278, 1983.

McMillan MC: Diseases of cage and aviary birds. *In* Petrak ML (ed): *Avian Radiology*, 2nd ed, pp 329–360. Lea & Febiger, Philadelphia, 1982.

Morgan JP, Silverman S: *Techniques in Veterinary Radiography*, 4th ed. Iowa State University Press, Ames, 1984.

Rubel GA, Isenbugal E, Wolvekamp P: *Atlas of Diagnostic Radiology of Exotic Pets*. WB Saunders, Philadelphia, 1991.

Silverman S: Avian radiographic technique and interpretation. *In* Kirk R (ed): *Current Veterinary Therapy VII*, pp 649–653. WB Saunders, Philadelphia, 1980.

INDEX